T0120491

WHAT YOU MUST KNOW ABOUT
WOMEN'S HORMONES

YOUR GUIDE TO NATURAL HORMONE TREATMENT FOR PMS, MENOPAUSE, OSTEOPOROSIS, PCOS, AND MORE

SECOND EDITION

PAMELA WARTIAN SMITH, MD, MPH

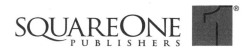

SQUAREONE
PUBLISHERS

EDITOR: Erica Shur
COVER DESIGNER: Jeannie Tudor
TYPESETTER: Gary A. Rosenberg

The information and advice contained in this book are based upon the research and the personal and professional experiences of the author. They are not intended as a substitute for consulting with a healthcare professional. The publisher and author are not responsible for any adverse effects or consequences resulting from the use of any of the suggestions, preparations, or procedures discussed in this book. All matters pertaining to your physical health should be supervised by a healthcare professional. It is a sign of wisdom, not cowardice, to seek a second or third opinion.

Square One Publishers

115 Herricks Road • Garden City Park, NY 11040

(516) 535-2010 • (877) 900-BOOK

www.squareonepublishers.com

Library of Congress Cataloging-in-Publication Data
Names: Smith, Pamela Wartian, author.
Title: What you must know about women's hormones : your guide to natural hormone treatments for PMS, menopause, osteoporosis, PCOS, and more / Pamela Wartian Smith.
Description: Second edition. | Garden City Park : Square One Publishers, 2022. | Includes bibliographical references and index.
Identifiers: LCCN 2021060436 (print) | LCCN 2021060437 (ebook) | ISBN 9780757005183 (paperback) | ISBN 9780757055188 (ebook)
Subjects: LCSH: Menopause—Hormone therapy—Popular works. | Middle-aged women—Diseases—Hormone therapy—Popular works. | Endocrine gynecology—Popular works.
Classification: LCC RG186 .S678 2022 (print) | LCC RG186 (ebook) | DDC 618.1/7506—dc23/eng/20211214
LC record available at https://lccn.loc.gov/2021060436
LC ebook record available at https://lccn.loc.gov/2021060437

Copyright © 2010, 2022 by Pamela Wartian Smith, MD, MPH

All rights reserved. No part of this publication may be reproduced, stored in a retrieval system, or transmitted, in any form or by any means, electronic, mechanical, photocopying, recording, or other-wise, without the prior written permission of the publisher.

Printed in the United States of America

10   9   8   7   6   5   4   3   2   1

Contents

Part III   Hormone Replacement Therapy

To my daughters, Autumn, Hollie, and Caitlin, Lynn and Sarah. I am blessed to have five daughters, all of whom have had their own unique hormonal experience.

To my husband Christopher, whose patience with me as I traveled along my own hormonal "journey" has been nothing short of wonderful.

Acknowledgments

To Dr. Lindsey Berkson, the author of 21 books including *Safe Hormones, Smart Women*. Dr. Lindsey Berkson has worked as a continuing education professor for doctors and pharmacists. She is a functional medicine specialist focusing on hormones, anti-aging, and medical nutrition, especially for breast cancer survivors. She has served as a hormone scholar at an environmental estrogen think tank at Tulane University and has published original peer-review research with Houston's University of Texas Medical School. Thank you, Lindsey, for all you have done to help women achieve optimal hormonal balance.

Special thanks to Rudy Shur, my publisher and mentor. I am blessed to be able to call him my friend.

I would also like to recognize my editor, Erica Shur, who has the gift of keeping me focused. I thank her for her hard work and dedication to this project.

Preface

What You Must Know About Women's Hormones is the second edition of this book. When this book was first written, the science was very new and hormone replacement therapy was controversial in the medical literature. I am happy to say that the science has now caught up to what we have always known clinically, in order to achieve and maintain optimal health, you have to be hormonally balanced no matter your age.

This book is for women of all ages. My husband and I have been blessed with five daughters. They are truly a gift from God. They have all experienced their own hormonal journey, as have my patients, other relatives, friends, and neighbors. I have had the great fortune in my life to be able to help patients around the world achieve hormonal balance as well as to be able to teach internationally.

With the completion of the Genome Project, medicine has changed. The science is now here to individualize treatment—this includes hormonal therapies. How you metabolize medication, including hormones, or the amount you need are very different from your mother, your sister, or your friend.

Much of this book is written in a concise, bullet-style format, as opposed to long, literary prose. It was formatted as such for today's busy woman who does not want to wade through extraneous sentence structure. You can see the important points at a moment's glance. Consequently, some of the lengthy scientific explanations are not present in the body of this text. For those readers who want a further explanation of the principles contained in this book, please avail yourself of the numerous citations from the medical journals in the References section.

It is my hope that this book will serve as a guide for all women so that we can each receive the individualized care that we all deserve.

In good health,
Pamela W. Smith, MD, MPH, MS

Introduction

How would you like to live to be a healthy 100 years of age? Well, perhaps you can. We now have the scientific means to help you live to be at least 100 years of age. However, in order to live to that age, you need to be hormonally and nutritionally balanced. I hope that my book will help you to achieve this. It was written to provide you with hormonal and nutritional aspects of staying healthy and preventing disease.

All the hormones in the body are a symphony. Much like an orchestra must play in tune, your hormonal symphony must be in tune throughout your life in order for you to have optimal health. Hormonal dysfunction can occur at any age—it is not exclusive to older people. For example, if you have PMS, postpartum depression, fibroids, or fibrocystic breast disease, there is a good chance that your progesterone-to-estrogen ratio is too low.

Treatments for these kinds of ailments (or any hormonal abnormality, for that matter) may involve hormone replacement therapy (HRT), change in diet, exercise, and/or nutritional therapies. In the past, no matter what her symptoms or hormonal levels were, every woman would receive the same one-size-fits-all treatment. Today, medicine has changed, and the science is here to customize your healthcare.

Medicine is at a crossroads. Now, instead of just treating the symptoms of a disease, a new model of medicine has emerged that looks at the underlying cause of the problem. For example: why might a person suffer from depression? Antidepressants are wonderful medications—if you need them. Their purpose is to treat the symptoms of depression—not to uncover the cause of depression. In the new specialty of Precision Medicine/Anti-Aging Medicine, the reason *why* a person has depression would be examined. Depression may be a symptom of hypothyroidism, which is low thyroid function. Perhaps, it may be the result of the sufferer's body no longer making enough estrogen, progesterone, or testosterone. There may be a neurotransmitter imbalance or perhaps the GI tract is not functioning optimally. There are many different factors that can cause depression, and Precision/Anti-Aging Medicine aims to find and alleviate the cause instead of just treating the various symptoms. Just because two people are suffering the same problems does not mean they should receive the same treatment. Precision/Anti-Aging Medicine recognizes this and treats patients accordingly. To find a Precision/Anti-Aging specialist, see the Resources section of this book.

The copy in this book will explore the intricate web of your body's hormonal system, covering three areas.

Part I of the book explores the different hormones in your body, their functions, and the different side effects that can occur if these hormones are not at optimal levels. Additionally, the importance of hormonal levels and the ratio between them will be revealed. You will also learn the different causes that can create hormonal imbalances, which may help you eliminate an issue before it becomes a problem. The perfect levels of *all* of your hormones are needed for you to achieve optimal health.

I have organized Part I, The Hormones, in the order I felt would be most useful to women. While the order of importance for every woman may be different, understanding each hormone is key.

Part II, Ailments and Problems, focuses on the most common ailments and problems that arise from hormonal imbalances, such as perimenopause and menopause, PMS, postpartum depression, endometriosis, and fibrocystic breast disease, to name a few. You'll learn that even diseases that seemingly have nothing to do with hormones—like heart disease and osteoporosis—can be affected by a hormonal imbalance. Keeping your hormones at optimal levels is beneficial in preventing a wide array of health disorders, even ones you wouldn't suspect.

Part III, focuses on hormone replacement therapy. You'll learn the difference between synthetic and natural HRT, and how to get started should you decide HRT is the option for you. Different ways to have your hormone levels measured are discussed, along with a few examples of how hormone replacement therapy has been shown, in medical studies, to help prevent disease. Finally, you will learn how proper nutrition can benefit and boost the effects of HRT.

Fortunately, we do not have to suffer in silence like our grandmothers and mothers did! Science can help us. Not only can we have our symptoms resolved, but we now have a better chance of helping maintain our vision, memory, and mobility. This is not "Star Trek" medicine. It is here and available now. You too can have individualized and customized care. This book will help you discover how.

PART I

Hormones

INTRODUCTION

A hormone is a chemical substance produced in the body that controls and regulates the activity of certain cells or organs. The hormones in your body are a key component of your overall health. Endocrine glands, which are special groups of cells in the body, make hormones. The major endocrine glands are the pituitary, pineal, thymus, thyroid, adrenal, and parathyroid glands, as well as the glandular organ known as the pancreas. In addition, women make hormones in their ovaries. All the hormones in your body interact with each other. They form an interconnected web and must be balanced for you to feel great and experience optimal health.

This part of the book examines many of the hormones in your body. It discusses the sex hormones—estrogen, progesterone, and testosterone—and the importance of having a balanced ratio between these hormones. Your sex hormones interact with DHEA and cortisol, the hormone made in your adrenal glands that are located above your kidneys. All these hormones are made by pregnenolone, your memory hormone. Each of these hormones furthermore interfaces with insulin, the hormone that regulates your blood sugar.

Additionally, these hormones all interact with your thyroid hormone, which regulates many important functions in your body, including metabolism. The thyroid is the conductor of your hormonal symphony, so to speak. Just as the ratio between your sex hormones is important, thyroid levels that are too high or too low can have serious consequences. Moreover, your parathyroid glands surround your thyroid gland, producing and secreting parathyroid hormone, which plays a key role in regulating the amount of calcium in the blood and within bones. All these issues are discussed in this part of the book.

When your hormones are in balance, you feel fabulous. When your hormones are not in balance, you will likely experience symptoms. You will also be at an increased risk of developing various diseases, such as heart disease, osteoporosis (bone loss), and cognitive decline.

Your hormone levels change throughout your lifetime. The hormones your body makes, and the degree of fluctuation or change in hormone levels, are vital. There are many factors that influence the amount produced of a particular hormone by the body. For example, if you are stressed, take an antibiotic, deliver a baby, are near toxins, have an unhealthy diet, exercise too much or not enough, or take too few or too many vitamins, the quantity of hormones that your body produces will be affected.

I have chosen to organize the sections in Part I by order of importance instead of alphabetical order. This is the logical order of importance in a woman's body when symptoms, diseases, and other hormonal issues are taken into consideration. Of course, different women have different hormonal needs, and this format will not be the order of importance for every single woman.

Let us begin our hormonal journey.

ESTROGEN

Estrogen is a hormone that is produced in the ovaries and is essential to a woman's sexual development. There are receptor sites for estrogen practically everywhere in the human body: in the brain, muscles, bone, bladder, gut, uterus, ovaries, vagina, breasts, eyes, heart, lungs, and blood vessels, to name a few. Estrogen plays over 400 crucial roles in the body.

■ Functions of Estrogen in Your Body

- Acts as a natural calcium blocker to keep your arteries open
- Aids in the formation of neurotransmitters in your brain—such as serotonin—which decrease depression, irritability, anxiety, and pain sensitivity
- Decreases LDL (bad cholesterol) and prevents its oxidation
- Decreases lipoprotein A (a risk factor of heart disease)
- Decreases the accumulation of plaque on your arteries
- Decreases wrinkles
- Decreases your risk of developing colon cancer
- Dilates your small arteries
- Enhances energy
- Enhances magnesium uptake and utilization
- Enhances the production of nerve-growth factor
- Helps maintain the elasticity of your arteries
- Helps maintain your memory
- Helps prevent Alzheimer's disease
- Helps prevent muscle damage and maintain muscles
- Helps prevent tooth loss
- Helps regulate blood pressure
- Helps with fine motor skills
- Improves insulin sensitivity
- Improves mood
- Increases blood flow
- Increases concentration
- Increases HDL (good cholesterol) by 10 to 15 percent
- Increases reasoning
- Increases reasoning ability
- Increases sexual interest

- Increases the water content of your skin, which is responsible for your skin's thickness and softness

- Increases your metabolic rate, which helps your body run at a youthful level

- Inhibits platelet stickiness, which decreases your risk of heart disease

- Lowers homocysteine (a risk factor for heart disease)

- Maintains bone density

- Maintains the amount of collagen in your skin

- Protect against endothelial dysfunction by increasing endothelial nitric oxide

- Protects you against macular degeneration, an age-related eye ailment that may cause vision loss

- Reduces homocysteine (a risk factor for heart disease)

- Reduces vascular proliferation and inflammatory responses

- Reduces vascular proliferation and inflammatory responses, which decrease your risk of heart disease

- Reduces your overall risk of heart disease by 40 to 50 percent

- Reduces your risk of cataracts

- Regulates body temperature

Estrogen levels are lower in women who smoke. This may be why women who smoke experience more menopausal symptoms than women who do not smoke. In addition, low-fat diets decrease free estrogen (the amount of estrogen available for the body to use).

■ Signs and Symptoms of Estrogen Deficiency

- ❑ Acne

- ❑ Anxiety

- ❑ Arthritis

- ❑ Bladder problems (more infections, urinary leakage)

- ❑ Brittle hair and nails

- ❑ Chronic fatigue

- ❑ Decrease in breast size

- ❑ Decrease in dexterity

- ❑ Decrease in memory and focus

- ❑ Decrease in sexual interest/ function

- ❑ Depression

- ❑ Diabetes/insulin resistance

- ❏ Difficulty losing weight, even with diet and exercise
- ❏ Dry eye
- ❏ Elevated cholesterol
- ❏ Fibromyalgia
- ❏ Food cravings
- ❏ Heart attack
- ❏ Hypertension/elevated blood pressure
- ❏ Increase in facial hair
- ❏ Increase in insulin resistance, which can lead to diabetes
- ❏ Increase in tension headaches
- ❏ Increased cholesterol
- ❏ Infertility
- ❏ Joint pain
- ❏ Low energy, especially at the end of the day
- ❏ More frequent migraines
- ❏ More wrinkles (aging skin)
- ❏ Oily skin
- ❏ Osteoporosis/osteopenia
- ❏ Panic attacks
- ❏ Polycystic ovarian syndrome
- ❏ Restless sleep
- ❏ Stress incontinence
- ❏ Strokes
- ❏ Thinner skin
- ❏ Thinning hair
- ❏ Urinary stress incontinence/leakage
- ❏ Urinary tract infections
- ❏ Vaginal dryness
- ❏ Vulvodynia (vaginal pain)
- ❏ Weight gain around the middle

Most young women who suffer estrogen-related problems are estrogen dominant. However, as women grow older, most develop estrogen deficiency. It is extremely important that estrogen be replaced when it declines after menopause, provided you do not have a hormonally related breast cancer, since many studies have shown that estrogen helps to prevent heart disease and cognitive decline. (See Part III on page 363.) In addition, not all women lose estrogen at menopause. Estrogen is stored in fat cells; therefore, if a woman is overweight, she may not need estrogen for several years after she stops cycling.

■ Causes of Estrogen Deficiency

- ● Hormonal dysregulation following delivery
- ● Hypothalamic dysfunction

- Hypothyroidism
- Insulin resistance
- Perimenopause/menopause
- Pituitary dysfunction

- Polycystic ovarian syndrome (PCOS)
- Premature ovarian decline/ premature ovarian failure
- Synthetic hormone replacement
- Turner syndrome

■ Foods That Can Increase Your Estrogen Levels

If you would like to boost your estrogen levels naturally, dietary choices may be the answer. Similarly, if your estrogen levels are consistently high, the cause of this issue may be found on your plate. You may be consuming large amounts of foods that are known to increase this hormone in the body, such as the following examples.

VEGETABLES

- Artichoke
- Asparagus
- Bamboo shoots
- Beet
- Bell pepper (red, green, yellow, orange)
- Brussels sprouts
- Cabbage
- Carrot
- Cauliflower
- Celery
- Chives
- Corn
- Cucumber
- Eggplant
- Garlic
- Green beans
- Lettuce
- Mustard greens
- Okra
- Onion
- Parsley
- Pea seedlings
- Potato (all kinds)
- Pumpkin
- Radish
- Seaweed
- Shallot
- Spinach
- Tomato
- Turnip
- Yam

FRUITS

- Apple
- Apricot
- Banana
- Cherry
- Date
- Grape
- Grapefruit
- Lemon
- Muskmelon
- Orange
- Peach
- Pear

- Pineapple
- Plum
- Pomegranate
- Strawberry
- Watermelon

CEREALS AND GRAINS

- Barley
- Corn
- Rice
- Rye
- Wheat (bran, flour, whole)

LEGUMES (BEANS)

- Chickpeas
- Kidney
- Pea
- Peanut
- Soybean

SEEDS AND NUTS

- Almond
- Cashew
- Coconut
- Pecan
- Pine nut
- Pistachio
- Sesame seed
- Sunflower seed
- Walnut

OILS

- Coconut
- Corn
- Linseed (flaxseed)
- Olive
- Peanut
- Rice bran
- Safflower
- Sesame seed
- Soybean
- Sunflower
- Walnut
- Wheat germ

As mentioned, most young women with estrogen issues have too much estrogen in their bodies, not too little. Dr. John Lee coined the phrase "estrogen dominance" to describe the symptoms of excess estrogen in the body.

■ Signs and Symptoms of Excess Estrogen

- ❏ Bloating
- ❏ Brain fog
- ❏ Cervical dysplasia
- ❏ Decrease in sexual interest
- ❏ Depression with anxiety or agitation
- ❏ Elevated risk of developing breast cancer
- ❏ Fatigue

❏ Fibrocystic breasts

❏ Headaches

❏ Heavy periods

❏ Hypothyroidism (increases the binding of thyroid hormone, which causes low thyroid hormone levels)

❏ Increased risk of developing autoimmune diseases

❏ Increased risk of developing uterine cancer

❏ Irritability

❏ Mood swings

❏ Panic attacks

❏ Poor sleep

❏ Swollen breasts

❏ Uterine fibroids (non-cancerous tumors of the uterus)

❏ Water retention

❏ Weight gain (especially in the abdomen, hips, and thighs)

■ Causes of Excess Estrogen

● Diet low in grains and fiber

● Environmental estrogens

● Excessive doses of estrogen replacement therapy

● Foods that can increase your estrogen level

● Impaired elimination of estrogen through the liver/GI tract

● Lack of exercise

■ Methods That Can Lower Excess Estrogen Levels

● Exercise

● Eat foods that can decrease estrogen levels

● Improve the health of your gastrointestinal tract

● Improve phase I and phase II detoxification of the liver

● Lower your dose of estrogen replacement

● Lose weight if you are overweight

■ Foods That Can Decrease Your Estrogen Levels

If you would like to lower your estrogen levels naturally, the right dietary choices may prove helpful in this situation as well. There are a number of foods that are known to decrease estrogen in the body, including the following examples.

VEGETABLES

- Cruciferous vegetables
- Bok choy
- Broccoli
- Brussels sprouts
- Cabbage

- Cauliflower
- Collard greens
- Kale
- Rutabagas
- Turnips

- Mushrooms
  - Baby button
  - Cremini
  - Portobello
  - Shitake

FRUITS

- Pomegranate
- Red grapes

SEEDS AND NUTS

- Chia
- Flax
- Seeds that contain polyphenols
- Sesame

BEVERAGES

- Green tea

NATURAL ESTROGENS

When referring to natural estrogens, the term "natural" means biologically identical to the chemical substance made by your own body. Your body makes many kinds of estrogen. The three main estrogens are E1, called estrone; E2, called estradiol; and E3, called estriol.

■ Estrone (E1)

Although serum estradiol (E2) levels decrease significantly after natural menopause, a considerable amount of estrone (E1) still exists in women after this phase of life. It is derived from estradiol. High levels of E1 stimulate breast and uterine tissue, and many researchers believe this action increases the risks of developing breast cancer and uterine cancer.

E1 is considered a reserve source for estrogen. If your estrogen levels get too low, your body can draw from and use this stored amount. Estrone produced in adipose tissues may have a role in modulating the loss of bone mass occurring after menopause.

Before menopause, E1 is made by your ovaries, adrenal glands, liver, and fat cells. It is converted into E2 in your ovaries. After menopause, very little E1 becomes E2 since the ovaries stop working. In later years, E1 is made in your fat cells and, to a lesser degree, in your liver and adrenal glands. Therefore, the more body fat you have, the more E1 you make. Consequently, obese women tend to have an increased E1-to-E2 ratio. In addition, routine alcohol consumption decreases ovarian hormone levels and increases levels of E1, which can lead to an increased risk of breast cancer.

■ Estradiol (E2)

Estradiol is the strongest form of estrogen. It is twelve times stronger than E1, and eighty times stronger than estriol (E3). It is the main estrogen produced by the body before menopause. Most of your body's E2 is made in your ovaries. High levels of E2 are associated with an increased risk of breast and uterine cancer.

■ Functions of E2 in Your Body

- Decreases fatigue
- Decreases LDL (bad cholesterol)
- Decreases platelet stickiness
- Decreases total cholesterol
- Decreases triglycerides (transdermal, on the skin, administration of E2 only)
- Helps maintain memory
- Helps maintain potassium levels
- Helps maintain your bones
- Helps with the absorption of calcium, magnesium, and zinc
- Improves sleep
- Increases endorphins
- Increases growth hormone
- Increases HDL (good cholesterol)
- Increases serotonin
- Works as an antioxidant

E2 is the form of estrogen you lose at menopause. However, two-thirds of postmenopausal women up to the age of eighty continue to make some E2. Women who have had a surgical procedure that affected their ovaries tend to have lower levels of E2 than other women. (See the section on surgical menopause on page 274.)

■ Signs and Symptoms of Estradiol Decline

- ❏ Aching joints
- ❏ Anxiety attacks that worsen around menstrual cycle
- ❏ Bladder changes, such as more infections, pain during urination, more frequent urination, and urinary leakage
- ❏ Bone loss in spine, resulting in slumped posture
- ❏ Decline in collagen, resulting in dry, crawly, looser skin and more wrinkles
- ❏ Difficulty having an orgasm
- ❏ Difficulty losing weight, even with diet and exercise
- ❏ Dry, brittle nails
- ❏ Dry eye
- ❏ Fibromyalgia pain syndrome
- ❏ Food cravings
- ❏ Increase in facial hair
- ❏ Increase in tension headaches
- ❏ Loss of energy, or feeling too tired to get through the day
- ❏ Loss of sexual interest
- ❏ Memory and concentration problems that worsen before menstruation

- ❏ Mood swings, episodic tearfulness for no reason, irritability, angry outbursts, and spells of depression, especially pre-menstrual
- ❏ More irritable bowel problems prior to and during menstruation
- ❏ Muscle soreness or stiffness
- ❏ Palpitations, especially those that get worse a few days prior to menstruation and during the cycle
- ❏ Premenstrual migraines or more frequent migraines
- ❏ Restless sleep, difficulty sleeping (especially prior to menstruating), or multiple awakenings during the night
- ❏ Spiking blood pressure or blood pressure that is higher than normal
- ❏ Thinner hair and more scalp hair loss
- ❏ Vaginal dryness, resulting in pain during intercourse
- ❏ Weight gain around the middle
- ❏ Worsening allergies, such as sensitivities to chemicals or perfumes
- ❏ Worsening PMS

■ Estriol (E3)

Estriol (E3) has a much lesser stimulatory effect on the breast and uterine lining than E1 or E2. E3 does not promote breast cancer. In fact, considerable evidence exists to show that it protects against breast cancer. In Western Europe, E3 has been used for this purpose for more than sixty years.

Estrogen has two main receptor sites to which it binds in the body: estrogen receptor-alpha and estrogen receptor-beta. Estrogen receptor-alpha increases cell growth and estrogen receptor-beta decreases cell growth, helps to prevent breast cancer development, and promotes beneficial estrogenic effects on skin, bone, brain, and other tissues. E2 equally activates estrogen receptors alpha and beta. E1 activates estrogen receptor-alpha selectively at a ratio of five-to-one. Therefore, E1 prefers to bind with the alpha receptor type, which increases cell proliferation. In contrast, E3 binds preferentially to estrogen receptor-beta at a three-to-one ratio. It is believed that this selective binding to estrogen-beta receptor sites imparts to E3 a potential for breast cancer prevention.

One of the wonderful things about E3 is that it is an adaptogen, meaning it adapts to the specific environment of the body it is in. When given by itself, E3 does exert strong estrogenic effects. When given in a tenfold amount in relationship to E2, E3 antagonizes the effect of E2, which may be another reason why E3 helps decrease the risk of breast cancer.

Studies over the last forty years have revealed that E3 given experimentally to women with breast cancer has decreased a reoccurrence of the disease. This includes one study in the 1970s in which women with metastatic breasts were given E3. Of the women, 37 percent experienced remission—their cancer did not spread any further.

However, E3 does not offer the bone, heart, or brain protection that E2 provides. E3 does, however, have some positive effects on heart health by lowering cholesterol. It is also effective in controlling symptoms of menopause, including hot flashes, vaginal dryness, and frequent urinary tract infections.

I usually begin by prescribing 20 percent E2 and 80 percent E3 for an estrogen prescription if tests reveal that a patient's estrogen levels are low. Then the percentages of E2 and E3 are adjusted according to lab results of each patient. The combination of E2 and E3 together is called "biest," which is a prescription that a compounding pharmacist (a pharmacist who puts together medications in customized dosages) can formulate for you. Any percentage of these two estrogens can be used, since the dosage is personalized.

■ Functions of E3 in Your Body

- Benefits the vaginal lining
- Blocks E1 by occupying the estrogen receptor sites on your breast cells
- Controls symptoms of menopause, including hot flashes, insomnia, and vaginal dryness
- Decreases LDL (bad cholesterol)
- Helps reduce pathogenic bacteria
- Helps restore the proper pH of the vagina, which prevents urinary tract infections (UTIs)
- Helps your gut maintain a favorable environment for the growth of good bacteria (Lactobacilli)
- Increases HDL (good cholesterol)

Before you begin HRT, it is necessary that you have your levels of all three estrogens measured. You should also have them measured regularly thereafter, to help your healthcare provider ensure you maintain the optimal amount of each type of estrogen. See Part III of this book for further discussion.

Estriol is also now being used to treat multiple sclerosis (MS), which is associated with a progressive decrease in gray matter in the brain. This decrease in gray matter leads to cognitive impairment, which is seen in a high percentage of MS patients. In a phase 2 trial of estriol treatment in women with relapsing-remitting multiple sclerosis, increased levels of estriol were linked to improvements in cognitive impairment.

■ Estrogen Detoxification

Estrogen synthesis, estrogen metabolism, and estrogen detoxification are of paramount importance in order to maintain optimal health. The effect of estrogen on your body is not related solely to its function but also to how it is detoxified in the liver and in other tissues.

Toxins are poisonous substances that are either produced by the body, inhaled, or ingested. When they build up, the health effects can be quite serious. This is why it is important to detoxify.

Detoxification is the process through which toxic substances—environmental pollutants, medications, byproducts of metabolism, and more—are removed from the body. This process is one of the major functions of the liver, gastrointestinal tract, kidneys, and skin, with the liver being one of the most important organs of detoxification. Studies have shown that the effectiveness of the body's ability to break down toxins varies from person to person.

Each year, over 2.5 billion pounds of pesticides are dumped on crop lands, forests, lawns, and fields. According to the U.S. Environmental Protection Agency, more than 4 billion pounds of chemicals were released into the ground in the year 2000, threatening our natural ground water sources.

■ Toxin Buildup

Toxicity can affect your endocrine, immune, and neurological systems. Endocrine toxicity affects reproduction, menstruation, libido, metabolic rate, stress tolerance, and glucose regulation. Immune toxicity may be a factor in asthma, allergies, skin disorders, chronic infections, and cancer. Neurological toxicity also affects cognition, mood, and neurological function.

■ Signs and Symptoms of Toxin Buildup

- ❏ Allergies
- ❏ Bloating
- ❏ Chemical sensitivities
- ❏ Clammy hands
- ❏ Constipation
- ❏ Depression
- ❏ Difficulty tolerating exercise
- ❏ Disturbed sleep
- ❏ Fatigue
- ❏ Flatulence
- ❏ Fluid retention
- ❏ Headaches
- ❏ Intolerance to fat, alcohol, caffeine
- ❏ Irritability
- ❏ Itchy skin
- ❏ Jaundice (eyes and skin may be yellow in severe cases)
- ❏ Lethargy
- ❏ Muscle aches and pains
- ❏ Nausea
- ❏ Trouble breathing

Additionally, there are some situations that can increase your exposure to toxins.

■ Some Situations That Can Increase Your Exposure to Toxins

- Chronic inflammation
- Chronic infections
- Chronic use of medication
- Drinking tap water
- Excessive consumption of alcohol
- Excessive consumption of caffeine
- Excessive consumption of processed foods and fats
- Intestinal (gut) dysfunction
- Kidney problems
- Lack of exercise
- Liver dysfunction
- Living or working near areas of high traffic of industrial plants
- Occupational or other exposure to pesticides, paints, or other toxic substances without adequate protective equipment
- Recreational drug use
- Tobacco use
- Using pesticides, paint, or other toxic substances without adequate protective gear

In addition to the previous issues, genetic factors and aging also affect your liver's ability to detoxify the body.

In terms of exposure to toxins, you are exposed to estrogen-like compounds, known as xenoestrogens, every day. Xenoestrogens have estrogenic activity and can interfere with or mimic your own hormone synthesis. Consequently, they can be disruptive to your own hormone production.

THE DETOXIFICATION PROCESS

Detoxification is a process by which your body transforms toxins and medications into harmless molecules that can be eliminated. This process takes place primarily in the liver and to a smaller degree in other tissues, such as your gastrointestinal tract, skin, kidneys, and lungs.

There are three major phases of detoxification that your body undergoes. The first two take place in your liver. In phase I, enzymes change toxins into intermediate compounds. In phase II, the intermediate compounds are neutralized through the addition of a water-soluble molecule.

Phase III is accomplished by multiple organs systems, namely your gut, kidneys, and lymphatic system, after which the body is able to eliminate the transformed toxins through the urine or feces.

It is very important for you to detoxify estrogen completely in your body. The good news is that all three phases of detoxification can be measured to see if your liver and GI tract are able to adequately detoxify substances.

Phase I Detoxification: Your First Line of Defense

In phase I detoxification, enzymes in the cytochrome P450 system use oxygen to modify toxic compounds, medications, and steroid hormones. This is your first line of defense for the detoxification of all environmental toxins, medications, supplements (for example, vitamins), and many waste products that your body produces.

The cytochrome P450 system is a group of over sixty enzymes that your body uses to break down toxins. Most of these enzymes are located in your liver. Three of the twelve cytochrome P450 gene families share the main responsibility for drug metabolism in your body. In other words, many of the medications that you take are broken down through this system. The cytochrome P450 system is also involved in other processes in your body, such as the conversion of vitamin D into more active forms.

Phase I occurs in the liver, where estrogen goes through the cytochrome P450 system. This influences the amount of estrogen that is exposed to your other cells. If you do not completely detoxify the intermediates of estrogen metabolism, it can result in an increase in estrogen activity in your body.

Within your own genetic makeup, there are variations called "single nucleotide polymorphisms" (SNPs, pronounced "snips"). These SNPs in your genes code for a particular enzyme that can increase or decrease the activity of that enzyme. Both increased and decreased activity may be harmful to you. Furthermore, if you increase phase I clearance (elimination) without increasing phase II clearance, it can lead to a buildup of intermediates that may be more toxic than the original substance.

Decreased phase I clearance will cause toxic accumulation in your body. Sometimes, the body completes phase I but builds up a toxic metabolite that phase II is unable to eliminate from the system. Adverse reactions to medications are often due to a decreased capacity for clearing them from your system.

■ Nutrients Required for Phase I Detoxification

- Copper
- Flavonoids
- Folic acid
- Magnesium
- Niacin
- Vitamin B_2
- Vitamin B_3
- Vitamin B_6
- Vitamin B_{12}
- Vitamin C
- Zinc

Phase II Detoxification: Conjugation of Toxins

In phase II detoxification, large water-soluble molecules are added to toxins, usually at the reactive site formed by phase I reactions. After phase II modifications, the body is able to eliminate the transformed toxins in the urine or the feces. Phase II detoxification has six stages.

Stage I: Glutathione conjugation. Glutathione is the strongest antioxidant that your body makes. It plays an important role in the detoxification of carcinogens and other environmental toxins. This stage of detoxification requires glutathione and vitamin B_6.

Stage II: Amino acid conjugation. In this stage, amino acids combine with toxins to neutralize them. Glycine and taurine are amino acids used for this pathway, along with glutamine, arginine, and ornithine.

Stage III: Methylation. Methylation is needed for many reactions in the body including detoxification of estrogen and breakdown of homocysteine. It requires folic acid, choline, methionine, trimethylglycine (TMG), and s-adenosyl-methionine (SAMe).

Stage IV: Sulfation. The sulfation pathway is required in the detoxification of food additives, steroid hormones, thyroid hormones, estrogen hormones, and toxins from intestinal bacteria. It requires cysteine, methionine, and molybdenum.

Stage V: Acetylation. The acetylation pathway detoxifies substances known as amines, such as histamine and tyramine, as well as compounds such as caffeine and choline. It requires acetyl CoA and Vitamin B_5. Sluggish acetylation has been associated with an increased risk of bladder cancer.

Stage VI: Glucuronidation. This pathway is responsible for metabolizing drugs and estrogens, and also conjugates bilirubin. It requires glucuronic acid. Calcium D-glucarate supports the glucuronidation pathways and metabolism of estrogen.

Phase III Detoxification: Antiporter System

Recent scientific study suggests the existence of a third detoxification phase, which is located primarily in the small intestine. It is called the antiporter system, or simply phase III, and makes use of antiporter proteins for its detoxification activity. These proteins can be increased, boosting detoxification, or inhibited, decreasing detoxification. The most studied of these proteins is known as P-glycoprotein.

P-glycoprotein is found in the intestines, liver, kidneys, and capillary endothelial cells, which form the blood–brain barrier and blood-testis barrier. It helps in the elimination of toxins from these areas of the body.

Inflammation of the gut can hinder the functioning of phase III, leading to a decrease in the functioning of phase II and then a buildup of the metabolites created in phase I. This domino effect can result in oxidative damage and impair your body's entire detoxification system. In light of this fact, in order to evaluate your body's ability to rid itself of dangerously high levels of certain substances, including estrogen, a phase I/phase II liver detoxification test and a GI health test should be performed. Fostering a healthy GI tract and reducing inflammation in the gut allows your detoxification system to bind toxins and eliminate them.

Detoxification and Nutrition

The detoxification process is dependent on nutrients. All three phases of detoxification are fueled by vitamins, minerals, and other key food components. Therefore, if you are undernourished and lacking key vitamins or nutrients, you may not be able to break down estrogen properly. In addition, if your gastrointestinal tract is not functioning optimally, you will not metabolize estrogen effectively. This can leave estrogen available to cause cell transformation in the breasts and predispose you to breast cancer. Consequently, adequate nutrition is essential for effective detoxification.

SYNTHETIC ESTROGEN

Estrogen replacement comes in many forms. The most commonly prescribed hormone replacement in the world remains a drug that contains horse estrogens (equilin and equilenin) and additives that are synthetic. These additives and coatings may cause their own side effects, including burning in the urinary tract, allergies, joint aches, and pains.

In addition, endothelial nitric oxide synthase is a crucial enzyme involved in the production of nitric oxide in endothelial cells. A study showed that compared to natural estrogen, gene transcription of endothelial nitric oxide synthase was 30 to 50 percent lower in response to synthetic estrogen.

Synthetic estrogens contain many forms of estrogen that do not fit into the estrogen receptors in your body. It is unknown what happens to the estrogens that do not fit into your receptors. The estradiol (E2) molecules your body makes are eliminated from your body through urine within a day. Conversely, equilin (estrogen derived from the urine of horses) has been shown to stay in the body for up to thirteen weeks. This is because your enzymes are designed to metabolize your own estrogen and not equilin.

How you take estrogen is also important. I recommend using estrogen by the transdermal route, which means applying it to the skin. Estrogen used vaginally is also an effective form. Orally used estrogen can have major side effects.

■ Side Effects of Taking Estrogen Orally

- Decrease in growth hormone (the hormone that keeps you younger)
- Elevated liver enzymes
- Increase in C-reactive protein (a marker of inflammation)
- Increase in gallstones
- Increase in sex hormone-binding globulin (SHBG), which can decrease testosterone
- Increased blood pressure
- Increased carbohydrate cravings
- Increased estrone (E1)
- Increased prothrombic effects (blood clots)
- Increased triglycerides
- Interruption in metabolism of tryptophan and serotonin, neurotransmitters that keep you calm and happy
- Weight gain

Therefore, estrogen creams are the preferred method of replacing this hormone, which has so many functions. Many studies have been conducted on transdermal application of estradiol (E2). One study revealed that, when compared with no hormone therapy, the use of oral conjugated equine estrogen or oral estradiol was associated with excess risk of venous thromboembolism (blood clot). In contrast, the use of transdermal estradiol was not associated with excess venous thromboembolism.

When applied, it is important that you rub the estrogen in for two minutes and rotate sites. Discuss with your healthcare practitioner the best location on your skin to apply the estrogen, since it is best absorbed when applied to areas that contain fat cells—except for the abdomen.

■ Therapeutic Benefits of Estrogen

The benefits of estrogen are many. It can help to prevent or improve:

- Cardiovascular disease
- Cataracts
- Cognitive decline
- Colon cancer
- Depression
- Diabetes mellitus
- Glaucoma
- Improve symptoms of menopause

- Inflammation
- Macular degeneration
- Metabolic syndrome
- Multiple sclerosis (estriol)
- Obesity
- Osteoarthritis
- Osteopenia/osteoporosis (bone loss)

In addition to these benefits, estrogen can also strengthen your immune system. Research suggests that estrogen deficiency puts you in a state of accelerated aging. Furthermore, a meta-analysis of twenty-seven studies showed a 28 percent reduction in mortality in menopausal women under age sixty who used hormone replacement therapy. The participants also displayed improved quality of life.

Unfortunately, the study known as the "Study of Women's Health Across the Nation" revealed the number of women with low estrogen to be greater than previously acknowledged. In light of their findings, the authors of this study proposed the use of estrogen replacement therapy. Part III of this book examines hormone replacement therapy and discusses in detail the role of estrogen in the prevention of age-related issues such as heart disease and memory loss.

PROGESTERONE

Progesterone is one of your sex hormones. It plays a role in menstruation, pregnancy, and the formation of embryos. Progesterone is made in the ovaries up until menopause. After menopause, it is made in the adrenal glands. Progesterone is made from pregnenolone and performs many functions in your body. In addition, progesterone works together with estrogen in your body to help you achieve optimal hormonal balance.

■ Functions of Progesterone in Your Body

- Acts as a diuretic
- Acts as an anti-inflammatory
- Aids in ovulation
- Balances estrogen
- Effects the potentiation of GABA
- Enhances the action of thyroid hormones
- Has a positive effect on sleep
- Helps build bone
- Helps maintain bladder function
- Helps maintain pregnancy
- Helps prevent anxiety, irritability, mood swings
- Helps promote implantation of the egg
- Helps restore proper cell-oxygen levels
- Helps the body use and eliminate fats
- Increases metabolic rate
- Increases scalp hair
- Induces conversion of E1 to inactive E1S form
- Lowers LDL
- Modulates oxytocin receptor binding in the hypothalamus
- Promotes Th2 immunity
- Promotes the formation of myelin sheaths
- Protects breast health
- Relaxes smooth muscle
- Relaxes the smooth muscle of the gut to aid in breaking down food
- Supports immune system

Progesterone levels in the body can drop below optimal levels at different times in your life. There are many reasons why this can happen. (See

"Causes of Progesterone Deficiency" listed below). When progesterone levels decline, there can be side effects, some more serious than others. A study measured blood levels of progesterone in almost 6,000 women that were premenopausal. Women with the highest levels of progesterone who had regular cycles had an 88 percent reduction in the risk of developing breast cancer. In another study, over 1,000 women who had undergone treatment for infertility were evaluated for over thirty years. The trial was done to look at subsequent breast cancer risk. Women who were deficient in progesterone had a 5.4 times increased risk of developing premenopausal breast cancer and were ten times as likely to die from any cancer.

■ Signs and Symptoms of Progesterone Deficiency

- ❑ Anxiety
- ❑ Decreased HDL levels
- ❑ Decreased libido
- ❑ Depression
- ❑ Excessive menstruation (lasting longer than seven days and very heavy bleeding)
- ❑ Hypersensitivity
- ❑ Insomnia
- ❑ Irritability
- ❑ Migraine headaches prior to menstrual cycles
- ❑ Mood swings
- ❑ Nervousness
- ❑ Osteoporosis
- ❑ Pain and inflammation
- ❑ Weight gain

As mentioned, a progesterone deficiency may be caused by a variety of factors.

■ Causes of Progesterone Deficiency

- ● Antidepressants
- ● Aging
- ● Hypothyroidism (decreased thyroid hormone)
- ● Deficiencies of vitamins A, B_6, C, and zinc
- ● Excessive arginine consumption
- ● Impaired production
- ● Increased prolactin production
- ● Low luteinizing hormone (LH)
- ● Saturated fat intake
- ● Stress
- ● High sugar intake

Just as your body can have too much estrogen, it can also have too much progesterone. Too much progesterone can lead to a variety of signs and symptoms.

■ Signs and Symptoms of Excess Progesterone

❑ Anxiety

❑ Decreased glucose tolerance, which can lead to an increase in blood sugar

❑ Decreased growth hormone

❑ Incontinence (leaky bladder)

❑ Increased appetite

❑ Increased carbohydrate cravings

❑ Increased cortisol

❑ Increased fat storage and weight gain

❑ Increased insulin and insulin resistance

❑ Increased the risk of gallstones

❑ Irritability

❑ Laxity of ligaments to relax, which can lead to backaches, leg aches, and achy hips

❑ Mood swings

❑ Relaxation of smooth muscles of the gut, which may cause bloating, fullness, or constipation

❑ Suppressed immune system

Unlike excess estrogen, which can be caused by a variety of factors, high progesterone levels occur less commonly—the major reason being too high a dose of progesterone prescribed by a healthcare provider.

NATURAL PROGESTERONE

Natural progesterone means that the progesterone that you are taking is the same chemical structure as the progesterone that you were born with. It is usually made from yams or soy. Synthetic progesterone, which will be discussed later in this section, is not the same chemical structure.

The process of producing natural progesterone was discovered by Russell Marker, a Pennsylvania State College chemistry professor. Back in the 1930s, Marker discovered that by using a chemical process, diosgenin (a plant steroid) could be turned into a form of progesterone that is an exact biological duplicate of the progesterone produced by the human body.

Natural progesterone, since it is biologically identical to the progesterone produced by the human body, has plenty of good effects not seen with synthetic progesterone. Consequently, many of these effects are similar to the effects of the progesterone that is produced by the body itself.

■ Effects of Natural Progesterone

- Balances estrogen levels
- Balances fluids in the cells
- Decreases the rate of cancer on all progesterone receptors
- Does not change the good effect estrogen has on blood flow
- Enhances the action of thyroid hormones
- Has a natural calming effect
- Helps restore proper cell oxygen levels
- Helps you sleep
- Helps your body use and eliminate fats
- Increases beneficial effects estrogen has on blood vessel dilation (hardened arteries)
- Increases metabolic rate
- Increases scalp hair
- Induces conversion of E1 to the inactive E1S form (E1S does not increase the risk of breast cancer)
- Is a natural antidepressant
- Is a natural diuretic (water pill)
- Is an anti-inflammatory
- Leaves the body quickly
- Lowers cholesterol
- Lowers high blood pressure
- May protect against breast cancer by inhibiting breast tissue overgrowth
- Normalizes and improves libido.
- Prevents migraine headaches that are menstrual cycle-related
- Promotes a healthy immune system
- Promotes myelination, which helps protect nerves from injury
- Relaxes smooth muscle
- Stimulates the production of new bone

One of the most commonly asked questions about hormones is, "Does natural progesterone increase the risk of developing breast cancer?" Studies have shown that progesterone does not induce estrogen-stimulated breast cell proliferation (growth). In fact, natural progesterone has been shown in clinical trials to decrease the risk of developing breast cancer. One study looked at 80,000 postmenopausal women who used different kinds of hormone replacement therapy over eight years. It found that women who had used estrogen in combination with synthetic progestin had a 69 percent increased risk of developing breast cancer when compared with women who had never taken HRT. Women who had used progesterone in combination with estrogen had no increased risk of developing breast cancer when compared with women that had not used HRT, they also had a decreased risk of developing breast cancer when compared with women who had used progestin. Another study done by the same researchers found a 40 percent increased risk of developing breast cancer in women who had used estrogen with progestin. In women who had used estrogen combined with progesterone, there was a trend toward a decreased risk of developing breast cancer.

SYNTHETIC PROGESTERONE

Synthetic progesterone is called "progestin." It is very different from natural progesterone since it does not have the same chemical structure as the progesterone that your body makes on its own. Consequently, progestins do not reproduce the actions of natural progesterone (which have similar effects on the body as the progesterone the body produces itself). For example, progestins do not help balance the estrogen in the body. They interfere with the body's production of progesterone and may attach themselves to many of your body's receptor sites, not just the progesterone receptors. Furthermore, progestins stop the protective effects estrogen has on your heart and can cause spasms of your arteries.

There are now many studies that show that progestins increase breast cancer replication and growth due to the stimulation of estrogen receptors by progestin, supporting the research that progestins increase the risk of breast cancer. In addition, one study revealed that estrogen plus progestin increased breast cancer incidence with cancers more commonly node positive. Moreover, breast cancer mortality also appears to be increased with combined estrogen plus progestin use.

Progestins may have other side effects that do not occur with natural progesterone. These include the following:

■ Possible Side Effects of Progestins

- Acne

- Bloating

- Breakthrough bleeding/
spotting

- Breast tenderness

- Counteracts many of the
positive effects estrogen has on
serotonin

- Decrease in energy

- Decrease in sexual interest

- Decreased HDL (good
cholesterol)

- Depression

- Fluid retention

- Hair loss

- Headaches

- Inability to help produce
estrogen and testosterone

- Increased appetite

- Increased LDL (bad cholesterol)

- Insomnia

- Irritability

- Nausea

- Protects only the uterus from
cancer (not the breasts)

- Rashes

- Remains in your body longer
than natural progesterone,
which can prevent it from
balancing with other hormones

- Spasms of the coronary arteries

- Weight gain

There are, however, a few positive effects of progestins, all of which are also effects of natural progesterone. For example, both build bone, help the thyroid hormone function, protect against fibrocystic breast disease and endometrial cancer, and normalize zinc and copper levels.

Aside from these few common positive effects, it is clear from this discussion that natural progesterone offers a safer approach to HRT than synthetic progesterone (progestin) does. It is also very important that you have your levels of progesterone measured before you begin HRT, and then on a regular basis afterwards to confirm that you are taking an optimal dose for you. (See the section on testing on page 376.)

Progesterone can be used orally or transdermally (on the skin). After receiving your prescription, you'll need a compounding pharmacist in order to get it filled. As mentioned, natural progesterone is made from yams or soy. Your compounding pharmacist will add an enzyme to convert the hormone from these plants (disogenin) into progesterone.

Over-the-counter progesterone, which you can buy without a prescription, frequently does not contain this enzyme.

If you're suffering from insomnia and you need to take progesterone, you should opt for the pill form. The pill affects the GABA receptors in your brain. GABA is an amino acid that acts as a neurotransmitter. It has a calming effect on your brain, which helps you sleep.

Natural progesterone is also available as Prometrium, which is a pill derived from peanut oil made by a pharmaceutical company. The absorption rate of oral progesterone may change over the years, so you need less medication as you grow older. As women age, progesterone orally is most often used. Some women experience side effects from oral progesterone, such as nausea, breast swelling, dizziness, drowsiness, and depression, due to its effects on the liver and gastrointestinal tract. If you develop any of these symptoms, you should contact your healthcare provider in order to have your hormone levels measured and, if needed, a gut-health test done to determine if your GI tract is functioning optimally.

Many women who have had a complete hysterectomy wonder if they still need progesterone. The answer is categorically yes. Natural progesterone has many positive effects on the body, as previously discussed.

Last, adrenaline also interacts with progesterone. When a person feels stressed, adrenaline surges, which can block progesterone receptors. This can prevent progesterone from being used effectively by the body.

■ Therapeutic Benefits of Progesterone

- Acts as an anti-inflammatory

- Decreases risk of breast cancer (balances estrogen)

- Helps in weight loss (increases metabolic rate, helps the body use and eliminate fats, and is also a diuretic)

- Helps against hair loss (increases scalp hair)

- Helps against hypercholesterolemia

- Helps against hypertension

- Helps against insomnia

- Helps against multiple sclerosis (promotes myelination)

- Helps against osteopenia/ osteoporosis

- Improves sexual dysfunction

- Mitigates anxiety disorders

- Prevents heart disease (increases beneficial effects estrogen has on blood vessels)

- Protects the myelin sheath post stroke
- Reduces depression

ESTROGEN/PROGESTERONE RATIO

You've already learned about estrogen and progesterone. But did you know that it is important that the two hormones remain in a specific ratio within your body? The increase in inflammatory agents in today's world are enhancing estrogen levels (or estrogen mimics), fueling estrogen dominance, which has increased greatly over the years.

As you will discover, there is an increased risk of breast cancer if estrogen metabolism favors the 16-hydroxyestrone pathway or the 4-hydroxyestrone pathway. There is also a higher risk for breast cancer if you have a low progesterone-to-estrogen ratio, meaning that the estrogen and progesterone ratio in your body is out of balance. Having a low progesterone-to-estrogen ratio can have other effects on the body as well.

■ Effects of a Low Progesterone-to-Estrogen Ratio

- Abnormal bleeding during peri- and post-menopause
- Increase in some autoimmune diseases
- Increased risk of breast cancer
- Increased risk of uterine cancer
- Infertility

Estrogen and progesterone work together in your body. E2 (one of the forms of estrogen your body makes) lowers body fat by decreasing the amount of lipoprotein lipase, an enzyme, in your fat cells. Progesterone increases body fat storage by increasing the amount of lipoprotein lipase.

Estrogen and progesterone also work in concert to balance your body's release of insulin. E2 increases insulin sensitivity and improves glucose tolerance. Progesterone decreases insulin sensitivity and can cause insulin resistance. For this reason, women who have diabetes need to make sure that their estrogen/progesterone ratio is normal.

An estrogen/progesterone ratio that is too high in progesterone will break down protein and muscle tissue, which will make diseases (like fibromyalgia, an autoimmune disease that causes muscle pain) worse.

There are other side effects of a high progesterone-to-estrogen ratio.

■ Possible Effects of a High Progesterone-to-Estrogen Ratio

- Anxiety
- Decrease in sexual interest
- Depression
- Fatigue
- Gut disturbances
- Heart racing

- Incontinence
- Insomnia
- Insulin resistance/diabetes
- Irritability
- Mood swings
- Weight gain

If you use progesterone for too long without adequately using estrogen, there can be negative effects on the body.

■ Side Effects of Progesterone Without Adequate Estrogen Use*

- Decreased HDL (good cholesterol)
- Decreased libido
- Depression
- Fatigue

- Increased insulin resistance (can predispose you to diabetes)
- Increased LDL (bad cholesterol)
- Increased total cholesterol
- Increased triglyceride levels
- Weight gain

See the list on page 30 to learn what can happen if you have too much estrogen and not enough progesterone.

When you have a salivary test or blood spot test done to measure your hormone levels, your healthcare practitioner or pharmacist will also receive a measure of the estrogen/progesterone ratio. Your healthcare provider will then prescribe the appropriate treatment according to the lab results.

TESTOSTERONE

Testosterone falls into a class of hormones called "androgens." Androgens are commonly referred to as "male" hormones, but they are present in women as well. The reason they are called male is because the human characteristics they stimulate and control are considered to be masculine characteristics.

Testosterone is made in the adrenal glands and ovaries. For most women as they age, the ovaries produce less testosterone. Of this testosterone, only one percent is free, meaning it is available for the body to use. The rest is bound to sex-hormone binding globulin (SHGB).

Women who have increased levels of androgens have higher levels of free testosterone. Therefore, it is important for these women to measure their salivary levels and not just their total testosterone blood hormone levels (see page 377 for salivary testing). This is also paramount since your hormone levels fluctuate throughout your cycle. Also, salivary or blood spot levels are a measure of the hormones in your entire body and not just the levels in your blood.

Testosterone performs many important functions in the body.

■ Functions of Testosterone in Your Body

- Aids in pain control
- Decreases bone deterioration
- Decreases excess body fat
- Elevates norepinephrine in the brain (has the same effect as taking an antidepressant)
- Helps maintain memory
- Increases muscle mass and strength
- Increases muscle tone (so your skin doesn't sag)
- Increases sense of emotional well-being, self-confidence, and motivation
- Increases sexual interest (86 percent of woman say they experience a decrease in sexual interest with menopause)

Women of any age can experience a deficiency of testosterone, which is indicated by a variety of symptoms.

■ Signs and Symptoms of Testosterone Deficiency

❑ Anxiety

❑ Decline in muscle tone

- Decreased HDL (good cholesterol)
- Decreased sex drive
- Droopy eyelids
- Dry, thin skin with poor elasticity
- Dry, thinning hair
- Fatigue
- Hypersensitive, hyperemotional states
- Fewer dreams
- Loss of pubic hair
- Low self-esteem
- Mild depression
- Muscle wasting (despite adequate calorie and protein intake)
- Saggy cheeks
- Thin lips
- Weight gain

SHBG is a carrier protein for testosterone and DHT, and somewhat for estradiol (E2). If SHBG levels are high, there is less E2 and testosterone available for use by the body. Likewise, low SHBG levels mean there is more E2 and testosterone available for use. In addition, low SHBG levels may be a marker for low thyroid function. High insulin levels and high prolactin levels also change the levels of SHBG.

■ Causes of Testosterone Deficiency

- Adrenal stress or burnout
- Birth control pills, which increase SHBG (see page 379)
- Chemotherapy
- Childbirth
- Depression
- Endometriosis
- HMG-CoA-reductase inhibitors (cholesterol-lowering medication)
- Menopause
- Psychological trauma
- Surgical menopause

If you are taking estrogen orally, it can increase your SHBG by 50 percent. If you are taking Premarin (equine estrogen), your SHBG levels can increase by 100 percent. Topically applied estrogen nominally increases SHBG, unless you have been overdosed.

▪ Ways to Increase Testosterone Levels Without Medication

- Decrease your calorie intake
- Exercise
- Get enough sleep (at least seven hours a night is an adequate amount)
- Increase the amount of protein in your diet
- Lose weight if you are overweight
- Practice stress-reduction techniques
- Take arginine, leucine, or glutamine (amino acids)
- Take zinc, which helps metabolize testosterone

Like other hormones, you can have too much testosterone in your body. Excess production of androgens is usually due to overproduction by your adrenal glands, but this can also be from your ovaries. Androgen dominance is the most common hormonal disorder in women. Many women have had or will have a form of androgen imbalance in their lifetime. In younger woman, adrenal imbalance is commonly related to PCOS. (See page 299.) As women go through menopause, about 20 percent of them will experience high testosterone levels that will not decline with age. It is paramount to work with your healthcare provider to lower this level.

▪ Signs and Symptoms of Excess Testosterone

- Acne or oily skin
- Agitation
- Anger
- Anxiety
- Changes in memory
- Decreased HDL (good cholesterol)
- Depression
- Fatigue
- Fluid retention
- Hair loss
- Hirsutism (facial hair)
- Hypoglycemia
- Increased insulin resistance
- Increased risk of developing breast cancer
- Infertility
- Irregular periods
- Mood swings
- Poor prognosis if you have breast cancer
- Salt and sugar cravings
- Weight gain

■ Causes of Elevated Testosterone Levels

- Aggressive exercise program

- High DHEA levels, which may raise testosterone

- Perimenopause/menopause

- Polycystic ovarian disease (PCOS)

- Prescribed a dose of testosterone that is too high

Dihydrotestosterone (DHT) is a byproduct of testosterone. High DHT levels can cause hair loss in women. You can have your DHT levels measured by taking a blood test. In the body, DHT makes androstanediol, another androgen. Androstanediol levels can be measured with a urine sample. (See the section on urine tests on page 378.) Elevated urinary androstanediol has been observed in people who have PCOS, hirsutism, and visceral obesity, and in postmenopausal women who have breast cancer. Likewise, higher DHT levels in women were associated with an increased risk of all-cause mortality as evidenced in a medical study.

5-alpha-reductase is an enzyme that is present in the conversion of testosterone to androstanediol. High levels of 5-alpha-reductase are associated with insulin resistance, obesity, high-protein diets, sodium (salt) restriction, licorice (a supplement or a food), hyperthyroidism (high thyroid levels), and DHEA supplementation. Lower levels of this enzyme are seen in vegetarians, people who use progesterone, epigallocatechin gallate (EGCG, which is in green tea), flaxseed ligans, medications such as *Proscar* and *Propecia*, and the intake of saw palmetto, pygeum, and stinging nettles.

■ Ways to Lower Testosterone Levels

- Saw palmetto: 240 to 260 mg twice a day

- Spironolactone: 100 mg twice a day. This is the least favorite of these methods. (It is a prescription and may have side effects, so other methods are suggested first)

- *Urtica dioica* (nettle): 300 mg twice a day. The root binds to and increases SHBG, which decreases the amount of bioavailable testosterone

- *Camellia sinensis* (green tea): 270 mg works by increasing SHBG

- *Glycyrrhiza glabra* (licorice root): 3.5 g licorice containing 7.6 percent glycyrrhizic acid decreases testosterone synthesis

- Spearmint tea lowers testosterone levels and may raise FSH and LH

- White peony (*Paeonia laterflora*) increases progesterone, reduces elevated testosterone, modulates estrogen, and modulates prolactin

Any attempt to reduce testosterone levels should be done under the guidance of a healthcare professional. If none of the above-referenced methods are successful, then discuss the matter with your healthcare provider further. Glucophage (Metformin) is a medication that is used to lower blood sugar, but it can also lower testosterone in women with elevated testosterone levels. Depending on your personal healthcare needs, your doctor may prescribe this treatment.

TESTOSTERONE AND ESTROGEN

Research shows that for testosterone to work optimally, E2 must also be optimized. Without enough estrogen present, testosterone cannot attach to your brain receptors. Therefore, estrogen plays a role in how well testosterone works in your body.

If testosterone is taken with E2, it lowers your cardiac risk. If your estrogen levels are low and you take testosterone alone, it can increase plaque formation in the vessels of your heart, which increases your risk of developing heart disease.

NATURAL AND SYNTHETIC TESTOSTERONE

Natural testosterone is the preferred method of testosterone replacement. Synthetic testosterone, or methyltestosterone, has been associated with an increased risk of liver cancer. Natural testosterone is effective when taken as a pill or applied as a cream, but it is much more commonly used as a cream. However, if you are using it as a cream, remember to rotate application sites. Applying the cream to the same location all the time will result in an increase in hair growth in that area. Interestingly, a study showed improvement in scalp hair with testosterone use in women with low testosterone levels. The fact that no individual complained of hair loss as a result of treatment casts doubt on the presumed role of testosterone causing female scalp hair loss as was previously thought by healthcare providers.

■ Therapeutic Benefits of Testosterone

- Mitigates anxiety disorders

- Reduces depression

- Improves aging skin

- Increases sexual interest in women with low testosterone levels

- Improves memory

- Reduces risk of osteopenia/ osteoporosis (bone loss)

- Helps in weight loss

DHEA

DHEA is another sex hormone. It is made by your adrenal glands, but a small amount is also made in your brain and skin. DHEA also makes your estrogen and testosterone.

DHEA production declines with age, starting in the late twenties. By the age of seventy, your body makes only one-fourth of the amount it made earlier. Furthermore, DHEA levels change if you are stressed long-term. When you begin to experience stress, DHEA levels increase. Over-time, if you remain stressed, DHEA levels start to drop and can become too low in the body.

■ Functions of DHEA in Your Body

- Decreases allergic reactions

- Decreases cholesterol

- Decreases formation of fatty deposits

- Has anti-inflammatory properties

- Helps you deal with stress

- Helps your body repair itself and maintain tissues

- Increases bone growth

- Increases brain function

- Increases growth hormone levels

- Increases lean body mass

- Increases nitric oxide
- Increases sense of well-being
- Is an antioxidant
- Lowers triglycerides
- Prevents advanced glycation end-products (AGE) formation

- Prevents blood clots
- Promotes weight loss
- Reduces blood sugar and spikes in blood sugar
- Supports your immune system

Low DHEA levels can occur at any age.

■ Signs and Symptoms of DHEA Deficiency

- ❑ Decreased energy
- ❑ Decreased muscle strength and lean body mass
- ❑ Difficulty in dealing with stress
- ❑ Increased risk of infection
- ❑ Insomnia

- ❑ Insulin resistance
- ❑ Irritability
- ❑ Joint soreness
- ❑ Osteopenia/osteoporosis
- ❑ Weight gain

There are many factors that can contribute to suboptimal and low levels of DHEA, which can occur at any age.

■ Causes of DHEA Deficiency

- Aging
- Decreased production of DHEA
- Menopause

- Smoking (nicotine inhibits the production of 11-beta-hydroxylase, an enzyme needed to make DHEA)
- Stress

If your body has a low DHEA level, it would be a good idea to consider DHEA replacement. There are many benefits of replacing DHEA, which can be supplemented orally or with a cream. For example, DHEA has been shown to have a protective effect against cancer, diabetes, obesity, high cholesterol, heart disease, and some autoimmune diseases.

In studies conducted at the University of Tennessee, supplementation with DHEA produced a 30 percent reduction in insulin levels when compared to taking the diabetes drug Metformin alone. Importantly, the supplements also tripled patients' sensitivity to insulin. This result may be related to the idea that diabetics may have lower levels of DHEA in their bodies than people who have normal blood sugar levels.

In the elderly, DHEA exerts an immunomodulatory action, increasing the number of monocytes, T cells expressing T-cell receptor gamma/delta, and natural killer cells, all of which affect the immune system. DHEA also improves physical and psychological well-being, muscle strength, and bone density, and reduces body fat and age-related skin atrophy, stimulating procollagen/sebum production. Moreover, DHEA modulates cardiovascular-signaling pathways and exerts anti-inflammatory, vasorelaxant, and anti-remodeling effects. Therefore, low levels of DHEA correlate with increased cardiovascular disease and all-cause mortality. In addition, DHEA appears to be protective against asthma and allergies by attenuating allergic inflammation and reducing eosinophilia and airway hyperreactivity. Eosinophilia refers to a high eosinophil (a kind of white blood cell) count that occurs with infection or allergy. Furthermore, in women, DHEA improves sexual satisfaction, fertility, and age-related vaginal atrophy (thinning, drying, and inflammation of the vaginal walls).

However, like most other hormones, you can have too much DHEA in your body.

■ Signs and Symptoms of Excess DHEA

- Acne
- Anger
- Deeper voice
- Depression

- Facial hair
- Fatigue
- Insomnia
- Irritability

- Mood changes
- Restless sleep
- Sugar cravings
- Weight gain

■ Causes of Excess DHEA

- Long-term stress
- Taking too much DHEA

- Tumor in the adrenal glands

■ Recommended Daily Dosage of DHEA

Women are more sensitive to the effects of DHEA than men, and therefore they need less DHEA than men, until they are above the age of sixty-five. Work with your healthcare provider to determine which dose of DHEA is best for you. It is usually taken in the morning.

■ Possible Side Effects and Contraindications of DHEA

It is contraindicated in patients with a history of hormonally related cancers, such as breast, ovarian, and uterine cancers.

■ Therapeutic Benefits of DHEA

- Helps in weight loss
- Helps against rheumatoid arthritis
- Helps against ankylosing spondylitis
- Helps against hypercholesterolemia
- Helps against hypertriglyceridemia
- Helps against insomnia
- Helps against insulin resistance/diabetes
- Helps against lupus
- Helps against sexual dysfunction
- Helps to reduce the risk of coronary heart disease
- Improves memory
- Improves the stress response
- Mitigates symptoms of menopause
- Post-traumatic stress disorder (PTSD)
- Reduces depression
- Reduces the risk of osteopenia/ osteoporosis

CORTISOL

Cortisol is the only hormone in your body that increases with age. It is also one of your sex hormones. Like DHEA, cortisol is made by your adrenal glands, which make all your sex hormones after menopause. Cortisol levels are regulated by adrenocorticotropic hormone (ACTH), which is synthesized by the pituitary in response to corticotropin-releasing hormone (CRH). CRH is released by the hypothalamus. Cortisol is commonly known as the "stress hormone" due to its involvement in your response to stress.

Low levels of cortisol are characterized as hypocortisolism, hypoadrenalism, or adrenal fatigue. High levels of cortisol are characterized as hypercortisolism or hyperadrenalism. When no cortisol is produced, Addison's disease is indicated. When extremely high levels of cortisol are produced, Cushing's disease or an adrenal tumor is indicated.

■ Functions of Cortisol in Your Body

- Acts as an anti-inflammatory
- Affects pituitary/thyroid/adrenal system
- Balances blood sugar
- Balances DHEA
- Controls weight
- Improves mood and thoughts
- Influences estrogen/testosterone ratio
- Participates with aldosterone in sodium reabsorption
- Promotes good sleep hygiene
- Regulates bone turnover rate
- Regulates immune system response
- Regulates the stress reaction
- Supports protein synthesis

Abnormal cortisol levels that are too high or too low can be associated with many medical conditions.

■ Conditions Associated With Abnormal Levels of Cortisol

- Alzheimer's disease
- Anorexia nervosa
- Breast cancer
- Chronic fatigue syndrome
- Coronary heart disease
- Depression
- Diabetes
- Exacerbations of multiple sclerosis
- Fibromyalgia
- Generalized memory loss
- Heart disease
- Impotence
- Infertility

- Insulin resistance
- Irritable bowel syndrome (IBS)
- Menopause
- Osteoporosis
- Panic disorders
- PMS
- Post-traumatic stress disorder (PTSD)
- Rheumatoid arthritis
- Sleep disorders
- Weight gain

There is a strong interrelationship between activation of the hypothalamic-pituitary-adrenal (HPA) axis and energy balance. Individuals with abdominal obesity tend to have elevated cortisol levels. Furthermore, stress and glucocorticoids (steroid hormones made in the adrenal glands) act to control both food intake and energy expenditure. Glucocorticoids are known to increase the consumption of foods high in fat and sugar in animals and humans. In women, high-cortisol individuals eat more in response to stress than low-cortisol, leading to increased food intake and reduced energy expenditure, and thus a predisposition to obesity. Therefore, cortisol responsiveness may be used as a marker to identify people who are at risk of weight gain and subsequent obesity.

The optimal method of measuring cortisol for the purposes of balancing your hormones (not for the diagnosis of Addison's disease or Cushing's disease) is salivary testing. An assay for cortisol levels will not be accurate if you have been on steroids within the last thirty days. Contact your healthcare provider to discuss steroid use and cortisol measurement if you are taking prescription steroids. If you require long-term steroid treatment for another medical problem, your doctor can take this information into account when interpreting the results of the saliva test. If you are on steroids short-term, then usually your healthcare provider will not have you do saliva testing within one month of your using a prescription for a steroid medication (such as an asthma inhaler).

When you are stressed, your cortisol levels increase. When you are stressed for a long time, then your cortisol levels can actually become too low. You require cortisol, however, to survive. Therefore, when cortisol becomes too low, your body will take pregnenolone to make cortisol, no matter what age you are, even if it means depleting your body of pregnenolone.

When your adrenal glands do not produce enough cortisol, your body is in a state of emergency, and consequently you do not feel well. You may turn to coffee, soft drinks, or sugar as a source of energy, but this will only make the situation worse. Consuming any of these items will temporarily make you feel better or more energetic, but the negative effects far outweigh the temporary fix. If your adrenal glands stay stimulated when they are in a state of emergency, they may weaken and "burn out." When this happens, your cortisol and DHEA levels will drop. This is called adrenal fatigue, or hypoadrenalism.

If the adrenals become totally depleted, this condition is called Addison's disease. If you have Addison's disease, your body makes no cortisol at all. Adrenal fatigue is not a total depletion of cortisol, but it does bring cortisol levels down low enough to prevent optimal functioning of the body. Adrenal fatigue is one of the most pervasive and underdiagnosed syndromes of modern society. A deficiency of cortisol that is not Addison's disease is usually caused by stress.

■ Signs and Symptoms of Adrenal Fatigue (Cortisol Deficiency)

- ❏ Allergies (environmental sensitivities and chemical intolerance)

- ❏ Decreased immunity

- ❏ Decreased sexual interest

- ❏ Digestive problems

- ❏ Drug addiction

- ❏ Emotional imbalances

- ❏ Emotional paralysis

- ❏ Fatigue

- ❏ Feeling overwhelmed

- ❏ General feeling of "unwellness"

- ❏ Hypoglycemia (low blood sugar)

- ❏ Increased PMS, perimenopausal, and menopausal symptoms

- ❏ Increased risk of alcoholism and drug addiction

- ❏ Lack of stamina

- ❏ Loss of motivation or initiative

- ❏ Low blood pressure

- ❏ Poor healing of wounds

- ❏ Progressively poorer athletic performance

- ❏ Sensitivity to light

- ❏ Unresponsive hypothyroidism (low thyroid function that doesn't respond to treatment)

■ Causes of Low Cortisol

- Chronic inflammation
- Chronic pain
- Depression
- Dysbiosis
- Hypoglycemia
- Long-term stress
- Nutritional deficiencies
- Overly aggressive exercise
- Poor sleep
- Severe allergies
- Toxic exposure

If your cortisol level is too low due to adrenal fatigue from long-term stress, begin your therapy with stress reduction techniques. Your doctor will also start you on a multivitamin. Your adrenal glands need vitamin C, B vitamins, calcium, magnesium, zinc, selenium, copper, sodium, and manganese. Adaptogenic herbs are also very beneficial, such as ashwagandha, *Panax ginseng, Rhodiola rosea,* and *Cordyceps sinensis.* Calming herbs such as chamomile and lemon balm can be very beneficial. If you are not improving, your healthcare provider may take discontinue the adaptogenic herbs and begin you on adrenal extracts after approximately six months.

If your cortisol level is still low after another three to six months, then your doctor may add licorice root to your therapy regimen. Licorice root decreases the amount of hydrocortisone that is broken down by the liver, which reduces the demand on the adrenals to produce more cortisol. Licorice root can raise your blood pressure, so it should not be taken if you have hypertension. If you develop high blood pressure while taking it, then discontinue its use.

If your DHEA level is low, your healthcare provider can prescribe you DHEA. It is important that you also take the herbal therapies, otherwise when your DHEA is measured again the level may be even lower despite your taking it. If all other therapies fail and your cortisol level is still low, then your healthcare provider may prescribe Cortef to take for six months. It is the therapy of last resort. Your doctor will keep you on adrenal extract or adaptogenic herbs while you are taking the Cortef so that you have a therapy available for your body to use when it comes time to wean yourself off Cortef, which can take at least a month.

Usually it takes six months of constant stress or more for adrenal fatigue to settle in. However, once you start treatment for your exhausted adrenals, it takes one to two years for your glands to heal completely.

There are other things you can do to help treat adrenal fatigue. Restful sleep (sleeping until 9 AM or later), resolving a stressful situation, lying down during a break from work, going to bed early (around 9 PM), and avoiding eating fruit in the morning can all help. Clearly, trying these options before things get out of hand is a good idea. If adrenal fatigue can be helped or improved, the overall healing time will be shortened.

Many women who have adrenal fatigue also have a thyroid that isn't functioning to its full potential (hypothyroidism). It is important to always work on fixing the adrenal glands before thyroid medication is instituted; otherwise, the symptoms of adrenal fatigue may be made worse.

Adrenal fatigue is a symptom that can dramatically affect your health and can be reversed with proper treatment. Lifestyle changes, good nutrition, dietary supplements, and stress reduction techniques have all proven to be affective.

CORTISOL AND STRESS

When you are stressed, cortisol levels rise. As stress decreases, levels come back down. However, in today's world, a lot of people are stressed a lot of the time. Overbooking is an issue with almost everyone. If you have too many tasks on your plate or you multitask all the time, your body will remain in a state of constant stress. One study showed that as many as 75 percent to 90 percent of visits to primary care doctors are related to stress. In fact, chronic stress has been shown to contribute to accelerated aging and premature death. Another study revealed that chronic stress accelerated the aging process and was associated with shortened telomeres.

The most important thing you can do to get rid of your stress is to gain control of your time. Learn to say "no" kindly. Know how much work and responsibility you can take on without feeling overwhelmed, and do not take on more than you can handle. It is also useful to practice some relaxing techniques that you can turn to in times of stress. Running a hot bath, drinking a cup of coffee or tea, listening to your favorite song, or curling up with a good book are all effective ways to reduce stress. Figure out what works for you and turn to it if you feel your stress levels rising.

Carl Sandberg, a famous American poet, once wrote:

Time is the coin of your life. It is the only coin you have,
and only you can determine how it will be spent.
Be careful lest you let other people spend it for you.

Stress can be harnessed to fuel success and achievement. However, if your stress is to the point of "distress," then that is a problem. Magnesium, potassium, B vitamins, vitamin C, zinc, carbohydrates, and other nutrients are used up when you are stressed.

Your brain is one of the body parts that is most affected by stress. When you are stressed and your cortisol levels increase, your body produces more free radicals. This damages your neurons and decreases your ability to think and remember things. When this happens, your body's ability to change short-term memories into long-term memories is affected. Your ability to recall and retrieve information is also impacted by stress. High levels of cortisol are associated with deterioration of the hippocampus, the part of your brain that processes memory.

Other Signs of Stress

By this point, you have learned that stress greatly affects cortisol levels, causing them to elevate. Elevated cortisol levels can have many negative consequences. (See page 47.) Over the years, I have compiled a list of common signs of stress, which can be divided into four categories.

Behavioral symptoms may be seen in the way you act. Some behavioral symptoms include bossiness, compulsive eating or gum chewing, excessive smoking, grinding your teeth at night, alcohol abuse, and an inability to focus on and complete tasks.

Cognitive symptoms are those that affect the way you think. If you are stressed, you may experience constant worry, forgetfulness, memory loss, or a lack of creativity. Additionally, you may have difficulty making decisions, lose your sense of humor, or have thoughts of running away.

Emotional symptoms affect your mood and feelings. If you're stressed, you may find that you are easily upset. Additionally, you may experience a range of emotions, including anger, boredom, edginess, loneliness, nervousness, anxiety, and unhappiness. Finally, people who are stressed commonly feel like they are under pressure, and they often feel powerless to change anything.

Last, there are some physical symptoms of stress that can affect your body. These include back pain, dizziness, headaches, a racing heart, restlessness, indigestion, stomachaches, tiredness, sweaty palms, a stiff neck or shoulders, ringing in the ears, and difficulty sleeping.

If you find that you are experiencing any of these symptoms, it would be a good idea to try and lower your levels of stress. (Some suggestions for how you can do this are on page 45.) You will greatly benefit in the long run.

In addition to stress, cortisol levels also increase with depression, high progestin intake, use of birth control pills, infections, inadequate sleep, inflammation, hypoglycemia (low blood sugar), toxic exposure, pain, and toxic exposure.

■ Signs and Symptoms of Elevated Cortisol

❑ Binge eating

❑ Compromised immune system

❑ Confusion

❑ Fatigue

❑ Favors the development of leaky gut syndrome

❑ Impaired hepatic conversion of T4 to T3 (see thyroid section on page 000)

❑ Increased blood pressure

❑ Increased blood sugar

❑ Increased cholesterol

❑ Increased insulin and insulin resistance

❑ Increased risk of developing osteoporosis/osteopenia

❑ Increased susceptibility to bruising

❑ Increased susceptibility to infections

❑ Increased triglycerides

❑ Irritability

❑ Low energy

❑ Night sweats

❑ Shakiness between meals

❑ Sleep disturbances

❑ Sugar cravings

❑ Thinning skin

❑ Weakened muscles

■ Effects of Stress on the Immune System

● Decreased release of antibodies

● Inhibition of the proliferation of T cells

● Increased inflammatory cytokines

● Inhibition of the release of certain interleukins

● Latent virus activation

● Shift from Th1 to Th2 cytokine expression

Lowering your cortisol level, if it is elevated, is very important. Stress-reduction techniques and a multivitamin are key components to start you on your way to normalizing your cortisol level. As previously mentioned, adaptogenic herbs such as ashwagandha, *Panax ginseng, Rhodiola rosea, Cordyceps sinensis,* and *Ginkgo biloba* are very beneficial if you feel stressed, and calming herbs such as lemon balm and chamomile are helpful if you feel wired. If cortisol is high in the evening, then add phosphatidylserine (300 mg) which may be taken at any point during the day.

Adaptogenic Herbs for Chronic Stress

Plant adaptogens are compounds that increase the ability of an organism to adapt to environmental factors and to avoid damage from these factors. The beneficial effects of multi-dose administration of adaptogens are mainly associated with the hypothalamic-pituitary-adrenal (HPA) axis, a part of the stress-system that is believed to play a primary role in the reactions of the body to repeated stress and adaptation.

The best adaptogens to treat chronic stress are ashwagandha, bacopa, cordyceps, and holy basil. Each of these herbal therapies has a different mechanism of action. Some herbs can be used for both acute and chronic stress.

Grown in India, Pakistan, and Sri Lanka, ashwagandha (*Withania somnifera*) is part of the nightshade family. The roots of ashwagandha are known to improve resistance to emotional and physical stress and to benefit the body in other ways, as well. Ashwagandha is available in capsule form or can be made into a tea. Recommended capsule dosages range from 500 to 2,000 milligrams daily. Recommended dosages of dried root prepared in tea range from 3 to 4 grams daily.

■ Functions of Ashwagandha in Your Body

- Activates the immune system

- Enhances endurance and strength

- Has antibacterial properties

- Has anti-inflammatory properties

- Has cytotoxic (cell-killing) and tumor-sensitizing actions

- Helps preserve adrenal function

- Helps with stress reduction

- Increases libido and sexual performance
- Increases muscle mass
- Is an antioxidant

- Lowers cholesterol
- Protects the liver

■ Therapeutic Benefits of Ashwagandha

- Anxiety
- Asthma
- Back pain
- Constipation
- Coronary heart disease
- Depression
- Fever
- Fibromyalgia
- Hiccups
- Hypocholesterolemia (high cholesterol)
- Hypothyroidism (underactive thyroid)

- Infection (antibacterial and antifungal)
- Inflammation
- Insomnia
- Insulin resistance
- Memory loss
- Mood swings
- Osteoarthritis
- Stress
- Tardive dyskinesia
- Weakness

■ Possible Side Effects and Contraindications of Ashwagandha

- Diarrhea
- Nausea

- Vomiting

Bacopa (*Bacopa monnieri*) has been used for many years in Ayurvedic medicine to revitalize nerves, brain cells, and the mind. Bacopa helps to strengthen the adrenal glands and purify the blood. Studies have shown that it may have beneficial effects for anxiety and mental fatigue.

■ Functions of Bacopa in Your Body

- Is effective against H. Pylori
- Enhances acetylcholine
- Improves transmission of nerve impulses
- Increases the body's utilization of nitric oxide
- Regulates dopamine production
- Regulates serotonin production

Bacopa can intensify the activity of thyroid-stimulating drugs or inhibit the effectiveness of thyroid-suppressant drugs. Bacopa can have a sedative effect therefore use caution when combining it with other sedatives. Possible side effects can occur, particularly if taken on an empty stomach.

■ Side Effects and Contraindications of Bacopa

- Bloated stomach
- Cramping
- Dry mouth
- Fatigue
- Nausea

A study revealed that bacopa was able to provide protective effects against multitasking. In addition, bacopa improved both cognitive performance and mood in 1 to 2 hours. The recommended dosage ranges from 320 to 650 mg.

■ Therapeutic Benefits of Bacopa

- ADHD
- Allergies
- Alzheimer's disease
- Anxiety
- Diabetic neuropathy
- Epilepsy
- Hypertension
- Improves focus
- Irritable bowel syndrome (IBS)
- Pain relief
- Protects the kidneys
- Stress

Cordyceps (*Cordyceps sinsensis* and *Cordyceps militaris*) is a fungus that has long been used in traditional Chinese and Tibetan medicine. Because natural cordyceps is difficult to obtain and is expensive when available, most supplements are made with cordyceps that has been created in a laboratory (Cordyceps CS-4).

Cordyceps is nutritionally rich, containing various types of essential amino acids; vitamins B_1, B_2, B_{12}, and K; carbohydrates; and trace elements. Studies have indicated that cordyceps can boost energy and oxygen during exercise, improve heart health, and combat inflammation, cancer, diabetes, and aging.

The recommended dosage is 400 milligrams twice a day. Be sure to use a pharmaceutical grade product, as some lower-grade products have been found to contain lead.

■ Functions of Cordyceps in Your Body

- Has antibacterial properties
- Has anti-cancer properties
- Has anti-inflammatory properties
- Has antimicrobial properties
- Has antioxidant properties
- Improves cardiac output
- Improves heart rhythm
- Improves kidney function
- Improves lung capacity
- Increases energy levels
- Lowers blood sugar levels
- Lowers cholesterol levels
- Lowers fibrinogen (a clotting factor)
- Modulates the immune system
- Protects the nervous system
- Provides adrenal support for stress

■ Therapeutic Benefits of Cordyceps

- Asthma
- Bronchitis
- Cancer
- Cardiac arrhythmia (irregular heartbeat)
- Chronic kidney disease (use only a healthcare provider's direction)
- Congestive heart failure
- Coughs
- Diabetes
- Hepatic cirrhosis
- Hepatitis B
- High cholesterol
- Infection
- Sexual dysfunction
- Stress due to adrenal fatigue

■ Possible Side Effects and Contraindications of Cordyceps

● Can cause problems when taken with medications such as predniso-lone, as well as with antiviral or diabetic medications.

● May increase the risk of bleeding if you have a bleeding disorder or are taking medications that change bleeding time.

● Discontinue use two weeks before surgery.

● Do not take cordyceps if you are allergic to mold, have an autoimmune disease, or are pregnant or breastfeeding.

Holy basil (*Ocimum sanctum*) is also known as tulsi. It is an aromatic plant that has been used for thousands of years. It is considered by many practitioners to be the best of the adaptogens in Ayurvedic medicine.

Holy basil can be used as a raw fresh whole herb. As dried leaves the dose is 300 to 600 mg a day for prevention, and 600 to 1,800 mg in divided doses as a therapy. There are no reported toxicities or adverse effects and no interactions have been described.

■ Functions of Holy Basil in Your Body

● Acts as a diuretic

● Enhances the immune system

● Has anti-anxiety properties

● Helps protect against heavy metal toxicity

● Helps protect from gamma radiation

● Helps protect from radioactive iodine

● Helps with fatigue

● Improves blood pressure if it is too low

● Is an adaptogen

● Is an antibacterial, antifungal, antimalarial, anti-parasitic, and antiviral agent

● Is an anticoagulant

● Is an antidepressant

● Is an anti-inflammatory

● Is an antioxidant

● Is an aphrodisiac

● Lowers blood sugar

● Lowers cholesterol

● Lowers temperature if elevated

● Promotes cognitive enhancement

- Protects against cancer
- Protects the liver

- Reduces of stress from noise

◼ Therapeutic Benefits of Holy Basil

- Allergy
- Anti-androgenic
- Anxiety
- Arthritis
- Asthma
- Asthma
- Back pain
- Bioremediation of contaminated air and soil
- Cardiopathy
- Cataracts
- Cough
- Diabetes
- Diarrhea and dysentery

- Earache
- Eye diseases
- Fever
- Food and herb preservation
- GI tract disorders
- Hand sanitizer
- Hiccups
- Indigestion
- Infertility
- Insect, snake, and scorpion bites
- Ischemic heart disease
- Leukoderma (loss

of pigmentation of the skin)
- Malaria
- Metabolic syndrome
- Mouthwash
- Pain control
- Ringworm
- Skin disorders
- Stroke
- Ulcers
- Urinary diseases
- Vomiting
- Water treatment
- Wound healing

◼ Possible Side Effects and Contraindications of Holy Basil

Avoid using Holy basil if you are allergic or sensitive to members of the Lamiaceae (mint) family. Possible side effects to this herb are an upset stomach. Also use with caution if you have low blood sugar.

Adaptogenic Herbs for Acute Stress

A single-dose application of an adaptogen is important in situations that require a rapid response to tension or a stressful situation. In this case, the effects of the adaptogen are associated with another part of the stress system, namely, the sympatho-adrenal-system (SAS), which provides a rapid-response mechanism mainly to control the acute reaction of the organism to a stressor. SAS-mediated stimulating effects of single doses of adaptogens have been associated with *Rhodiola rosea, Schisandra chinensis,* and *Eleutherococcus senticosus.* Furthermore, these adaptogens effectively increase mental performance and physical working capacity in humans.

Eleutherococcus (or simply Eleuthero), Rhodiola, and Schisandra have all been found to be effective. Rhodiola is the most active of the three plant adaptogens, producing within thirty minutes of administration a stimulating effect that continues for at least 4 to 6 hours. In addition, a combination of herbal therapies can be beneficial for acute stress. Each of these herbal therapies has a different mechanism of action.

Eleuthero (*Eleutherococcus senticosus*)—a species of shrub found in China, Korea, Japan, and Russia—has long been used by natural healers to increase energy, enhance endurance, and boost immunity. For many years, it was called Siberian ginseng because its effect are similar to those of ginseng. That name is now rarely used in the United States because it implies that the herb is part of the Panax genus (like American and Asian ginseng), while it actually belongs to the genus Eleutherococcus. Regardless of the controversy over its name, this herb is used to treat a variety of ailments. The recommended dosage ranges from 500 to 1,000 milligrams daily. Eleuthero can be taken for three months, followed by three to four weeks off.

■ Functions of Eleuthero in Your Body

- Acts as a stimulant

- Acts as an adaptogen to help your body manage stress

- Aids the immune system by increasing T-cell and natural killer cell activity

- Improves endurance

- Improves learning ability

- Increases mental awareness

- Increases physical performance and stamina

- Increases tolerance to excessive heat, noise, and workload

- Is an anti-inflammatory

- Is an antioxidant

- Promotes healing

■ Therapeutic Benefits of Eleuthero

- Anxiety
- Chronic fatigue
- Common cold and flu
- Crohn's Disease
- Diabetes
- Fibromyalgia
- Herpes simplex type 2 infection
- Hypercholesterolemia (high cholesterol)
- Inflammation

- Insomnia
- Joint pain
- Kidney disease
- Liver disease
- Memory loss
- Osteoarthritis
- Premenstrual syndrome (PMS)
- Rheumatoid arthritis
- Stress

■ Possible Side Effects and Contraindications of Eleuthero

- Can also interact with medications taken to treat an autoimmune disease, drugs taken after organ transplant, steroids, digoxin, lithium, and sedatives (especially barbiturates).

- Can lower blood sugar levels. If you are being treated for insulin resistance or diabetes, monitor your blood sugar levels often to make sure they don't get too low.

- Do not use if you have a history of heart disease, hypertension, sleep apnea, narcolepsy, mania, or schizophrenia, or if you are pregnant or breastfeeding.

- Has a blood-thinning effect. If you have a bleeding disorder or are taking a medication or supplement that may thin your blood, do not take this herb. If you are planning to have surgery, discontinue this herbal therapy two weeks before the procedure.

- Women who have a history of estrogen-sensitive cancers or uterine fibroids should avoid eleuthero, as it has mild estrogenic effects.

Rhodiola (*Rhodiola rosea*) grows in cold, mountainous regions of Asia and Eastern Europe. Traditionally, this herb—which is known to contain more than 140 active ingredients—is used to treat anxiety, fatigue, and depression. It belongs to a group of plants known as adaptogens, which can help your body adapt to physical and environmental stress. Active compounds like rosoavin are able to balance the stress hormone cortisol.

The recommended dosage ranges from 200 to 600 milligrams a day in divided doses of standardized 3-percent rosavin and 1-percent salidroside.

■ Functions of Rhodiola in Your Body

- Decreases depression
- Has antibacterial properties
- Improves mental function
- Improves physical performance
- Is an adaptogen that helps the body manage stress
- Is an anti-inflammatory

- Is an antioxidant
- Is protective of the heart
- Is protective of the liver
- Is protective of the nervous system
- Lowers blood sugar levels
- Reduces anxiety

■ Therapeutic Benefits of Rhodiola

- Altitude sickness
- Anxiety
- Cognitive problems
- Depression

- Insulin resistance/diabetes
- Nicotine dependence
- Physical and mental stress

■ Possible Side Effects and Contraindications of Rhodiola

Rhodiola decreases the possible liver side effects associated with the chemotherapeutic drug Adriamycin. It has a synergistic effect with cyclophosphamide's anti-tumor effect and decreases the risk of developing liver toxicity. The side effects of Rhodiola use are usually mild. At high doses, they may include:

- Allergic symptoms
- Fatigue

- Insomnia
- Irritability

Schisandra is also an effective adaptogenic herb that has immediate action. It has many functions in the body.

■ Functions of Schisandra in Your Body

- Acts as an antibacterial
- Decreases allergies
- Decreases anxiety
- Decreases spasms in the GI tract
- Enhances exercise endurance
- Generates alterations in the basal levels of nitric oxide
- Has anti-cancer activity
- Helps protect the heart
- Helps to control blood sugar
- Improves bone mineralization
- Improves cortisol levels positively affects the blood cells, vessels, and central nervous system
- Improves erectile dysfunction

- Increases endurance and accuracy of movement
- Increases mental performance
- Increases working capacity
- Inhibits leukotriene formation
- Is a platelet-activating factor antagonist
- Is an anti-inflammatory
- Is an antioxidant
- Is kidney protective
- Is liver protective
- Is neuroprotective
- Lowers cholesterol
- Modulates neurotransmitter function
- Promotes weight loss
- Regulates immune system

■ Therapeutic Benefits of Schisandra

- Acute gastrointestinal diseases
- Alcoholism
- Allergic dermatitis
- Asthenia (lack of energy)
- Asthma

- Cardiovascular disorders
- Chronic cough
- Chronic sinusitis
- Depression
- Dyspnea

- Hypotension (low blood pressure)
- Impaired visual function
- Influenza
- Insomnia
- Irritability
- Liver dysfunction
- Mediterranean fever
- Memory maintenance
- Neuritis

- Neurosis
- Night sweats
- Otitis (ear infection)
- Otosclerosis (inherited disorder)
- Palpitations
- Pneumonia
- Stomach and duodenal ulcers
- Stress
- Wound healing

■ Possible Side Effects of Contraindications of Schisandra

If you are on any medication, contact your healthcare provider before beginning this herb since it may interact with drugs that are metabolized by the CYP3A4 system. In addition, there may be an elevation of serum levels of drugs that are P-glycoprotein substrates when taken with this herb. *Schisandra* may produce mild gastrointestinal discomfort.

■ Combination Therapies for Acute Stress

A study showed that *Panax ginseng, Rhodiola rosea,* and *Schisandra chinensis* were adaptogens that had numerous functions, and their effects were found to be very different in patients, depending on circumstances such as age, gender, environment, and diet. Consequently, make sure your healthcare provider or pharmacist works with you on herbal therapies that you are thinking about taking.

■ Nutrients Associated With Increased Adrenal Function

- B vitamins
- Calcium
- Copper

- Magnesium
- Manganese
- Omega-3-fatty acids, such as fish oil

- Phosphatidylserine
- Selenium
- Sodium
- Vitamin C
- Zinc

As previously discussed, all the hormones in your body work together like a symphony. In order for you to have good health, they have to be balanced and at optimal levels. If your cortisol levels increase, your body's production of progesterone decreases. Cortisol competes with progesterone for common receptors. When cortisol levels are elevated, the thyroid gland is directly affected. The thyroid hormone produced may become stored, or bound, in the body, and therefore it will be unavailable for your body to use.

Having decreased levels of estradiol (E2) is also a stressor on your body because it causes cortisol levels to rise. Decreased E2 also causes a decrease in optimal functioning of norepinephrine, serotonin, dopamine, and acetylcholine, which are neurotransmitters responsible for communication between cells.

■ Factors Regulated by Neurotransmitters

- Appetite
- Memory
- Mood
- Muscle growth and repair
- Sexual interest
- Sleep
- Thirst
- Weight

The simplest way to stop your cortisol levels from increasing is to better manage your stress. However, as you get older, this becomes more difficult because your ability to bounce back after a stressful event is reduced. Each event takes a deeper and more lasting toll on your body. Premature aging and many age-related disorders can begin with excessive stress.

Of course, abnormal levels of cortisol can occur at any age, but there are certainly different factors that can affect stress levels. One such factor is your job. Some jobs create more stress than others.

■ Most Stressful Occupations According to the National Institutes of Health

- Construction worker
- Farm worker
- Foreman/supervisor
- House painter
- Laboratory technician
- Machine operator
- Midlevel manager
- Secretary
- Waiter or waitress

The jobs on this list have one thing in common: a lack of control. Remember, you may not be able to control the things that are stressing you, but you can control how you respond to the stress. In other words, the key is not to avoid stress, but to change your perspective and how you respond to stress.

■ Optimal Cortisol Levels Helps to Prevent or Improve These Diseases

- Alzheimer's disease and other forms of cognitive decline
- Anorexia nervosa
- Anxiety disorders
- Breast cancer
- Chronic fatigue syndrome
- Coronary heart disease
- Decreases risk of infection
- Depression
- Fibromyalgia
- Impotence
- Infertility
- Insulin resistance/diabetes
- Irritable bowel syndrome (IBS)
- Menopause
- Multiple sclerosis
- Osteopenia/osteoporosis
- Panic disorders
- Polycystic ovary syndrome (PCOS)
- Post-traumatic stress disorder (PTSD)
- Premenstrual syndrome (PMS)
- Rheumatoid arthritis
- Sleep disorders

As you have seen in this section, stress affects most every function in the body and is involved in almost all disease processes. A small amount of stress helps your body heal. Too much stress harms your body. Stress reduction techniques are a key component to healing. Prayer, meditation, tai chi (a Chinese form of martial arts), yoga, chi gong (a form of body and mind therapy), breathing exercises and techniques, exercise (not strenuous exercise if you have adrenal fatigue), music, acupuncture, and dancing have all been shown to be therapeutic.

In order to be healthy, you have to be physically healthy, emotionally healthy, and spiritually healthy. All these areas of your life must be optimally functioning in order for you to enjoy a stress-free existence.

PREGNENOLONE

Pregnenolone is synthesized from cholesterol. It makes estrogen, progesterone, testosterone, DHEA, and cortisol. Pregnenolone levels decline with age. By the age of seventy-five, most patients have 65 percent less pregnenolone than they did at age thirty-five. In addition to making the previously listed hormones, pregnenolone performs a variety of other functions in the body.

◼ Functions of Pregnenolone

- Blocks production of acid-forming compounds

- Enhances acetylcholine neurotransmission

- Enhances nerve transmission and memory

- Helps repair nerve damage

- Improves energy (both physically and mentally)

- Improves sleep

- Increases resistance to stress

- Modulates NMDA receptors (regulate pain control, learning, memory, and alertness)

- Modulates the neurotransmitter GABA (calming neurotransmitter)

- Promotes mood elevation

- Reduces pain and inflammation

- Regulates the balance between excitation and inhibition in the nervous system

- Stimulates formation of new brain cells

■ Signs and Symptoms of Pregnenolone Deficiency

❑ Arthritis

❑ Depression

❑ Fatigue

❑ Insomnia

❑ Lack of focus

❑ Memory decline

■ Causes of Pregnenolone Deficiency

● Aging

● Eating too much saturated fat and trans fat

● Having a severe illness or dealing with prolonged stress

● Hypothyroidism

● Low cholesterol levels (total cholesterol needs to be 140 ng/dL to make pregnenolone)

● Pituitary dysfunction

At any age, pregnenolone will make more cortisol and less of the other hormones to help the body deal with stress.

■ Recommended Daily Dosage of Pregnenolone

Your blood level of pregnenolone must be at least 50 ng/dL to help maintain memory. Work with your healthcare provider to determine what dose of pregnenolone is best for you. A common starting dose is 10 mg. It is usually taken in the morning.

■ Possible Side Effects and Contraindications of Pregnenolone

It is contraindicated in patients with a history of hormonally related cancers, such as breast, ovarian, and uterine cancers. Supplementation may decrease the seizure threshold in people with a history of seizure disorder. Therefore, commonly lower doses of pregnenolone are used in these individuals.

■ Signs and Symptoms of Excess Pregnenolone

❑ Acne

❑ Anger

❑ Anxiety

❑ Drowsiness

❑ Fluid retention

❑ Headache

❑ Heart racing/palpitations

❑ Insomnia due to overstimulation

❑ Irritability

❑ Muscle aches

■ Causes of Excess Pregnenolone

● Pituitary tumor

● Taking too high a dose of pregnenolone

■ Therapeutic Benefits of Pregnenolone

● Helps against ankylosing spondylitis

● Helps against arthritis

● Helps against endometriosis

● Helps against insomnia

● Helps against lupus

● Helps against multiple sclerosis

● Helps against psoriasis

● Helps against rheumatoid arthritis

● Helps against scleroderma

● Improves memory loss

● Improves spinal cord injuries

● May protect the brain from cannabis intoxication

● Mitigates allergic reactions

● Mitigates moodiness

● Reduces depression/bipolar depression

● Reduces fatigue

INSULIN

Insulin is the hormone responsible for the regulation of blood sugar in your bloodstream. Insulin is produced in the body with peak functioning of the pancreas along with optimal balancing of other hormones. It helps store glucose in your liver, fat, and muscles, and it helps regulate your body's metabolism of carbohydrates, fats, and proteins. Perfect insulin levels are a key to the best health possible. Insulin levels that are too high or too low can cause symptoms and increase the risk of developing insulin resistance, diabetes, as well as other diseases.

■ Functions of Insulin

- Affects glycogen metabolism by stimulation of glycogen synthesis

- Aids other nutrients to get inside cells

- Counters the actions of adrenaline and cortisol in the body

- Has an anti-inflammatory effect on endothelial cells and macrophages

- Helps convert blood sugar into triglycerides

- Helps the body repair itself

- Increases expression of some lipogenic enzymes

- Keeps blood glucose levels from rising too high

- Partially regulates protein turnover rate

- Plays a major role in the production of serotonin

- Stimulates the development of muscle (but at high levels it turns off the production of muscle and increases the production of fat)

- Suppresses reactive oxygen species (ROS)

Have your healthcare provider measure your fasting insulin level. Fasting serum insulin is used as an index of insulin sensitivity and resistance. The optimal fasting insulin level is 6 uIU/mL. Insulin levels that are too low or too high signify that insulin is not working optimally in your body. Commonly your doctor will measure your fasting blood sugar (FBS) and maybe also your hemoglobin A1c. Your hemoglobin A1c test tells you your average level of blood sugar over the past two to three months. It's also called HbA1c, glycated hemoglobin test, and glycohemoglobin. It is rare unless you are seeing a practitioner that specializes in Precision/Anti-Aging Medicine that you would have your fasting insulin level measured. Make sure you request this test from your doctor.

■ Signs and Symptoms of Insulin Deficiency

- ❑ Blurred vision
- ❑ Bone loss
- ❑ Confusion
- ❑ Depression

- ❑ Dizziness
- ❑ Fainting
- ❑ Fatigue
- ❑ Hunger

❑ Hypoglycemia

❑ Insomnia

❑ Insulin resistance

❑ Loss of consciousness (late stage)

❑ Palpitations

❑ Seizures (late stage)

❑ Sweating

■ Causes of Insulin Deficiency

- Eliminating carbohydrates from the diet

- Hypopituitarism

- Insulin resistance/diabetes

- Not eating enough

- Over-exercising without sufficient food and nutritional support

- Pancreatic diseases such as chronic pancreatitis, cancer of the pancreas, and cystic fibrosis

When you eat complex carbohydrates and simple sugars, your insulin levels climb. If you eat too much sugar, your body produces more and more insulin until the insulin level is elevated and it does not work as effectively as it should. The medical term for this is insulin resistance.

■ Conditions Associated With Excess Insulin Production

- Acceleration of aging

- Acne

- Acromegaly

- Asthma

- Cushing's syndrome

- Depression and mood swings

- Estrogen levels that are too low

- Heart disease

- Heartburn

- Hypercholesterolemia

- Hypertension

- Hypertriglyceridemia

- Increased risk of developing cancer

- Infertility

- Insomnia

- Insulin resistance/diabetes

- Irritable bowel syndrome

- Metabolic syndrome

- Migraine headaches

- Osteopenia/osteoporosis

- Weight gain

Insulin is part of the hormonal symphony in your body, so when it is not performing optimally, all the other hormones are affected. Your body will attempt to compensate for insulin's decreased effects by producing more and more insulin. This can result in high insulin levels all the time, which can cause the cells in your adrenal glands, called theca cells, to turn on an enzyme called 17, 20-lyase. This enzyme causes your body's hormones to stop making estrogens and instead make androgens. (Both estrogens and androgens are made from DHEA.) This shift in hormonal balance can cause you to gain weight around the middle. It may also promote further insulin resistance. In fact, prolonged levels of high insulin can lead to diabetes. Furthermore, most major processes that lead to hardening of the arteries are caused by the overproduction of insulin.

When you eat simple sugars and consume caffeine to help with fatigue, not only will your adrenal glands suffer, but this will contribute to an elevated level of insulin in your body. Additionally, this causes your body to produce gas and you may experience bloating. Water is pulled into your colon from the bloodstream to respond to the high sugar load, which can lead to loose stools. You may develop gluten sensitivity from overeating carbohydrates.

There are many habits that can elevate insulin besides eating a diet high in simple sugars. Having a lot of stress, which causes your cortisol levels to be abnormal, will have a negative impact on insulin production. The following list contains lifestyle choices that raise insulin, as per Dr. Diana Schwarzbein, an endocrinologist and author of *The Schwarzbein Principle* and *The Schwarzbein Principle II.*

■ Causes of Excess Insulin Production

- Cigarette smoking
- Consuming soft drinks
- Eating a low-fat diet
- Eating trans-fats (partially hydrogenated or hydrogenated)
- Elevated DHEA levels
- Excessive alcohol consumption
- Excessive caffeine intake
- Excessive or unnecessary thyroid hormone replacement
- Excessive progesterone replacement
- Increased testosterone levels (male or female)
- Lack of exercise
- Poor sleep hygiene
- Skipping meals

- Some over-the-counter cold medications (any that contain caffeine)
- Some prescription medications (these are the most common)
  - Beta-blockers
  - Levodopa
  - Oral contraceptives
  - Some medications for depression and psychosis
  - Steroids
- Thiazide diuretics
- Stress
- Taking diet pills
- Taking thyroid hormone replacement while not eating enough
- Use of artificial sweeteners
- Use of natural stimulants
- Use of recreational stimulants
- Yo-yo dieting

Elevated insulin levels can be lowered by eating a balanced diet of carbohydrates, proteins, and fats. The right amount of exercise (three or four times a week) can help to normalize insulin levels. Changing medications, quitting smoking, discontinuing stimulants, and decreasing or stopping caffeine consumption can also be beneficial. In addition, there are nutrients that can help insulin work more effectively in the body. Alpha lipoic acid, chromium, and vitamin D all do just this. However, these supplements can be very powerful, so if you are already taking a drug that lowers your blood sugar, you may need less medication with the use of these products. Make sure you monitor your blood sugar closely. Alpha lipoic acid has even been shown to prevent and treat diabetic neuropathy, a condition in which the body's nerves become damaged due to diabetes. (See "Insulin Resistance" on page 68 for further information.)

■ Therapeutic Benefits of Optimal Insulin Levels

- Helps to normalize weight
- Memory maintenance
- Prevention and treatment of insulin resistance and diabetes
- Prevention and treatment of polycystic ovary syndrome (PCOS)
- Prevention of coronary heart disease
- Prevention of hypertension
- Prevention of osteoporosis/ osteopenia
- Prevention of some cancers

■ Insulin Resistance

Insulin resistance is evident when cells do not properly absorb glucose, the body's preferred source of fuel, resulting in a buildup in the blood. If left untreated, insulin resistance may lead to prediabetes, a condition in which glucose levels are higher than normal but not high enough to be considered diabetes. Insulin resistance occurs when insulin is present but does not work as effectively in the body as it should. Consequently, levels start to rise to help the body compensate for less than effective insulin function.

More than 80 percent of the adult population in the United States has blood glucose levels that are too high. If a patient has a fasting blood sugar (FBS) that is high-normal (over 85 mg/dL), the risk of the patient dying of cardiovascular disease (heart disease) is increased by 40 percent. Furthermore, having a FBS that is high-normal increases the patient's risk of vascular death. Insulin also plays a profound role in cognitive function. High-normal levels of FBS may account for a decrease in the volume of the hippocampus and amygdala of 6 to 10 percent. Consequently, insulin resistance is a risk factor for cognitive decline. Also, the "Honolulu-Asia Aging Study" showed that the effect of hyperinsulinemia (high insulin levels) on the risk of dementia was independent of diabetes and blood glucose. Therefore, growing evidence supports the concept that insulin resistance is important in the pathogenesis of cognitive impairment and neurodegeneration.

■ Sign and Symptoms of Insulin Resistance

❑ Fuzzy brain

❑ Infertility

❑ Irregular menstrual cycles

❑ Irritability

❑ Loose bowel movements alternating with constipation

❑ Water retention

❑ Weight gain

■ Causes of Insulin Resistance

Insulin resistance has many possible causes. Here are some reasons why individuals with insulin resistance are not able to effectively use insulin.

● Abuse of alcohol

● Decreased estrogen

● Eating processed foods

● Elevated DHEA levels

- Excessive caffeine intake
- Excessive dieting
- Excessive progesterone in females (prescribed)
- Genetic susceptibility
- Hypothyroidism
- Increased stress

- Increased testosterone due to PCOS, perimenopause, menopause, or too high a dose of prescribed testosterone
- Insomnia
- Lack of exercise
- Use of nicotine
- Use of oral contraceptives

Conventional therapies for insulin resistance involve exercise and a diet centered on consumption of foods with low glycemic index numbers. If an individual is overweight, then weight reduction is very beneficial. If these methods are not successful, then medications such as Glucophage may be added.

Precision/Anti-Aging Medicine has many therapies to improve and sometimes even reverse insulin resistance. The first one is exercise. Lack of exercise is a risk factor for the development of insulin resistance and diabetes in susceptible individuals. Exercising four days a week for an hour a day has been shown to be beneficial. Eating foods that are low on the glycemic index (GI) is important. The GI ranks carbohydrate-containing foods on a scale from 0 to 100 according to the speed with which they enter the bloodstream and raise glucose levels. Foods high on the list increase blood sugar and cause insulin to rise.

One study showed that insulin secretion was lower in people who were on a low glycemic index program for only two weeks. The glycemic index is affected by the size of the particles into which the food breaks down. Therefore, the more the processed the food or the longer it is cooked, the higher its glycemic index. The best carbohydrates that curb insulin are broccoli, lentils, and chickpeas. In addition, the fat content of a food influences its glycemic index ranking. Fat slows down sugar absorption and therefore lowers the glycemic index number.

The right balance of saturated to polyunsaturated to monounsaturated fats is important both for the prevention and treatment of insulin resistance and diabetes. Likewise, a high-fiber diet is crucial. Soluble fiber has been shown to lower insulin levels. Furthermore, getting enough protein in the diet decreases the absorption of sugars and consequently decreases your glycemic load. Weight loss has been shown to be helpful as well.

Moreover, getting a good night's sleep has been shown to be beneficial. If you do not sleep at least six and a half hours a night, then insulin levels may rise and lead to insulin resistance.

There are also many nutritional supplements and botanical nutrients that have clinical trials supporting their use in insulin resistance.

SUPPLEMENTS TO TREAT INSULIN RESISTANCE		
Supplements	**Dosage**	**Considerations**
Alpha lipoic acid	100 mg to 400 mg daily	Alpha lipoic acid improves blood sugar levels, so diabetics may be able to take less medication. Alpha lipoic acid also slows the development of diabetic neuropathy. Consult your healthcare provider if you are considering taking more than 500 mg in a day. Larger doses can negatively impact thyroid functioning.
Arginine	1,000 to 5,000 mg once a day	Do not take if you have kidney disease, liver disease, or herpes except under a doctor's supervision. Arginine can interact with some medications. Consult with your healthcare provider before beginning this therapy.
Asian ginseng*	50 to 200 mg of extract standardized to 4 percent ginsenosides twice a day	Always take with food. Use with caution if you have high blood pressure. Do not use if you are taking a blood thinner or if you have a hormonally related cancer such as breast, prostate, uterine, or ovarian.
B-complex vitamins	50 mg twice a day	I suggest taking a multivitamin along with your B-complex vitamins.
Berberine*	Start with 200 mg twice a day (You may go up to 500 mg three times a day)	Do not use this supplement during pregnancy. It can cause uterine contractions.
Bergamot	800 mg once or twice a day	It also blocks the rate-limiting step in cholesterol production. If you are on a cholesterol lowering medication, have your healthcare provider measure your cholesterol after three months. You may need a lower dose of the drug.
Carnitine*	2,000 to 3,000 mg once a day	Have your healthcare provider measure your TMAO levels before starting long-term supplementation with carnitine.

Supplements	Dosage	Considerations
Carnosine	2,000 mg once a day	Check with your doctor before starting carnosine therapy if you have diabetes, hypertension, kidney disease, or liver damage. Too much carnosine can result in hyperactivity.
Chromium	300 to 1,000 mcg once a day as chromium picolinate	Combining with the protein picolinate allows your body to absorb chromium more efficiently. However, some chromium picolinate supplements contain more chromium than necessary. Ask your healthcare provider for a recommendation on chromium consumption.
Coenzyme Q-10*	30 to 200 mg daily	If you are on blood-thinning medications, speak to your healthcare provider before using CoQ-10. Since some medications can cause a deficiency of this nutrient, speak to your healthcare provider to determine if you might need a larger dose.
Copper	2 to 3 mg once a day	Your copper-to-zinc ratio is very important for your health. Also, do not take copper supplement cupric oxide, which has a very low bioavailability.
Cysteine	500 mg once a day as n-acetylcysteine, or NAC	When taking NAC supplements, also take extra vitamin C, copper, and zinc.
D-ribose	15,000 mg three times a day	D-ribose can lower blood sugar levels, so check with your healthcare provider before taking this supplement with any diabetes medication, especially insulin.
EPA/DHA (fish oil)*	1,000 to 2,000 mg once a day	Choose a source that contains vitamin E to prevent oxidation.
Fenugreek*	50 mg of seed powder twice a day, or 2 to 4.5 ml of 1:2 liquid extract twice a day	Avoid fenugreek if you are allergic to chickpeas, peanuts, green peas, or soybeans. Fenugreek has mild blood-thinning effects. If you have a bleeding disorder or are taking a medication or supplement that may thin your blood, do not take this herb. Fenugreek may also negatively impact thyroid functioning.
Fiber, soluble	Suggested daily intake is 25 grams for women and 38 grams for men (Try to get most of your fiber from whole foods)	Choose a fiber supplement with no added sugar, and take with several glasses of water to prevent side effects.

This supplement can have a blood-thinning action.

Supplements	Dosage	Considerations
Ginkgo biloba*	120 mg once daily	Do not use with blood-thinning medications or supplements.
Green coffee bean extract	400 mg a day	Because green coffee contains caffeine, you should avoid taking this supplement if you are sensitive to caffeine.
Gymnema sylvestre	400 to 600 mg a day of an extract that contains 24 percent gymnemic acid	Stop taking this supplement two weeks before surgery, as it can interfere with blood sugar control during and after surgical procedures. At high doses, gymnema can cause gastric irritation or liver toxicity.
Inositol	2,000 to 4,000 mg once a day	May stimulate uterine contractions. Women who wish to become pregnant should consult their doctor regarding its use. Doses larger than 200 mg should be taken only under physician supervision.
Magnesium	400 to 800 mg once a day	Consult your healthcare provider for dosage if you have kidney disease. Discontinue use and see your doctor if you experience abdominal pain. Take a lower dose if it causes diarrhea.
Manganese	2 to 5 mg once a day	Use with caution if you have gallbladder or liver disease.
Olive leaf extract*	500 mg to 750 mg a day containing 20 mg of oleuropein per capsule	Olive leaf extracts can interact with many prescription medications, and may increase the effects of blood thinners. Consult your healthcare provider before using olive leaf extract if you are taking any medication. Don't use if you are pregnant or breastfeeding.
Quercetin*	300 mg three times a day	For best results, take with bromelain and vitamin C. Do not use with blood-thinning medications or supplements.
Selenium	200 mcg once a day	Do not exceed 200 mcg a day without consulting your healthcare provider.
Taurine	1,000 to 1,500 mg once a day	Take between meals. Discontinue use if you suddenly have feelings of chest or throat tightness or if you break out in hives. Do not take with aspirin. Have your healthcare provider measure levels before starting taurine therapy.

Supplements	Dosage	Considerations
Vanadium*	50 mcg once a day	Do not take more than 50 mcg a day without a doctor's supervision. Do not use if you are taking blood-thinning medications or supplements.
Vitamin B_6 (pyridoxine)	75 mg twice a day	Do not take more than 500 mg a day. If you are taking L-dopa for Parkinson's disease, do not take B_6 without first consulting your doctor. High doses can deplete your body of other vitamins in the B complex, so take a B-complex vitamin twice a day.
Vitamin B_7 (biotin)	8 to 10 mg once a day	Large doses of biotin can deplete your body of other vitamins in the B complex, so take B-complex vitamins twice a day. Biotin can also negatively impact thyroid function.
Vitamin B_{12} (cobalamin)	500 to 1,500 mcg twice a day	High doses can deplete your body of other vitamins in the B complex, so take with a B-complex vitamin twice a day.
Vitamin C	500 to 1,500 mg twice a day	Do not take high doses if you are prone to kidney stones or gout. High doses can also cause diarrhea.
Vitamin D_3	Have your blood levels measured by your healthcare provider, who will determine proper dosage	You can become vitamin D toxic. Therefore, have your healthcare provider measure your levels to determine the perfect dose for you.
Vitamin E*	400 to 800 IU once a day	Take mixed tocopherols, the more active type of vitamin E. Consult your healthcare provider first if you are taking a blood thinner.
Zinc	20 to 50 mg once a day as zinc picolinate or zinc citrate	Your copper-to-zinc ratio is very important to your health. If you are taking zinc and iron supplements, take one in the morning and one in the evening. (Taking them together reduces the efficiency of both.)

This supplement can have a blood-thinning action.

Many people in the United States and the remainder of the world have insulin resistance. The great news is that there are many therapies with proven clinical trials that have been shown to be effective in helping insulin to work more effectively in the body.

If insulin resistance occurs long enough, you can develop diabetes, which is discussed in Part II of this book. (See page 68.)

THYROID HORMONE

Your thyroid gland is your body regulator. Therefore, an imbalance of your thyroid hormone can affect every metabolic function in your body. Consequently, your thyroid gland has a has a lot of important tasks.

■ Functions of the Thyroid Gland and Thyroid Hormones in Your Body

- Affects tissue repair and development

- Aides in the function of mitochondria (energy makers of your cells)

- Assists in the digestion process

- Controls hormone excretion and balance of other hormones

- Controls oxygen utilization

- Modulates blood flow

- Modulates carbohydrate, protein, and fat metabolism

- Modulates muscle and nerve action

- Modulates sexual function

- Regulates energy and heat production

- Regulates growth

- Regulates vitamin usage

- Stimulates protein synthesis

TYPES OF THYROID HORMONE

It is common for thyroid problems to appear at menopause. Your ovaries have thyroid receptors, and your thyroid gland has ovarian receptors. Therefore, the loss of estradiol (E2) and testosterone from your ovaries that occurs at menopause can have an effect on your thyroid.

There are a few different types of thyroid hormones that your body produces. They are:

- Thyroid stimulating hormone (TSH), which is made in your pituitary gland located in your brain. Production of T3 and T4 are activated by TSH.

- Diiodothyronine (T2), which is produced from T3 and from reverse T3

- Triiodothyronine (T3), which is a byproduct of thyroxine (T4). It affects almost every physiological process in the body, including growth and development, metabolism, body temperature and heart rate.

- Thyroxine (T4), which is made in your thyroid gland.

T4 is 80 percent of the thyroid gland's production. Most of T4 is converted into T3 in your liver or kidneys. T3 is five times more active than T4. T4 can also be converted into reverse T3, which is an inactive (stored) form. Additionally, T2 increases the metabolic rate of your muscles and fat tissues and its levels decrease with advancing age.

Thyroid Hormone and Iodine

Iodine, a chemical element, is particularly important when considering thyroid function. Iodine is an antibacterial, anticancer, antiparasitic, antiviral, and mucolytic agent.

Iodine is needed to maintain healthy breast tissue and nerve function, and it protects against toxic effects from radioactive material. According to the World Health Organization, up to 72 percent of the world's population is affected by an iodine deficiency disorder.

Causes of Iodine Deficiency

- Diet high in pasta and breads with contain bromide (bromide binds to the iodine receptors)

- Diet low in salt

- Diet without ocean fish or sea vegetables such as seaweed

- Fluoride use (inhibits iodine binding)

- Ground depleted of iodine

- Medications that contain fluoride or bromide

- Sucralose (contains chlorinated table sugar)

- Vegan and vegetarian diets

Contrary to the foods that interfere with iodine, there are plenty of foods that are useful sources of iodine.

Food Sources of Iodine

- Beef
- Beef liver
- Bread, whole wheat
- Butter
- Cheese, cheddar
- Cheese, cottage
- Clams
- Cream
- Eggs
- Green peppers
- Haddock
- Halibut
- Lamb
- Lettuce
- Milk
- Oysters
- Peanuts
- Pineapple
- Pork
- Raisins
- Salmon
- Sardines (canned)
- Shrimp
- Spinach
- Tuna (canned)

Be aware, however, that if you intake too much iodine you can get acne. Excess iodine intake can also cause thyroiditis, an inflammation of the thyroid gland that results in overproduction of the thyroid hormone. Your healthcare practitioner can measure your iodine levels with a urine test.

If you need iodine replacement, it will most likely contain iodine and iodide. Iodine replacement comes in both a liquid and tablet form. About one-third of people treated for low thyroid function will need to have a lower dose of thyroid medication when the iodine deficiency is corrected.

Your body can produce too little or too much thyroid hormone. Too little thyroid hormone production is called hypothyroidism. Excessive thyroid hormone production is termed hyperthyroidism. See Part II of this book for an extensive discussion of these disorders.

Decreased production of T3 can cause high cholesterol, because low levels of T3 cause less cholesterol to be removed from your blood. This causes an increase in bad cholesterol. Individuals who have low thyroid levels have cholesterol levels that are 10 to 50 percent higher than people with normal thyroid function.

Moreover, inadequate thyroid function can stimulate CYP3A4, a part of the P450 system in the liver, which can cause an increase in production of 16-hydroxy estrone, which can increase your risk of developing breast cancer. It can also lead to a decrease in SHBG, which increases the bio-available amount of E2 and testosterone in your body.

Decreased thyroid hormone levels can be caused by a variety of factors. Sometimes, a deficiency of certain minerals or vitamins can lead to low T4 production.

■ Nutritional Deficiencies That Can Cause a Decrease in T4 Production

- Copper
- Vitamins A, B$_2$, B$_3$, B$_6$, and C
- Zinc

■ T4 to T3 Conversion

Your body also needs to be able to convert T4 to T3. T3 is the more active form of thyroid hormone. This conversion requires an enzyme called 5'diodinase.

The inability to convert T4 to T3 will lead to symptoms of thyroid hormone loss. As discussed earlier, T4 also sometimes converts into reverse T3, which can also lead to symptoms of thyroid loss.

■ Effects of Decreased T3 (or Increased Reverse T3)

- Aging
- Chronic fatigue
- Diabetes
- Fasting
- Fibromyalgia
- IL-6, TNF-alpha, IFN-2 (immune system factors)
- Increased catecholamines (epinephrine and norepinephrine)
- Increased free radicals
- Infections
- Prolonged illness
- Stress
- Toxic metal exposure
- Yo-yo dieting

As mentioned, the conversion of T4 to T3 cannot take place without 5'diodinase, an enzyme. There are many factors that can affect your body's production of this important enzyme.

Reverse T3

Reverse T3 is a measurement of inactive thyroid function. Reverse T3 has only 1 percent of the activity T3 does. It is an antagonist of T3, which means that the higher your reverse T3 level is, the lower your T3 level will be. T3 and reverse T3 bind to the same receptor sites, so they cannot both occupy these sites at the same time. This situation occurs due to a malfunction of the metabolism of T4. When your reverse T3 is high this is a medical syndrome now called "reverse T3 dominance."

The most common reason that reverse T3 levels become elevated is stress. When you are stressed, your cortisol levels rise. If you stay stressed all the time your cortisol levels will stay elevated (see page 45). This phenomenon can cause your body to produce more reverse T3.

Risk Factors and Causes of Reverse T3 Dominance

- Diet low in fruit
- Diet low in green vegetables
- Estrogen dominance
- High intake of red meat
- High-fat diet
- History of abuse
- Immune dysfunction
- Lack of exercise from an early age on
- Menstrual cycles that occur more frequently than every twenty-eight days, with menstrual bleeding lasting more than seven days.
- Mitochondrial dysfunction
- Naturally red hair
- Use of intrauterine devices (IUD)

When you have a high reverse T3 level, you can have any, or all of the symptoms of hypothyroidism (low thyroid function). The most common symptom that I see in my practice in patients who have high reverse T3 levels is weight gain and the second is fatigue. It is very difficult to lose weight and keep it off if your reverse T3 levels remain elevated. Unfortunately, weight gain is also very discouraging. It may make dealing with other problems seem more difficult.

Additionally, when your reverse T3 level is high your body temperature goes down. This slows the action of many enzymes in your body, which can lead to a syndrome called "multiple enzyme dysfunction."

Causes of Multiple Enzyme Dysfunction

- Exposure to environmental estrogens or estrogen disruptors (PCBs, weed killers, plastics, detergents, household cleaners, and tin can liners)

- Liver dysfunction

- Long-term exposure to dioxin (a class of toxic chemicals)

- Poor estrogen metabolism

- Prenatal exposure to high levels of estrogen

Consequently, it is very important to have your reverse T3 levels measured. Some scientists believe that the best indicator of thyroid function is the ratio between T3 and reverse T3 since this ratio examines the tissue levels of thyroid hormone.

High levels of reverse T3 can be treated in several ways. Taking the nutrients that aid the conversion of T4 to T3 (see page 81) are very beneficial. Selenium (if levels are low), zinc, vitamins B_6 and B_{12}, iron, vitamin D, and iodine, if levels are low, have all been found to be helpful. If you are taking T4 medication, discontinuing it can also increase T3 and lower reverse T3 levels. Always consult your healthcare provider before discontinuing any drug. In addition, taking T3 as a prescription will also increase T3 levels and decrease reverse T3. Furthermore, if you have an elevated cortisol level, lowering it to normal will also diminish your reverse T3. In addition, a high normal or elevated reverse T3 can be a sign of mitochondrial dysfunction, which causes ineffective transport of thyroid hormone to the cell. See the section on hypothyroidism in Part II of this book (see page 246) for further discussion.

■ Factors That Affect 5'diodinase Production

- Cadmium, mercury, or lead toxicity

- Chronic illness

- Decreased kidney or liver function

- Elevated cortisol

- Estrogen excess

- Herbicides, pesticides

- High carbohydrate diet

- Inadequate protein intake

- Oral contraceptives

- Polycyclic aromatic hydrocarbons

- Selenium deficiency

- Starvation

- Stress

There are other factors besides insufficient 5'diodinase levels that can lead to an inability to convert T4 to T3 effectively.

■ Additional Factors That Cause an Inability to Convert T4 to T3

- Aging

- Alpha-lipoic acid (600 mg a day or more)

- Calcium excess

- Certain medications (these are the most common)

  - Beta-blockers

  - Birth control pills

  - Chemotherapy

  - Estrogen

  - Lithium

  - Phenytoin

  - Theophylline

- Copper excess

- Deficiency in the following nutrients

  - Iodine

  - Iron

  - Selenium

  - Vitamins A, B_2, B_6, and B_{12}

- Zinc

- Diabetes

- Dietary factors

  - Cruciferous vegetables (too many)

  - Excessive alcohol intake

  - Low carbohydrate diet

  - Low fat diet

  - Low protein diet

  - Soy

  - Walnuts (excessive intake)

- Dioxins

- Fluoride

- Inadequate production of adrenal hormones (DHEA, cortisol)

- Lead

- Mercury

- PCBs

- Pesticides

- Phthalates (chemicals added to plastics)
- Radiation
- Stress
- Surgery

Moreover, iron deficiency and physical inactivity impair your body's response to T3. These factors will also cause you to have symptoms of hypothyroidism.

Conversely, there are factors that will increase the conversion of T4 to T3 if there is not enough T3 being made by your body.

■ Factors That Increase the Conversion of T4 to T3 *

- Ashwagandha
- Glucagon
- Growth hormone
- High protein diet
- Insulin
- Iodine
- Iron
- Melatonin
- Potassium
- Selenium
- Testosterone
- Tyrosine
- Vitamins A, B_2, and E
- Zinc

You may notice that some of the same things that decrease the conversion of T4 to T3 increase it. This is due to the fact that it is important to have the right amount of these nutrients, herbs, and hormones in your body. Too much or too little will affect thyroid production and, subsequently, function.

OTHER TESTS OF THYROID FUNCTION

Besides blood studies, your doctor can do some other tests to look at thyroid function.

- **Thyroid scan.** A thyroid scan is a common test that is done to determine if you have a thyroid nodule (a lump that arises on the thyroid gland) and if the nodule is hot or cold. If you have a goiter (enlargement of the thyroid gland) its size can be measured by a thyroid scan. If you have had thyroid cancer, then a thyroid scan can be used after surgery to see if you have a reoccurrence of cancer. A thyroid scan is also used to determine if you have thyroid tissue located outside of the neck. The scan is done by giving a radioisotope (like radioactive iodine) and letting the thyroid gland (or thyroid tissue outside of the thyroid) take up the isotope.

- **Thyroid ultrasound.** A thyroid ultrasound is another method of testing thyroid function and assessing thyroid nodules. With this study, sound waves are used to tell if a thyroid nodule is solid or a cyst. However, this test will not tell your doctor if the nodule is cancerous or benign (non-cancerous). If your healthcare practitioner needs more information, you may be sent for a biopsy of your thyroid gland.

- **Basal body temperature.** Some people will have normal or even optimal levels of thyroid hormone but still will have symptoms of hypothyroidism. For these individuals it is important to get a basal body temperature. A basal body temperature is the temperature underneath your arm taken before you get out of bed in the morning for ten minutes. You take your temperature for three consecutive days. If you are menstruating, then take your temperature during your menstrual cycle.

- **Thyroid binding globulin (TBG).** Thyroid binding globulin (TBG) can also be measured. Thyroxine-binding globulin is one of three major transport proteins, which are primarily responsible for binding to and transporting thyroid hormones to the necessary tissues. The other two serum transport proteins include transthyretin and human serum albumin. Thyroid binding globulin is produced by the liver and is affected by illness, liver disease, and some medications. Sometimes estrogens can raise TBG so this is another test that you doctor may order.

- **Thyroid releasing hormone (TRH).** Your healthcare provide may also order a thyroid releasing hormone (TRH) level which is a hormone made in the hypothalamus that stimulates the release of thyroid stimulating hormone (TSH) and prolactin from the pituitary. TRH expression is activated by energy demanding situations, such as cold and exercise and it is inhibited by negative energy balance situations such as fasting, inflammation, or chronic stress.

Some individuals have an autoimmune process where their body is literally trying to attack its own thyroid gland and the body produces a normal amount of thyroid hormone or not enough thyroid hormone. This is called Hashimoto's thyroiditis. If you have Hashimoto's thyroiditis, your test results will reveal that your thyroid antibody levels are high. Your thyroid antibodies can also be increased if you have a special kind of hyperthyroidism (over production of thyroid hormones) called Graves' disease. Both these diseases are discussed at length in Part II.

PARATHYROID HORMONE

The parathyroid glands are two pairs of small, oval-shaped glands. They are located next to the two thyroid gland lobes in the neck. Each gland is usually about the size of a pea. The parathyroid gland secretes parathyroid hormone (PTH), a polypeptide, in response to low calcium levels detected in the blood. PTH facilitates the synthesis of active vitamin D, calcitriol (1,25-dihydroxycholecalciferol, or vitamin D_3) in the kidneys. In conjunction with calcitriol, PTH regulates calcium and phosphate. PTH effects are present in the bones, kidneys, and small intestines. As serum calcium levels decrease, the secretion of PTH by the parathyroid glands increases. In contrast, increased calcium levels in the serum serve as a negative-feedback loop, signaling the parathyroid glands to stop the release of PTH. In addition, parathyroid hormone promotes the absorption of calcium and magnesium and inhibits the absorption of phosphate and bicarbonate. How parathyroid hormone works in the body is an intricate balance and the clinical ramifications of irregularities are significant. Therefore, the understanding of PTH is of paramount relevance and importance to help you achieve and maintain optimal health.

The three main functions of parathyroid hormone are its effects on the bones, kidney, and small intestine.

■ Effects of Parathyroid Hormone on Bones

In the bones, PTH stimulates the release of calcium in an indirect process through osteoclasts, which ultimately leads to resorption of the bones. However, before osteoclast activity, PTH directly stimulates osteoblasts, which increases their expression of RANKL, a receptor activator for nuclear factor kappa-B ligand, allowing for the differentiation of osteoblasts into osteoclasts. PTH also inhibits the secretion of osteoprotegerin, allowing for preferential differentiation into osteoclasts. Osteoprotegerin normally competitively binds with RANKL, diminishing the ability to form osteoclasts. Osteoclasts possess the ability to remodel the bones (resorption) by dissolution and degradation of hydroxyapatite and other organic material, releasing calcium into the blood.

■ Effects of Parathyroid Hormone on Kidneys

In the kidneys, parathyroid hormone has three functions in increasing serum calcium levels. Most of the physiologic calcium reabsorption in the nephron (kidney) takes place in the proximal convoluted tubule and additionally at the ascending loop of Henle. Circulating parathyroid hormone targets the distal convoluted tubule and collecting duct, directly increasing calcium reabsorption. Parathyroid hormone decreases phosphate reabsorption at the proximal convoluted tubule. Phosphate ions in the serum form salts with calcium that are insoluble, resulting in decreased plasma calcium. The reduction of phosphate ions, therefore, results in more ionized calcium in the blood.

■ Effects of Parathyroid Hormone on the Small Intestine

Starting at the kidneys, PTH stimulates the production of 1alpha-hydroxylase in the proximal convoluted tubule. This enzyme is required to catalyze the synthesis of active vitamin D 1,25-dihydroxycholecalciferol from the inactive form 25-hydroxycholecalciferol. Active vitamin D plays a role in calcium reabsorption in the distal convoluted tubule via calbindin-D, a cytosolic vitamin D-dependent calcium-binding protein. In the small intestine, vitamin D allows the absorption of calcium through an active transcellular pathway and a passive paracellular pathway. The transcellular pathway requires energy, while the paracellular pathway allows for the passage of calcium through tight junctions.

The body can produce too little parathyroid hormone, called hypoparathyroidism, or too much parathyroid hormone, called hyperparathyroidism. See part II of this book to take a further look at these diseases.

MELATONIN

Melatonin is a hormone produced in the pineal gland, retina, GI tract, and white blood cells, and is associated with sleep. In addition, there are melatonin receptors expressed all over the body—for example, in the intestines, fat tissue, kidneys, liver, lungs, adrenals, and other organs. The amount of melatonin the body produces decreases as one ages and depends on the activity of an enzyme called serotonin-N-acetyltransferase (NAT). The body's production of NAT, on the other hand, depends on its storage of vitamin B_6. Melatonin has many functions in your body.

■ Functions of Melatonin

- Acts as an antioxidant

- Aids the immune system

- Blocks estrogen from binding to receptor sites

- Decreases cortisol levels that are elevated

- Decreases platelet stickiness (decreases the risk of heart disease)

- Dilates and contracts blood vessels

- Effects the release of sex hormones

- Helps balance the stress response

- Helps prevent cancer and treat some cancers

- Improves mood

- Improves sleep quality

- Inhibits the release of insulin from beta cells in the pancreas

- Inhibits the release of prolactin, follicle stimulating hormone (FSH) and luteinizing hormone (LH)

- Is cardioprotective

- Promotes healthy cholesterol levels

- Protects against GI reflux

- Protects skin cells against UV damage

- Regulates skin pigmentation

- Relieves jet lag

- Stimulates the parathyroid gland

- Stimulates the production of growth hormone

■ Signs and Symptoms of Melatonin Deficiency

- ❑ Anxiety

- ❑ Compromised immune system

- ❑ Early morning awakening

- ❑ Fatigue

- ❑ Heart disease

- ❑ Immunological disorders

- ❑ Increased risk of cancer

- ❑ Insomnia

- ❑ Interrupted sleep

- ❑ Seasonal affective disorder

- ❑ Stress

■ Causes of Melatonin Deficiency

There are many etiologies of melatonin deficiency. Perhaps the most common cause of melatonin deficiency in today's world is electromagnetic fields. Other causes include the following.

- Acetaminophen
- Alcohol abuse
- Aspirin/indomethacin/ ibuprofen
- Caffeine abuse

- High glycemic index foods
- Some medications
- Tobacco
- Vitamin B_{12} deficiency

■ Therapeutic Benefits of Melatonin

The therapeutic benefits of melatonin are numerous. Melatonin is a hormone that does much more than regulate the sleep cycle.

Alzheimer's Disease. Some of the symptoms of low melatonin levels are also common to patients with Alzheimer's disease: disruption of the circadian rhythm of the body, mood changes, and delirium. One medical trial showed that melatonin levels in the CSF in patients over the age of eighty were one-half the level of younger, healthier individuals. Individuals in this study with Alzheimer's disease had even lower levels—only 20 percent of the amount observed in young healthy people. Fortunately, numerous studies have shown that supplementing with melatonin helps to protect against Alzheimer's disease. In addition, in animal and human trials a benefit in melatonin replacement in patients with early Alzheimer's disease was seen even before it was clinically evident. In fact, when melatonin was replaced early, the participants did not show pathological changes nor have symptoms of cognitive decline.

In addition, melatonin supplementation has been shown to decrease the damage caused by amyloid beta proteins and tau proteins. Moreover, medical trials revealed that using melatonin in patients with Alzheimer's disease resulted in better sleep patterns, less sundowning, and slower progression of cognitive loss. Likewise, melatonin has also been shown to guard against the harmful effects of aluminum, which has been shown to cause oxidative changes in the brain that are similar to those seen in Alzheimer's disease.

Cancer. Many studies have shown that melatonin is an effective therapy for breast cancer as an adjunct to traditional care. It has also been shown to be effective in the prevention and reduction of some of the side effects of chemotherapy and radiation including mouth ulcers, dry mouth, weight loss, nerve pain, weakness, and thrombocytopenia (low platelet count). Moreover, melatonin has been used as a therapy for other cancer forms such as brain, lung, prostate, head and neck, and gastrointestinal cancers.

Cerebral Vascular Accident (CVA). If a person has a low melatonin level, they have an increased risk of developing a cerebral vascular accident (stroke). The odds rise more than 2 percent for every 1 pg/mL decline in melatonin. In fact, in individuals with a calcified pineal gland, the risk of developing a CVA is increased by 35 percent. Moreover, melatonin supplementation has been shown to shrink the size of an infarct area in a patient with acute CVA. This may be due to melatonin's ability to neutralize free-radical production.

Melatonin may also decrease the risk of CVA by significantly lowering cholesterol and decreasing blood pressure. Furthermore, melatonin supplementation in lab animals decreased the damage after stroke and decreased seizure occurrence. In addition, melatonin has been shown to increase plasticity of neurons after CVA. Likewise, in animal studies, melatonin reduced the damage caused by stroke by decreasing the activation of "protein-melting" enzymes. Melatonin has also been shown to tighten the blood-brain barrier, reduce tissue swelling, and prevent hemorrhagic transformation in animal trials with experimentally induced stroke.

Closed Head Injury (CHI)/Traumatic Brain Injury (TBI). Supplementation with melatonin has been shown to minimize the brain swelling and dysfunction that occurs after a closed head injury. Melatonin supplementation has also been shown to help protect the brain in the case of traumatic brain injury. Likewise, studies employing lab animals have shown that giving melatonin after a TBI had the following results: maintained the integrity of the blood-brain barrier, prevented dangerous brain swelling in the hours and days after injury, and shrank the size of the bruised and injured tissue. Melatonin, likewise, reduced the mortality rate after burst aneurysm in laboratory studies.

COVID-19. Melatonin is now being used as an adjuvant treatment for COVID-19, since it has been shown to limit virus-related diseases. It has also been demonstrated to be protective against acute lung injury and adult respiratory distress syndrome caused by viruses and other pathogens due to is anti-inflammatory and anti-oxidative effects. Unfortunately, COVID-19 tends to take a more severe course in individuals with chronic metabolic diseases such as obesity, diabetes mellitus, and hypertension. Since COVID-19 complications frequently involve severe inflammation and oxidative stress in this population, melatonin is being suggested as an add-on therapy for patients that are diabetic and overweight.

Gastrointestinal Diseases. The enterochromaffin cells of the gastrointestinal tract secrete 400 times as much melatonin as the pineal gland. Consequently, it is not surprising that numerous studies have found that melatonin plays an important role in GI functioning. As mentioned, melatonin is a powerful antioxidant that resists oxidative stress due to its capacity to directly scavenge reactive species, increase the activities of antioxidant enzymes, and stimulate the innate immune response through its direct and indirect actions. In the gastrointestinal tract, the activities of melatonin are mediated by melatonin receptors, serotonin, and cholecystokinin B receptors, as well as through receptor-independent processes.

Let us now examine the use of melatonin in several disease processes of the GI tract. The prevalence of gastroesophageal reflux disease (GERD) is increasing with individuals experiencing symptoms such as heartburn, regurgitation, dysphagia, coughing, hoarseness, or chest pain. Fortunately, melatonin has been shown to have inhibitory activities on gastric acid secretion and nitric oxide biosynthesis. Nitric oxide has an important role in transient lower esophageal sphincter relaxation which is a major etiology of reflux in people with this disease process.

A study revealed that a combination of melatonin, L-tryptophan, vitamin B_6, folic acid, vitamin B_{12}, methionine, and betaine was beneficial for patients with GERD. In addition, the other components of the formula exhibit anti-inflammatory and analgesic effects. All patients that took the combination of nutrients and melatonin reported a complete regression of symptoms after forty days of treatment. However, only 65.7 percent of the omeprazole patients reported regression of symptoms in the same period. Numerous other studies have also revealed that melatonin has a role in the improvement of gastroesophageal reflux disease when used alone or in combination with the drug omeprazole.

In addition, melatonin can protect the GI mucosa from ulceration by its antioxidant action, stimulation of the immune system, limitation of gastric mucosal injury, and promotion of epithelial regeneration. Melatonin can also reduce the secretion of pepsin and hydrochloric acid and influence the activity of the myoelectric complexes of the gut via its action in the central nervous system. This hormone furthermore attenuates acute gastric lesions and accelerates ulcer healing via its interaction with melatonin receptors due to an enhancement of the gastric microcirculation.

Similarly, melatonin is a promising therapeutic agent or irritable bowel syndrome (IBS), with activities independent of its effects on sleep, anxiety, or depression due to its important role in gastrointestinal physiology. It regulates gastrointestinal motility, has local anti-inflammatory reaction, and moderates visceral sensation. Studies have consistently showed improvement in abdominal pain, some trials even revealed improvement in quality of life in these individuals. In fact, studies have regularly publicized that alteration of the circadian rhythm is associated with the development of digestive pathologies that are linked to dysmotility or changes in microbiota composition in irritable bowel syndrome and similar conditions.

Moreover, disruption of circadian physiology, due to sleep disturbance or shift work, may result in various gastrointestinal diseases, such as irritable bowel syndrome, gastroesophageal reflux disease, or peptic ulcer disease. In addition, circadian disruption accelerates aging, and promotes tumorigenesis in the liver and GI tract. Furthermore, identification of the role that melatonin plays in the regulation of circadian rhythm allows researchers and clinicians to approach gastrointestinal diseases from a chronobiological perspective. Recently, it has been postulated that disruption of circadian regulation may lead to obesity by shifting food intake schedules. Likewise, a study suggests that sensing of bacteria through toll-like receptor 4 (TLR4) and regulation of bacteria through altered goblet cells and antimicrobial peptides is involved in the anti-colitic effects of melatonin. Consequently, melatonin may have use in therapeutics for inflammatory bowel diseases such as Crohn's and ulcerative colitis.

Heart Health. Patients with coronary artery disease tend to have low nocturnal serum melatonin levels. In addition, patients who developed adverse effects post myocardial infarction (MI) were shown to have lower nocturnal melatonin levels than patients without adverse effects. Melatonin is cardioprotective due to its vasodilator actions and free radical-scavenging properties. It also inhibits oxidation of LDL-C. Likewise, melatonin has been shown to reduce hypoxia and prevent reoxygenation-induced damage in individuals with cardiac ischemia and ischemic stroke.

The "MARIA" study was a prospective, randomized, double-blind, placebo-controlled trial that used IV melatonin in patients following an acute MI (heart attack) that were having angioplasty. It decreased CRP and IL-6, two major markers of inflammation. Melatonin also attenuated tissue damage from reperfusion, decreased V tach and V fib after reperfusion, and reduced cellular and molecular damage from ischemia. Another study revealed that there is an inverse correlation between melatonin levels and CRP levels after acute MI. Moreover, melatonin has been shown to protect cardiac myocyte mitochondria after doxorubicin (used for chemotherapy) use.

Hypertension. Melatonin has been shown to decrease blood pressure in patients with hypertension. In fact, a study revealed that evening controlled-release melatonin, 2 mg for one month, significantly reduced nocturnal systolic blood pressure in patients with nocturnal hypertension.

Immune Builder. Melatonin has been shown to be a major regulator of the immune system. Consequently, disease states affecting a wide range of organ systems have been reported as benefiting from melatonin administration.

Insulin Regulation and Obesity. Melatonin is necessary for the proper synthesis, secretion, and action of insulin. In addition, melatonin acts by regulating GLUT4 expression via its G-protein-coupled membrane receptors, the phosphorylation of the insulin receptor, and its intracellular substrates that mobilize the insulin-signaling pathway. GLUT4 is the insulin-regulated glucose transporter found primarily in adipose tissues (fat tissue) and striated muscle (skeletal and cardiac). Furthermore, melatonin is responsible for the establishment of adequate energy balance by regulating energy flow and expenditure through the activation of brown adipose tissue and participating in the browning process of white adipose tissue. Likewise, melatonin is a powerful chronobiotic, meaning that it helps regulate the body's internal clock.

Consequently, the reduction in melatonin production that may occur with aging, shift work, or illuminated environments during the night commonly induces insulin resistance, glucose intolerance, sleep disturbance, and metabolic circadian changes that commonly lead to weight gain. A study using laboratory animals showed that melatonin supplementation daily at middle age decreased abdominal fat and lowered plasma insulin to youthful levels. A low melatonin level is a frequently overlooked cause for an individual's inability to lose weight effectively.

Longevity. Lab trials have shown that melatonin replacement increases SIRT1, which is a longevity protein. SIRT1 is also activated by caloric restriction.

Mild Cognitive Impairment. Mild cognitive impairment (MCI) is impairment that precedes actual dementia. In fact, 12 percent of people with MCI proceed to develop dementia each year. Studies have shown that people who supplemented with melatonin (3 to 24 mg daily) for 15 to 60 months did much better on cognitive tests.

Neurodegenerative Disorders. Studies have shown that low melatonin levels are associated with an increased risk of developing neurodegenerative diseases such as Alzheimer's disease, mild cognitive impairment, cerebral vascular disease (stroke), and traumatic brain injury.

Parkinson's Disease. Melatonin replacement has been shown to decrease the risk of developing Parkinson's disease. Moreover, animal trials have shown that melatonin can prevent and, to some extent, may even help reverse the motor and behavioral changes that are associated with this disease process.

In Parkinson's disease there is an accumulation of a protein called alpha-synuclein. Melatonin supplementation also attacks alpha-synuclein and makes it more available to be removed by the body. In addition, a lab study showed that melatonin can reverse the inflammatory changes that occur in Parkinson's disease. Moreover, an animal trial also showed that melatonin helps to restore the normal activity of a key enzyme that is involved in the synthesis of dopamine. Furthermore, in lab studies melatonin supplementation was shown to increase the survival of dopamine-producing cells. Consequently, more research needs to be done concerning melatonin's use in Parkinson's disease.

Preoperative Anxiety. When compared to placebo, melatonin given as premedication (tablets or sublingually), can reduce preoperative anxiety in adults. In fact, melatonin may be equally as effective as the standard treatment with midazolam in reducing preoperative anxiety. The effect of melatonin on postoperative anxiety in adults is mixed but suggests an overall attenuation of the effect compared with preoperative anxiety.

Sleep Hygiene. Melatonin has long been known to be beneficial for sleep. Melatonin has been shown to synchronize the circadian rhythms and improve the onset, duration, and quality of sleep. The good news is that exogenous melatonin supplementation is well tolerated and has no obvious short- or long-term adverse effects when used in small doses to improve sleep hygiene.

■ Other Sources of Melatonin

The following are common foods that contain melatonin.

- Asparagus
- Barley
- Black olives/green olives
- Black tea/green tea
- Broccoli
- Brussels sprouts
- Corn
- Cucumber
- Mushrooms

- Oats
- Peanuts
- Pomegranate
- Red grapes
- Rice
- Strawberries
- Tart cherries
- Tomatoes
- Walnuts

■ Possible Side Effects and Contraindications of Melatonin

Melatonin is an immune stimulator. Therefore, it should be used with caution in individuals that are pregnant or breast feeding, patients that have an autoimmune disease, leukemia, or lymphoma, people who suffer from mental illness, and anyone taking steroids.

■ Signs and Symptoms of Excess Melatonin

- ❑ Abdominal pain
- ❑ Daytime sleepiness/fatigue

- ❑ Depression
- ❑ Headaches

- ❏ Hypotension (low blood pressure)
- ❏ Increase in cortisol, which can increase fat storage
- ❏ Intense dreaming/nightmares

- ❏ Suppression of serotonin, which increases carbohydrate cravings
- ❏ Transient dizziness

■ Causes of Excess Melatonin

The most common reason that people have elevated levels of melatonin is that they take doses that are too large, or they take melatonin and do not need it. Likewise, an individual may also have high levels of melatonin if they eat too many foods that contain melatonin. Some medications such as desipramine, fluvoxamine, thorazine, and tranylcypromine may raise melatonin levels, as can St. John's wort supplementation. Ingesting the herb *Vitex agnus-castus* (chaste tree) can also lead to elevated melatonin levels. If melatonin levels are high, serotonin levels tend to decline. There-fore, it is important to test your melatonin levels, by salivary testing, if you are taking more than one mg of melatonin at night.

■ Melatonin Dosing Schedules

Generally, women are more sensitive to melatonin than men if melatonin is being suggested for insomnia. Some women may need only a very low dose, and hence the melatonin may need to be compounded. In addition, medical studies have also suggested that patients may need less mela-tonin for insomnia as they age. As previously mentioned, large doses of melatonin are used to treat breast cancer and other cancers. Likewise, very large doses of melatonin are now being employed as co-therapies for COVID-19 under a healthcare provider's direction. If melatonin is going to be used long-term for COVID, measuring levels is suggested by saliva testing.

Melatonin is a wonderful hormone that has so many functions in the body aside from regulating sleep. As you have seen, it has been shown to be an effective therapy for many disease processes along with a beneficial way to build the immune system.

PROLACTIN

Prolactin is a hormone made by the pituitary gland located in your brain. The central nervous system, the immune system, the uterus, and the mammary glands all are all capable of producing prolactin. It has several functions in the body. Nipple stimulation, light, olfaction, and stress can all contribute to the initiation of prolactin synthesis in these tissues. Other factors that stimulate prolactin production include thyrotropin-releasing hormone (TRH), estrogen (pregnancy), and dopamine antagonists (antipsychotics).

■ Functions of Prolactin

- Decreases ovarian hormone production after delivery

- Enhances dopamine secretion

- Immunoregulatory (there are prolactin receptors on T and B lymphocytes.)

- Regenerative role in post-injury recovery from brain injury

- Regulates nursing

- Suppresses ovulation

■ Signs and Symptoms of Prolactin Deficiency

- ❏ Amenorrhea

- ❏ Decreased libido

- ❏ Inability to nurse

- ❏ Infertility

■ Causes of Prolactin Deficiency

- Autoimmune disorders (SLE, antiphospholipid syndrome, rheumatoid arthritis, multiple sclerosis, systemic sclerosis, autoimmune thyroid disease, and celiac disease)

- Closed head injury

- Infection (such as tuberculosis or histoplasmosis)

- Infiltrative diseases (sarcoidosis, hemochromatosis, lymphocytic hypophysitis, which is an inflammation of the pituitary gland)

- Parasellar diseases. Several lesions, including tumoral, inflammatory vascular, and infectious diseases may affect the parasesllar region, which is located around the sella turcica in the brain. Although invasive pituitary tumors are the most common neoplasms encountered within the parasellar region, other tumoral (and cystic) lesions can also be detected.

- Pituitary tumor

- Sheehan's syndrome (postpartum pituitary necrosis)

■ Recommended Daily Dosage of Prolactin

None.

■ Side Effects and Contraindications of Prolactin

None.

■ Signs and Symptoms of Excess Prolactin Production

- ❏ Bone loss
- ❏ Breast enlargement
- ❏ Depression
- ❏ Headaches
- ❏ Infertility
- ❏ Menstrual irregularity

- ❏ Milky discharge from breast
- ❏ Muscle loss
- ❏ Suppressed ovarian function with a decrease in ovarian hormone production
- ❏ Weight gain

■ Causes of Excess Prolactin

- Chest wall injury or irritation of the chest wall
- Cocaine or opiate use
- Excessive exercise
- Hypothalamic illness
- Hypothyroidism

- Medications
  - Anticonvulsants: Depakote
  - Antidepressants: SSRIs, tri-cyclic antidepressants
  - Estrogen
  - H2 blockers
  - Methyldopa

- Neuroleptic medications: Haldol, Mellaril, Risperdal, Seroquel
- Verapamil
- Menopause
- Other diseases of the pituitary
- Prolactinoma (noncancerous tumor of the pituitary gland)
- Renal disease
- Stress

If your prolactin level is high, then have your doctor repeat the study in the morning after you have been fasting for eight hours. The following items can temporarily elevate prolactin levels, therefore avoid the following prior to your blood redraw: a high protein meal, intense breast stimulation, recent breast exam, recent exercise, and stress.

The following are some of the reasons to have a prolactin level drawn by your healthcare provider.

- Amenorrhea (lack of menstrual cycle)
- Cirrhosis
- Decreased libido
- Erectile dysfunction
- Galactorrhea (milky discharge from the nipple)
- Hypothyroidism
- Infertility
- Kidney disease
- Low progesterone levels
- Suspect a pituitary tumor

CONCLUSION

As you have seen in Part I of this book, there are numerous hormones produced by your body. Included in this section are the most important women's hormones. It is paramount that all your hormones are balanced, and stay balanced, for you to achieve and maintain optimal health throughout your life.

PART II

Ailments
and Problems

INTRODUCTION

For many years, science has ignored the role that hormonal function plays in the relationship between a woman and her body. Issues such as insomnia or anxiety may be related to hormonal levels. How well you maintain vision, memory, and mobility are also related to optimal hormonal function. Even your risk of heart disease and stroke can be related, in part, to your hormonal levels.

Recent research has brought about many new medications and treatments to decrease your risk factors for disease and to help you live a healthier and longer life. An example of this is Precision/Anti-Aging Medicine. It is not a complementary or alternative specialty. It is a specialty that looks at the metabolism of the body and how the body works. It takes into consideration that medical problems are highly individualized. The same symptoms in two different people may mean entirely different things.

Part II of this book takes a glimpse at the ailments and problems that can occur if your hormones are not all balanced. Many common problems that women experience—such as PMS, premenstrual dysphoric disorder (PMDD), postpartum depression, endometriosis, bladder problems, migraine headaches, and vulvodynia—will be discussed in this section.

One size does *not* fit all when it comes to your medical treatment. As always, working with a healthcare professional and pharmacist that are specially trained in this area is suggested. Additionally, when taking supplements, always consume them with a full glass of water and make sure you are taking pharmaceutical grade nutrients. Pharmaceutic grade supplements are ones that are bioavailable (are absorbed easily into your body) and are also free of toxins. There is no regulation on vitamins in some countries such as the United States. Consequently, it is always important to make sure you are taking vitamins and other nutrients that are pharmaceutical grade.

It is also imperative you note the following precautions, along with the considerations given for each supplement. The dosages listed are intended for adults without kidney or liver disease. If you have kidney or liver disease, you may need to take lower dosages of most supplements and you should consult your healthcare provider before embarking on any nutritional program. Similarly, if you are pregnant or nursing, consult your doctor before following any of these protocols. If you are taking *Coumadin* or any other blood thinner, your dosage of certain nutrients may be lower than what is commonly suggested. Please ask your physician or pharmacist for help determining the appropriate dosage. If you are having surgery, do not take any nutrients (except for the surgery pre- and post-operative protocol that your doctor gives you) for 10 days before and one week after your surgery date.

ACNE

See Polycystic Ovarian Syndrome (PCOS); Premenstrual Syndrome (PMS).

ABNORMAL CHOLESTEROL LEVELS

See Heart Disease.

ADENOCARCINOMA

See Diethylstilbestrol (DES) Babies.

ANXIETY

See Premenstrual Dysphoric Disorder (PMDD); Premenstrual Syndrome (PMS); Menopause and Perimenopause.

ARTERIOSCLEROSIS

See Heart Disease.

BLADDER PROBLEMS

There are three types of urinary leakage (incontinence) that you may experience.

Overflow incontinence is the inability to completely empty your bladder which leads to frequent or constant dribbling of urine.

Stress incontinence which occurs when physical activities like vigorous exercise, coughing, laughing, or sneezing puts pressure on the bladder and it releases urine.

Urge incontinence occurs when an overactive or hyperactive bladder causes a sudden and intense urge to urinate causing an involuntary loss of urine.

Causes of Bladder Problems

There are also many causes of incontinence. Weakened pelvic floor muscles due to surgery or childbirth is a common cause. Pelvic floor exercise, called Kegel exercises, has shown great benefit if this is the cause of your incontinence. Urinary stones, urinary tract infections, as well as constipation, and nerve damage may be the etiology of incontinence. Moreover, drinking caffeine for some people can also cause urgency (the sensation that you must urinate immediately) or incontinence. Dyes that contain tartrazine (such as FD&C yellow #5) in foods, drinks, and even medications or vitamins can also irritate the bladder. Therefore, it is certainly worth trying to cut down on the caffeine and avoid dyes to see if it improves your bladder symptoms.

Studies have also shown that women with higher levels of vitamin D have a lower risk of developing pelvic floor disorders which include urinary incontinence. Have your healthcare provider measure your vitamin D levels. Like the vagina, the bladder has estrogen receptors. When your estrogen levels start to decline, you may have incontinence. Estrogen replacement therapy may significantly help bladder symptoms as can the right amount of progesterone. In addition, magnesium relaxes many things in the body including muscles. Muscle spasm may make your incontinence worse. Try taking magnesium glycinate 400 mg a day to see if this resolves your symptoms. Last, yoga, meditation, and acupuncture may be helpful.

BLOATING

See Menopause and Perimenopause; Premenstrual Dysphoric Disorder (PMDD); Premenstrual Syndrome (PMS).

BLOOD CLOTS

See Heart Disease.

BONE FRACTURES

See Osteoporosis.

BREAST CANCER

In the United States, 1 in 8 women will be diagnosed with breast cancer in her lifetime. An increasing body of evidence indicates that breast cancer is the most common malignancy among women, representing 23 percent of all diagnosed cancer cases, and the second leading cause of cancer deaths among women worldwide.

Risk Factors for Breast Cancer

- Alcohol consumption
- Diet
- Elevated cholesterol
- Estrogen dominance
- GI health
- Inflammation

- Lack of exercise
- Lack of vitamin D
- Obesity
- Stress
- Sugar intake

Breast Cancer Risks: How Can They Be Reduced?

There are many factors that have been shown to increase your risk of developing breast cancer. Although, there is no sure way to prevent breast cancer, there are ways that you can help decrease your risk of developing this disease.

Alcohol Consumption. Alcohol is liquid sugar. The results of one study suggest that alcohol consumption might be associated with an increased risk of breast cancer at relatively high levels of intake. Moreover, several studies showed that alcohol consumption increases the risk of breast cancer, in particular ER-positive tumors in postmenopausal women. A recent study showed a positive association between alcohol consumption and endogenous estrogen levels and mammographic density in premenopausal women. Similarly, alcohol intake after breast cancer diagnosis is associated with both increased risk of recurrence and death.

In addition, daily alcohol consumption increases serum estrogen levels, particularly E1 but also E2 and other forms of estrogen. Furthermore, alcohol consumption is shown to increase levels of internal estrogens which are known risk factors for breast cancer. This hypothesis is further supported by data showing that the alcohol-breast cancer association is limited to women with estrogen-receptor positive tumors. Furthermore, products of alcohol metabolism are known to be toxic and are hypothesized to cause DNA modifications that lead to cancer. Recent research has focused on genes that influence the rate of alcohol metabolism, with genes that raise blood concentrations of acetaldehyde hypothesized to heighten breast cancer risk. Acetaldehyde is produced by the partial oxidation of ethanol by the liver enzyme alcohol dehydrogenase and is a contributing cause of hangover after alcohol consumption.

Likewise, mounting evidence suggests that antioxidant intake, such as folate, may reduce alcohol-associated breast cancer risk, because it neutralizes reactive oxygen species, a second-stage product of alcohol metabolism. Therefore, diets lacking sufficient antioxidant intake may further elevate the risk of breast cancer among women consuming alcohol. Another study suggested that reactive oxygen species, resulting from ethanol metabolism, may be involved in breast carcinogenesis by causing damage, as well as, by generating DNA and protein adducts. An additional study concluded that alcohol interferes with estrogen pathways in multiple ways, influencing hormone levels and effects on the estrogen receptors. Moreover, alcohol may increase the activity of ER signaling in breast tumors or may increase endogenous steroid hormone levels.

Drinking even small amounts of alcohol is linked with an increased risk of breast cancer in women. Alcohol can raise estrogen levels in the body, which may explain some of the increased risk. Avoiding or cutting back on alcohol may be an important way for many women to lower their risk of breast cancer. Overall, the amount of alcohol someone drinks over time, not the type of alcoholic beverage, seems to be the most important factor in raising cancer risk. It does not matter therefore, if the alcohol is in the form of beer, wine, liquors (distilled spirits) or other drinks. Most evidence suggests that it is the ethanol that increases the risk, not other things in the drink. For example, in one trial, among healthy postmenopausal women who were not on HRT and who consumed 15 to 30 grams of alcohol per day, concentrations of serum estrone sulfate were increased by 7.5 percent and 10.7 percent, respectively, compared with levels in postmenopausal women who did not consume alcohol. Therefore, if you drink alcohol try not to drink more than one drink a day. If you have a strong family history of breast cancer, you may want to consider not drinking any alcohol.

Diet. Studies have shown that eating cruciferous vegetables (broccoli, cauliflower, Brussels sprouts, cabbage, and kale) decreases your risk of developing breast cancer, since their consumption improves the breakdown of estrogen in your body into components that decrease your risk of breast cancer.

A Mediterranean diet (a diet high in omega-3 fatty acids and vegetables) has been associated with a decreased risk in many diseases, including breast cancer. One study found that women who consume olive oil have a 25 percent lower risk of developing breast cancer. The intake of dietary lignans found in flaxseed have also been known to decrease breast cancer risk.

Estrogen Metabolism. How estrogen is broken down is one of the main risk factors for the development of breast cancer as discussed in the section on estrogen metabolism (see page 103). Estrogen is metabolized in two major pathways, the 2-OH and 16-OH estrogen, and the minor pathway, the 4-OH estrogen. The 2-OH is the "good estrogen." Methoxyestrogens, including 2-methoxyestradiol (types of estrogen), have been shown to inhibit carcinogenesis by suppressing cell proliferation and estrogen oxidation due to effects on microtubule (help support and shape the cell) stabilization. It acts as a cytostatin having anti-metastatic activity by inhibiting mitosis. Your body needs a small amount of 16-OH estrogen to maintain bone structure.

Results of a prospective study support the hypothesis that the estrogen metabolism pathway favoring 2-hydroxylation over 16 alpha-hydroxylation is associated with a reduced risk of invasive breast cancer risk in premenopausal women. Another study investigated the extent of estradiol 16 alpha-hydroxylation in relation to the risk of developing breast cancer in human breast tissue. They reported that 16 alpha-hydroxyestrone levels were eight-fold higher in cancerous mammary tissue than nearby mammary fat tissue. This suggests that 16 alpha-hydroxyestrone production may play an important role in breast cancer induction, 4-hydroxylated catechol estrogens possess carcinogenic potential due to their ability to cause DNA damage by forming adducts, which in turn, generate mutations with subsequent oxidative damage and initiation of breast cancer.

In addition, it has been shown that the ratios of quinone-estrogen DNA adducts to their parent or conjugated catechol estrogens were significantly higher in women with breast cancer or at high risk of breast cancer compared with women that were in the control group. To be more specific, individual variation in estrogen metabolism may also influence the risk of breast cancer and could provide clues to mechanisms of breast carcinogenesis. Recent medical studies have confirmed that more extensive 2-hydroxylation of parent estrogens is associated with lower risk, and less extensive methylation of potentially genotoxic 4-hydroxylation pathway catechols is associated with higher risk of postmenopausal breast cancer. See the section in Part I of this book on estrogen metabolism for a longer discussion on this topic along with ways to raise your 2-OH estrogen level in your body.

Exercise. A study found the lifestyle factor most strongly and consistently associated with both breast cancer incidence and breast cancer recurrence risk is physical activity. Another study supports the concept that moderate recreational physical activity (about 3 to 4 hours walking per week) may reduce breast cancer incidence. In addition, women with early-stage breast cancer who increased or maintain their physical activity may have lower recurrence risk as well.

Physical activity is recommended to avoid excessive weight gain. For example, the beneficial effects on the risk of breast cancer could be achieved by walking half an hour per day. Three to five hours per week of moderate physical exercise therefore should be considered for optimizing the reduction of the risk of cancer. For most women, moderate to intense activity, such as heavy housework, brisk walking, or dancing, could provide an effective level of activity to keep reduce the risk of breast cancer.

GI Health. The health of your GI tract has a great deal to do with whether you develop breast cancer and whether you are able to beat breast cancer. Seventy percent of your immune system is in your GI tract. In fact, the human microbiome in the gut plays an integral role in physiology, with most microbes considered benign or beneficial. However, some microbes are known to be detrimental to human health, including organisms linked to cancers and other diseases characterized by inflammation. Dysbiosis, a state of microbial imbalance with harmful bacteria species outcompeting benign bacteria, can lead to maladies including cancer. A study investigating differences in gut microbiome composition among postmenopausal women showed a less diverse fecal microbiome and a statistically significantly altered composition in newly diagnosed breast cancer patients (87 percent had ER-positive tumors) compared with healthy controls. These findings suggest an unrecognized link between dysbiosis and breast cancer which has potential diagnostic and therapeutic implications.

The gut bacterial microbiome includes an estrobolome. The estrobolome is the "the aggregate of enteric bacterial genes whose products are capable of metabolizing estrogens." It has a key influence on a women's lifetime exposure to major estrogens. The bacterial composition of the estrobolome in turn is likely affected by age and ethnicity, as well as lifetime environmental influences including diet, alcohol, and antibiotic use, which all affect bacterial populations. Some of these factors have also been independently linked to breast cancer risk.

Looking further at estrogens and their metabolism by the body, estrogens are primarily produced in the ovaries, adrenal glands, and adipose tissue and circulate in the bloodstream in free or protein-bound form and first undergo metabolism in the liver, where estrogens and their metabolites are conjugated. Conjugated estrogens are eliminated from the body by metabolic conversion to water-soluble molecules, which are excreted in urine or in bile into the feces. The conjugated estrogens excreted in the bile can be deconjugated by bacterial species in the gut with beta-glucuronidase activity (constituents of the 'estrobolome'), subsequently leading to estrogen reabsorption into the circulation. Especially relevant are gut bacteria possessing beta-glucuronidases and beta-glucosidases, hydrolytic enzymes involved in the deconjugation of estrogens. There are sixty bacterial genera that colonize the human intestinal tract that encode beta-glucuronidase.

Moreover, circulating estrogens exert effects on other tissues including the breast, which stimulate cell growth. By balancing the enterohepatic circulation (the circulation of biliary acids, bilirubin, drugs, or other substances from the liver to the bile, followed by entry into the small intestine, and transport back to the liver) of estrogens, the estrobolome affects both the excretion and circulation of estrogens. In other words, conjugated estrogens are excreted in bile, urine, and feces. Studies indicate that approximately 65 percent of estradiol, 48 percent of estrone, and 23 percent of estriol are recovered in bile. Approximately 10 percent to 15 percent of estradiol, estrone, and estriol are found in conjugated form in feces. Therefore, a significant proportion of estrogens are reabsorbed in the circulation.

In addition, an imbalance of the less desirous and good bacteria in the gut (dysbiosis) contributes to health problems including cancer.

Accordingly, gut microbiota are capable of modulating estrogen serum levels. Conversely, estrogen-like compounds may promote the proliferation of certain species of bacteria. Therefore, a crosstalk between microbiota of the GI tract and both endogenous hormones and estrogen-like compounds might provide protection from breast cancer. However, it may also increase the risk of developing hormone-related autoimmune diseases.

Recent research suggests that the microbiota (set of living organisms that inhabit the intestine) of women with breast cancer differs from that of healthy women, indicating that certain bacteria may be associated with cancer development and with different responses to therapy. Moreover, the microbiota-mediated regulation of innate and adaptive immune responses to tumors, and the consequences on cancer progression and whether tumors subsequently become resistant or susceptible to different anticancer therapeutic regiments is related to the ratio of healthy to non-healthy bacteria in the GI tract. In addition, interventions that may include use of prebiotics, probiotics, or antimicrobial agents could be designed specifically to target gut bacterial species with beta-glucuronidase activity to decrease estrogen-related cancer risk or become components of future therapies. Ultimately, understanding how gut dysbiosis impacts host response and inflammation will be critical to creating an accurate picture of the role of the microbiome in cancer development.

Hypercholesterolemia (Elevated Cholesterol). Hypercholesteremia is a risk factor for ER-positive breast cancer (cancer cells grow in response to estrogen). The cholesterol metabolite 27-hydroxycholesterol (27HC) has been shown to possess estrogenic activities and to promote breast tumor growth in animal and human trials in both pre- and post-menopausal women via several mechanisms. In addition, vitamin D supplementation has been shown to decrease circulating 27-hydroxycholesterol (27HC) in breast cancer patients most likely by inhibiting CYP27A1 (protein coding gene). Inhibition of CYP27A1, the enzyme responsible for the rate-limiting step in 27-hydroxycholesterol biosynthesis, significantly reduces metastasis in several studies. Moreover, oxidative modification of the lipoproteins and HDL glycation activate different inflammation-related pathways, thereby enhancing cell proliferation and migration and inhibiting apoptosis (cell death). Consequently, work with your healthcare provider to optimize your cholesterol level.

Inflammation. Breast cancer is an inflammatory disease process. Lowering the level of inflammation in your body decreases your risk of developing breast cancer. There are many articles that extensively demonstrate the direct relationship between chronic inflammation and cancer. In fact, inflammation is often associated with the development and progression of cancer. The cells responsible for cancer-associated inflammation are genetically stable and thus are not subjected to rapid emergence of drug resistance. Therefore, the targeting of inflammation represents an attractive strategy both for cancer prevention and for cancer therapy.

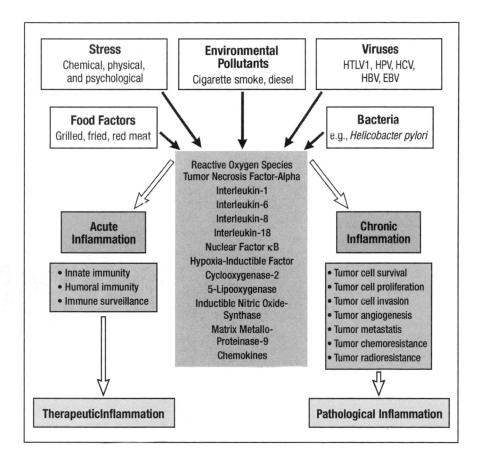

Tumor-extrinsic (occurs from outside the body) inflammation is caused by many factors, including bacterial and viral infections, autoimmune diseases, obesity, tobacco smoking, asbestos exposure, and excessive alcohol consumption, all of which increase cancer risk and stimulate malignant progression. In contrast, cancer-intrinsic (produced in the body) can be triggered by cancer-initiating mutations and can contribute to malignant progression through the recruitment and activation of inflammatory cells. Both extrinsic and intrinsic inflammations can result in immunosuppression, a compromised immune system, thereby providing a preferred background for tumor development.

These are the different faces of inflammation and its role in tumorigenesis described by Signh and others in the medical literature.

Chronic inflammation induced by biological, chemical, and physical factors, are associated with increased risk of human cancer at various sites. Chronic inflammatory processes induce oxidative/nitrosative stress and lipid peroxidation (LPO), which then generates excess reactive oxygen species (ROS), reactive nitrogen species (RNS), and DNA-reactive aldehydes.

Nitrosative stress (overproduction of nitric oxide) has been linked to the regulation of signal transduction, gene expression, and cell growth and apoptosis, and thus may be widely implicated in both physiological and pathological actions of nitric oxide.

The following are the consequences of nitrosative stress:

- Consumes important antioxidants such as melatonin and glutathione
- Disrupts important detoxification enzymes
- Disrupts the breakdown of cholesterol
- Disrupts neurotransmitter synthesis
- Disturbs hormone synthesis
- Disturbs the heme synthesis pathway
- Inhibits energy production in the mitochondria
- Interferes with the cell cycle and can lead to cell death
- Leads to DNA damage

While acute (sudden onset) inflammation is a part of the defense response, chronic inflammation can lead to cancer, diabetes, cardiovascular, pulmonary, and neurological diseases. Several pro-inflammatory gene products have been identified that mediate a critical role in suppression of apoptosis, proliferation, angiogenesis, invasion, and metastasis. Among these gene products are TNF and members of its superfamily: IL-1alpha, IL-1beta, IL-6, IL-8, IL-18, chemokines, MMP-9, VEGF, COX-2, and 5-LOX. The expression of all these genes is mostly regulated by the transcription factor NF-kappa B, which is constitutively active in most tumors and is induced by carcinogens (such as cigarette smoke), tumor promoters, carcinogenic viral proteins, chemotherapeutic agents, and gamma-irradiation. Consequently, several studies have identified nuclear factor-kappa B as a key modulator in driving inflammation to cancers. These observations suggest that anti-inflammatory agents, that suppress NF-kappa B or NF-kappa B-regulated products should have a potential in both the prevention and treatment of cancer. It has been found that chronic inflammation—caused by biological, chemical, and physical factors—increase the risk of developing cancer, including breast cancer.

Further data have expanded the concept that inflammation is a critical component of tumor progression, especially breast cancer. Many cancers arise from sites of infection, chronic irritation, and inflammation. Infection and inflammation account for approximately 25 percent of cancer-causing factors according to several medical studies. Furthermore, epigenetic alterations, such as DNA methylation and microRNA dysregulation, play vital roles in carcinogenesis, especially in inflammation-related cancers such as breast cancer.

Moreover, obesity is an inflammatory process and increases the risk of many cancer types. Obesity is also associated with poor outcomes. Furthermore, inflammatory processes induce oxidative stress and reduce cellular antioxidant capacity. In addition, overproduced free radicals react with cell membrane fatty acids and proteins impairing their function long-term.

In addition, free radicals can lead to mutation and DNA damage that can be a predisposing factor for cancer and age-related disorders. Likewise, as you have just seen, microbes, both commensal and pathogenic, are critical regulators of the host immune system and, ultimately, of inflammation. Consequently, microbes have the potential power to influence tumor progression as well, through a wide variety of routes, including chronic activation of inflammation, alteration of tumor microenvironment, induction of genotoxic responses, and metabolism. Therefore, have a healthy GI tract, as discussed in a previous section, decreases your risk of developing breast cancer, and helps to build your immune system.

In clinical trials, lifestyle modifications, including healthy diet, exercise, alcohol, and smoking cessation, have proven effective in ameliorating inflammation and reducing the risk of cancer-related deaths. Since breast cancer is inflammatory, work with your healthcare practitioner to consider taking low-dose naltrexone (LDN) if you have breast cancer. A few oncologists are even suggesting the use of LDN to prevent breast cancer if you have a strong family history of this disease process. It has been reported that lower doses of the opioid antagonist naltrexone are able to reduce tumor growth by interfering with cell signaling as well as by modifying the immune system. The results of increasing studies indicate that LDN exerts its immunoregulatory activity by binding to opioid receptors in or on immune cells and tumor cells. These new discoveries indicate that LDN may become a promising immunomodulatory agent in the therapy for cancer and many immune-related diseases.

Low-Dose Naltrexone (LDN). Low-dose naltrexone operates as a novel anti-inflammatory agent in the central nervous system, via action on microglial cells. These effects are unique to low dosages of naltrexone and appear to be entirely independent from naltrexone's better-known activity, at higher doses, on opioid receptors used for drug overdose and treatment for drug addiction.

As you have seen, chronic inflammatory diseases, such as cancer, are complex to treat. Due to the difficulty of treating cancer and other inflammatory processes, patients often seek off-label, complementary, or alternative medications. Low-dose naltrexone (LDN) is now being prescribed, off-label, for treatment of the inflammatory component of cancer, including breast cancer. It is an adjunct therapy and not designed to replace conventional treatment of cancer. As a daily oral therapy, LDN is inexpensive and well-tolerated.

Potential short-term side effects of LDN include insomnia, vivid dreams, fatigue, loss of appetite, nausea, hair thinning, mood swing, and mild disorientation. Insomnia is the most common possible side effect which for many people resolves after the first night. Potential long-term side effects are rare and include possible liver and kidney toxicity, possible tolerance to the beneficial rebound effect, and other unknown sequelae (an aftereffect of a disease). You cannot take LDN if you have acute hepatitis, liver failure, or have recent or current opioid use or if you abuse alcohol.

Melatonin. One of the many functions of melatonin, as you have seen in Part I of this book, is that it is a strong immune builder. In fact, many studies have shown that melatonin is an effective therapy for breast cancer as an adjunct to traditional care. If you are going to take more than 1 mg of melatonin at night, then have your healthcare provider or pharmacist measure your melatonin level by saliva testing.

Methylation. Think of methylation like the spark plug in a car that evokes certain chemical reactions. For example, methylation helps convert serotonin into melatonin. It helps change "strong" estrogens to milder, less aggressive estrogens. The disruption of normal methylation patterns has been found to be an important event in carcinogenesis. Cancer initiation and progression is driven by the accumulation of inherited or acquired DNA mutations. These alterations may be genetic or epigenetic in nature. Epigenetic modifications are changes in DNA structure that do not involve sequence changes but are stably inherited from cell to cell. These include DNA methylation, histone modifications (phosphorylation, acetylation, methylation) and microRNAs.

■ Signs and Symptoms of Hypomethylation (Methylation Pathway Not Functioning Optimally)

❑ Addictive behavior

❑ Adverse reaction to benzodiazepines

❑ Calm demeanor, yet high inner tension

❑ Competitiveness in sports

❑ Delusions

❑ Elevated histamine levels

❑ Family history of overachieving

❑ Frequent headaches

❑ High libido

❑ History of perfectionism

❑ Increased risk of developing major diseases

❑ Low pain tolerance

❑ Obsessive/compulsive tendencies (OCD)

❑ Phobias

❑ Poor long-term concentration

❑ Responds to antihistamines

❑ Ritualistic behaviors

❑ Seasonal allergies

❑ Self-motivated during school years

❑ Social isolation

❑ Sparse body hair

❑ Tears easily

❑ Underweight

❑ Very strong willed

Elevated levels of homocysteine—an amino acid—are often used as an indicator of methylation status. The estrogen metabolism test is also used as a marker of the body's ability to methylate. Methylation testing is furthermore available, measuring the entire methylation pathway.

Not everyone should take methylated vitamins. You can be over-methylated which also can cause you symptoms and increase your risk of developing various diseases. Over-methylation, or excessive methylation, is generally associated with oversaturation of methyl-related byproducts, including monoamines (serotonin, norepinephrine, dopamine). Abnormally high concentrations of monoamines can impair cognition, motivation, libido, and cause weight gain.

■ Signs and Symptoms of Over-Methylation

❑ Absence of seasonal allergies

❑ ADHD

❑ Adverse reaction to SAMe

❑ Adverse reaction to SSRI's

❑ Antihistamine intolerance

❑ Anxiety

❑ Artistic ability

❑ Behavior disorders

❑ Copper overload

❑ Depression

❑ Estrogen intolerance

❑ Food and chemical sensitivities

❑ High creativity

❑ High energy

❑ Hirsutism

❑ Histamine intolerance or low histamine levels

❑ Improvement with benzodiazepines

❑ Low libido

❑ Musical

❑ Pacing

❑ Panic attacks

❑ Rapid speech

❑ Restless legs

❑ Restlessness

❑ Schizophrenia

❑ Self-mutilation

❑ Sensitivity to environmental toxins

❑ Sleep disorders

❑ Tendency to be overweight

❑ Tinnitus

Obesity. Adiposity—being overweight—has been associated with higher circulating estrogen levels in postmenopausal women, as well as with increased breast cancer risk. A meta-analysis of 50 prospective observational studies confirmed a relationship between adult weight gain in women and risk for cancer; each 5 kg increase in weight was associated with increases in postmenopausal breast (+11 percent), ovarian (+13 percent), and endometrial cancers (+39 percent). In postmenopausal women, obesity and excess adiposity may lead to increased circulating estrogens through the peripheral aromatization of androgens. Several androgens are found normally in women, including dehydroepiandrosterone, dehydroepiandrosterone-sulfate, testosterone, dihydrotestosterone, and androstenedione. However, it also can induce insulin resistance, increase insulin-like growth factor (IGF)–1, and suppress production of hepatic hormone-binding proteins, thereby increasing total and bioavailable estrogens.

Moreover, data suggests that adult weight gain and central obesity increase the risk of pre-menopausal breast cancer as well as postmenopausal breast cancer. Obesity, likewise, at the time of diagnosis is thought to be significant as a poor prognostic factor. In fact, obesity is associated with adverse outcomes in both pre- and post-menopausal women with breast cancer, including women diagnosed with early-stage breast cancer. Dozens of studies demonstrate that women who are overweight or obese at the time of breast cancer diagnosis are at increased risk of cancer recurrence and death compared with leaner women. Also, some evidence suggests that women who gain weight after breast cancer diagnosis may also be at increased risk of poor outcomes. Therefore, weight management should be an integral part of any strategy to prevent and improve the outcome of breast cancer.

Stress. When you are stressed, your immune system becomes compromised, and you increase your risk of developing breast cancer. See the chapter in Part I of this book on cortisol, your stress hormone, for more information on the hormone and how to normalize the level if it is abnormal.

Sugar Intake. Many major researchers and authors have examined the relationship between cancer and high sugar intake in the past. Furthermore, studies have shown that people that consume more sugar have an increased risk of developing cancer, particularly breast cancer. Likewise, in older women a strong correlation was found between breast cancer mortality and sugar consumption.

Epidemiological studies have also shown that dietary sugar intake has a significant impact on the development of breast cancer. One proposed mechanism for how sugar impacts cancer development involves inflammation. Another mechanism that is suggested for the increased risk of breast cancer development with high sugar ingestion is a study suggesting that dietary sugar induces 12-LOX signaling to increase the risk of breast cancer development and metastasis.

Specific types of cancer, like triple-negative breast cancer (TNBC), are both responsive to dietary factors and very difficult to treat. Therefore, preventative care through dietary intervention in at risk populations is a must. One study showed a link between increased dietary fructose consumption, development of metabolic disturbances, and increased incidence of triple-negative breast cancer.

Vitamin D. Several studies have shown that there was a significant association found between low serum 25(OH)D levels and risk of breast cancer development. In these studies, the majority of patients suffering from breast cancer were vitamin D deficient. Moreover, results from a case-control study support the protective effect of higher serum concentration of 25(OH)D against breast cancer. Likewise, dietary but not total intake of vitamin D was associated with decreased risk of breast cancer.

In a prospective study, African American women in the lowest quartile of cumulative predicted 25(OH)D were estimated to have a 23 percent increased risk of breast cancer compared to those with relatively high levels. Consequently, preventing vitamin D deficiency may be an effective means of reducing breast cancer incidence in African American women. The same is true of a study of Saudi Arabian women. In this cohort of women with elevated risk, high serum 25(OH)D levels and regular vitamin D supplement use were associated with lower rates of incident, postmenopausal breast cancer over 5 years of follow-up. Yet another trial revealed the same association of low vitamin D levels and breast cancer risk among pre- and postmenopausal Hispanic women. These results may help to establish clinical benchmarks for 25(OH)D levels; in addition, they support the hypothesis that vitamin D supplementation is useful in breast cancer prevention when vitamin D levels are optimal.

- Vitamin D deficiency: less than 20ng/mL (50 nmol/L)
- Vitamin D insufficiency: less than 40 ng/mL (100 nmol/L)

- Optimal vitamin D status: 55 to 80 ng/mL (120 to 160 nmol/L)

- Vitamin D excess: serum levels greater than 80 to 100 ng/mL (200 nmol/L)

A study came out recently from Denmark examining almost a quarter of a million patients. This trial confirmed that low vitamin D levels were associated with an increase in mortality, but paradoxically high vitamin D levels were also found to be associated with higher mortality rates. The researchers found that the optimal level of vitamin D (with the exception of patients with hypersensitivity syndrome) was 70 nmol/L (about 30ng/mL). Patients with hypersensitivity syndrome include individuals with hyperparathyroidism, active cancer, and granulomatous diseases such as sarcoid, TB, and Crohn's disease. In these people, an optimal level of vitamin D may not be achievable without calcium levels elevating, which is detrimental to your health.

In summary, there are many risk factors for breast cancer related to: the body's ability to metabolize estrogen, your sugar and alcohol intake, whether you are obese and if you exercise, your melatonin level, whether your cholesterol level is elevated, if you methylate properly, if you have an optimal level of vitamin D, how healthy your GI tract is, and if your body is inflamed. A wide array of chronic inflammatory conditions predisposes susceptible cells to neoplastic transformation. In general, the longer the inflammation persists, the higher the risk of cancer.

Fortunately, as you have seen, there are also many methods to help you decrease your risk of developing breast cancer and/or reoccurrence if you have already had this disease. A great motto to live by is the following: *Life is not about how to survive the storm, but how to dance in the rain.* The great news is that you can mitigate most, or all, of these twelve risk factors.

IMPROVING BREAST HEALTH

As you have seen, there are many things you can do to prevent or decrease your risk of developing this disease.

As stated earlier, optimal levels of vitamin D in your body decrease your risk of developing breast cancer. Studies have shown that a lower intake of vitamin D and calcium can result in denser tissue (as revealed by mammography). This can also increase your risk of developing breast cancer.

Studies have shown that vigorous exercise decreases your risk of developing breast cancer by 30 percent.

Taking EPA/DHA (fish oil) may help prevent cancer, according to a clinical trial comparing women with invasive breast cancer and women with benign breast conditions. Women in this trial who had invasive breast cancer had much lower levels of DHA than women without breast cancer.

As discussed previously, prolonged stress is a risk factor for many cancers—but this is especially true of breast cancer. Stress that occurs for a long time reduces methylation of estrogens so that they are not broken down in the body into the "good" estrogens. This occurs because the methyl groups that are involved in methylation get used up by the body to make adrenaline when you are stressed. Some foods have been found to be helpful in improving methylation. Green leafy vegetables, legumes, citrus, berries, and nuts would be good choices.

See also Cancer.

BREAST SWELLING/TENDERNESS

See Fibrocystic Breast Disease; Menopause and Perimenopause; Premenstrual Dysphoric Disorder (PMDD); Premenstrual Syndrome (PMS).

CALCIUM DEFICIENCY

See Osteoporosis.

CANCER

Cancer is a disease in which abnormal cells divide without control and spread to other tissues. These cells can invade other parts of the body through the blood and lymph systems. Cancer is not a single disease, but many diseases.

This section is not designed to be an extensive, exhaustive look at the prevention of every type of cancer. Consequently, the focus in this section is on the cancers that most often affect women. The most common types of cancer women experience are breast, ovarian, uterine, and cervical cancers.

Risk Factors for Cancer

There are many elements of daily life that can serve as risk factors for various types of cancer.

- **DES.** Women who took DES—Diethylstilbestrol—(see page 132) have a higher risk of developing cancer. Additionally, other studies have shown that daughters of women who took DES have an increased risk of cervical, breast, and vaginal cancers.

- **Diet.** According to numerous medical studies, following a high glycemic index diet can increase the risk of many types of cancer, including breast, endometrial, stomach, and colorectal. The glycemic index ranks carbohydrates in the diet according to their effect on blood sugar levels. Make sure you always eat a low glycemic index program.

- **Enzymes.** High levels of certain enzymes can also increase your risk of developing cancer. Some cancers—such as endometrial, cervical, breast, ovarian, colon, lung, and glioma—are associated with high levels of COX and LOX, enzymes that are part of the inflammatory pathway. Nutrients such as ginkgo, curcumin, kaempferol, and quercetin decrease your levels of COX and LOX.

- **Nutrition.** Nutritional deficiencies of some vitamins have been associated with an increased risk of several types of cancers. For example, if you have a higher vitamin D level you have a markedly reduced risk of developing cancer of the breast, uterus, ovary, cervix, colon, esophagus, pancreas, rectum, bladder, kidney, or lung. You also have a reduced risk of developing non-Hodgkin's lymphoma and multiple myeloma. Consequently, a deficiency in vitamin D increases your risk of developing the types of cancer mentioned. However, medical studies have shown that your vitamin D level must be optimal and not just normal in order to reap this nutrient's benefits. An optimal level of vitamin D is 55 nanograms per milliliter (ng/mL) or greater. If all people had vitamin D levels of 55 ng/mL, it is projected that in North America alone, 85,000 cases of breast cancer and 60,000 cases of colon cancer would be prevented annually.

  Some researchers believe cancer may be linked to a dysfunction of the mitochondria, which are the "engines" of your cells. Many cancer patients have low levels of coenzyme Q-10, one of the main nutrients that fuels the mitochondria. Raising Q-10 levels in cancer patients has been associated with an increase in survival rate. Therefore, you want to make sure that your body has enough coenzyme Q-10. Coenzyme Q-10 levels decrease with true exercise, aging, and some medications. True exercise is doubling your pulse for twenty minutes. Exercising is great for you, but your body needs fuel to exercise, and coenzyme Q-10 is one of the fueling sources used. The body requires tyrosine, phenylalanine, vitamins C, B_2, B_3, B_5, B_6, B_{12}, and folate to make coenzyme Q-10. Consequently, a deficiency in any of these nutrients may lead to low coenzyme Q-10 levels in your body.

- **Stress.** Prolonged stress has been shown to be a risk factor for many cancers. The people who are most likely to suffer stress are those who avoid conflict, are overly nice, and use denial as a coping mechanism. These types of people tend to suppress their emotions, especially anger.

- **Weight.** Furthermore, being overweight increases your risk of many kinds of cancers. One study, which followed over 900,000 women and men over a sixteen-year period, showed that the heavier participants were, the higher their death rate for all forms of cancer was. Overweight women had a 62 percent higher death rate than those with "normal" weights, and overweight men had a 52 percent higher death rate. Being overweight can also increase your levels of estrogen and insulin, which may increase the rate of cancer cell growth. Endometrial and gallbladder cancer risks are five times greater if you are overweight.

■ Preventing Cancer

Because many elements of daily life serve as risk factors for cancer, it should come as no surprise that studies have shown most cancers are preventable by making lifestyle changes.

Exercising has been shown to decrease the risk of all cancers by almost 50 percent. Furthermore, exercise can help with some other risk factors for cancer, such as poor diet, being overweight, and smoking.

Vitamin D affects at least 200 genes. Some of these genes regulate cancer cell growth and differentiation. They also regulate cancer cell death and limit the growth of tumor blood supplies (angiogenesis).

SUPPLEMENTATION TO PREVENT CANCER		
Supplements	Dosage	Considerations
Vitamin D	About 1,000 international units (IU) a day, but the dosage is best determined by a lab measurement	Can reduce the risk of developing cancer by 60 to 77 percent

See also Breast Cancer; Cervical Cancer; Ovarian Cancer; Uterine Cancer.

CARCINOMA-IN-SITU

See Cervical Dysplasia (Abnormal Pap Smear).

CARDIOVASCULAR DISEASE

See Heart Disease.

CERVICAL CANCER

Cervical cancer is the fifth leading cause of cancer deaths in women overall. However, it is the second most common cancer women between the ages of fifteen and thirty-four suffer from. Since the development of the Papanicolaou (Pap) smear in the 1940s as an effective screening tool, the incidence of cervical cancer in the United States has decreased by 75 percent and the death rate continues to decline as well. After the long application of pap smear and histology, new technologies to assist in the screening for cervical cancer have now been developed. HPV typing has become an important tool in primary screening for further clinical management. However, each year, more than half a million women are diagnosed with cervical cancer and the disease results in over 300,000 deaths worldwide commonly in low-income areas where access to healthcare is limited.

■ Preventing Cervical Cancer

Cervical cancer remains the fourth most common cancer, affecting women worldwide with large geographic variations in cervical cancer incidence and mortality rates. Immunization by vaccine programs is certainly the best way to prevent cervical cancer. An immunization that covers all oncogenic HPV types, for a total prevention of this cancer, is the best strategy to prevent the infection of all high oncogenic risk types of the virus. The secondary prevention strategy for cervical cancer is based on screening strategies to detect precursor lesions, called intraepithelial neoplasia (CIN) alterations. The WHO recommends that screening for cervical cancer should be performed at least in the target age group (30 to 60), through cytology and visual inspection with the use of acetic acid. In women, who test negative on cytology or visual inspection, the screening interval should be every 3 to 5 years. In women, who test negative on an HPV test, rescreening should be done after a minimum interval of 5 years. Likewise, abstinence or being in a monogamous relationship will dramatically decrease your risk of getting cervical cancer.

■ Foods and Drinks That Decrease Your Risk of Developing Cervical Cancer

● Low glycemic index (GI) eating program. Diets rich in high-GI carbo- hydrates have been associated with an increased risk of several types of cancer. This link is likely to be related to the ability of high-GI foods to stimulate the production of insulin and insulin-like growth factor

Risk Factors for Cervical Cancer

The biggest risk factor to the development of cervical cancer is to be infected with the human papillomavirus. There are several other major risk factors that have been elucidated that increase your risk of developing cervical cancer.

- Age
- Being a DES baby
- Birth control pill use
- Having a child before the age of sixteen
- Immunosuppression (compromised immune system)

- Intercourse before the age of eighteen
- Multiple sexual partners
- Nutritional deficiencies
- Smoking

■ **Age.** Age plays a role in the development of cervical cancer along with how invasive the cancer may be. The risk of developing invasive cancer of the cervix increases after age twenty-five. Also, your odds of dying of cervical cancer increase as you age.

■ **Birth control pills.** These deplete the body of important nutrients, such as vitamin B_6 and beta-carotene, vitamin C, folate, riboflavin, vitamin B_{12}, magnesium, selenium, and tyrosine. The use of birth control pills has been

(IGF), two hormones that have been shown to promote tumor proliferation, progression, and spreading within the body.

● Eat cruciferous vegetables such as cauliflower, cabbage, broccoli, Brussels sprouts, and kale. The cancer-fighting properties of cruciferous vegetables largely attributable to indole-3-carbinol (I3C), a natural compound that occurs in cruciferous vegetables when they are chopped, crushed, or chewed. Indole-3-carbinol has been shown to promote the detoxification of many harmful substances, including carcinogens, and to have strong antioxidant properties. In addition, indole-3-carbinol has anti-estrogenic activities which may provide additional protection against cervical cancer.

● Curcumin can spice up your life. In India recently discovered that curcumin appears to arrest the development of cervical cancer by inactivating the HPV that lurks inside cervical cancer cells.

associated with an elevated risk of developing cervical dysplasia (precancerous lesion of the cervix). Clinical trials have shown that women who use birth control pills for more than five years may have an increased risk of cervical cancer. Some of the increased risk may be secondary to nutritional deficiencies caused using birth control pills. Therefore, if you are taking oral contraceptives, make sure that you supplement with a pharmaceutical-grade multivitamin and/or a good B complex vitamin. B vitamins are water soluble. Consequently, they should be taken twice a day.

■ **Nutritional deficiencies.** Some nutritional deficiencies are linked to the development of cervical cancer. A clinical trial showed that women with low vitamin C intake were 10 times more likely to develop cervical cancer than women who ate foods that were higher in vitamin C. Other studies have shown that if you eat a diet low in vitamins B_1, B_2, and B_{12}, you may have an increased risk of developing cervical dysplasia. The same study also showed that women who were at high risk for developing cervical cancer or who were diagnosed with the disease had much lower levels of beta-carotene, lycopene, canthaxanthin, and alpha-tocopherol (a kind of vitamin E) than the control group.

■ **Smoking.** Smoking increases your risk of developing cervical cancer. In fact, women who smoke are twice as likely to develop cervical cancer than those who do not smoke.

- Scientific studies suggest that ellagic acid can effectively eliminate cervical cancer-causing substances by activating certain detoxifying enzymes in the body. Furthermore, ellagic acid prevents carcinogens from attaching to cellular DNA. Moreover, ellagic acid has been shown to stimulate the immune system to destroy cancerous cells and to induce normal self-destruction of human cancer cells. Ellagitannin—which is converted into ellagic acid by the body—is found in some red fruits and berries, raspberries being one of the best dietary sources. Also, some nuts, such as walnuts and pecans, contain this important nutrient.

- Omega-3-fatty acids, which are abundant in fatty fish, flaxseed, and walnuts, are believed to have a protective effect against cervical cancer.

- Drinking green tea has been shown to prevent cervical cancer.

- Beta-glucans, a group of glucose polymers that are derived from the cell wall of fungi and bacteria decrease the risk. It has been shown that beta-glucans have some anti-cancer properties, which are due to their impact on adaptive and innate immunity. As well as the impact on immunity, these molecules could be used as drug carriers. Beta-glucans have complicated structures and because of that, they have several pivotal roles in the human body, such as increasing resistance to infectious challenges, anti-carcinogenic activities, anti-tumor effects, and activating leukocytes, T helpers, and NK cells, anticoagulant effects, and antibiotic impacts. Beta-glucans have an anti-cancer property because of their immunomodulation role on T cells and antigen-presenting cells, such as dendritic cells, macrophages, and B lymphocytes. As a result, beta-glucans also might be effective in reducing cervical cancer progression through modulating both innate and adaptive immunity.

See also Cancer.

CERVICAL DYSPLASIA (ABNORMAL PAP SMEAR)

Cervical dysplasia is the term used to describe abnormal cells on the surface of the cervix (the lowest part of the uterus). Each year in the U.S., 250,000 to 1 million women are diagnosed with cervical dysplasia. Cervical dysplasia can occur at any age with the mean age being 25 to 35 years.

Risk Factors for Cervical Dysplasia

Repeated HPV infection is the most common and important risk factor for cervical dysplasia. However, there are several risk factors besides HPV.

- **Cigarette smoking.** Smokers have a threefold increased risk compared to people who do not smoke. One study showed an increased risk of up to seventeen-fold in women that were 20 to 29 years of age if they smoked. Smoking may increase the risk of developing cervical dysplasia or cancer due the following: smoking compromises the immune system, causes vitamin C deficiency, and cervical cells may concentrate nicotine.

- **Diet.** Diet plays a role in the risk factors for cervical cancer. Deficiencies of certain nutrients can increase your risk of developing cervical cancer, but proper levels of other nutrients can help decrease your risk. If your diet is rich in fruits, vegetables, and fiber, you will have a lower risk for this type of cancer. One study showed that vegetable consumption and circulating cis-lycopene may be protective against HPV persistence.

- **Infections such as herpes, chlamydia, HIV or HPV, genital warts.** Most cervical cancer is associated with persistent HPV infection which is usually sexually transmitted. It may be a few weeks or years between time of exposure and when the patient develops an abnormal pap smear or lesion. Not all individuals that are infected with HPV get cervical dysplasia. This finding suggests that if the patient has a strong immune system, then it helps the body defend against the development of actual disease. Some studies suggest that up to 80 percent of people that are adults may be infected. HPV has been shown to be the etiology of cervical cancer in 99.8 percent of the 500,000 cases of cervical cancer that occur worldwide annually. Sexually transmitted disease has long been recognized as a major risk factor for cervical dysplasia and/or cancer. Exposure to HPV can also occur via examination tables, doorknobs, tanning beds, and other objects which is hard to document. In addition, since HPV is a sexually transmitted disease, it is important to also treat the sexual partner.

- **Long-term use of oral contraceptives.** Some studies have shown an association between cervical dysplasia and oral contraceptives, and some studies have not. Oral contraceptives cause nutritional depletions that may compromise the immune system which may be part of the problem.

Nutritional depletions caused by oral contraceptives include vitamins C, B_6, B_{12}, folic acid, riboflavin (B_2), and zinc.

- **Multiple sexual partners and sexual intercourse at an early age**. Multiple sexual partners (2 to 5) increase the risk 3.46-fold. First intercourse before age 18 increases the risk 2.76-fold.

- **Nutritional deficiencies.** Deficient dietary B-carotene (<5,000 IU/day) increases the risk almost 3-fold. Deficient dietary vitamin C (<30 mg/day) increases the risk over 6-fold.

- **Vitamin Deficiency.** Numerous vitamin deficiencies have been associated with cervical dysplasia and cervical cancer. One study focusing on people with untreated cervical cancer revealed that at least 67 percent of the patients studied had at least one abnormal vitamin level. Of those patients, 38 percent had multiple vitamin deficiencies.

Other Risk Factors

- Maternal history of exposure to DES

- MTHFR 677C>T polymorphism (genetic inheritance)

- Pregnancy

- Taking medications that suppress the immune system

The changes in the cells are classified as mild, moderate, or severe. Mild dysplasia is called CIN I. Moderate to marked dysplasia is called CIN II. Finally, severe dysplasia to carcinoma-in-situ is called CIN III. (Carcinoma-in-situ is the term used to describe an early stage of a tumor or cancer involving only the place in which it began.)

Cervical dysplasia is considered a pre-cancerous condition. It manifests prior to the development of cervical cancer. Left untreated, cervical dysplasia can lead to cervical carcinoma-in-situ, and eventually cervical cancer.

For the most part, there are no symptoms associated with cervical dysplasia. Therefore, it's imperative for women to get routine Pap smears, which will show the abnormality and allow for early diagnosis and treatment. An abnormal Pap smear can be seen as soon as a few weeks post-infection, or it can occur many decades after the infection.

Abnormal Pap smears can be a result of inflammation or infections.

Some nutritional deficiencies are also linked to abnormal Pap smears. However, the most common cause of an abnormal Pap smear is HPV (human papillomavirus).

The best time to catch and begin treatment for cervical dysplasia is in the beginning stages, before the cells become cancerous. A Pap smear or colposcopy (examination of the cervix and vagina) are the best ways of discovering a problem.

▪ Therapies for Cervical Dysplasia

Conventional Therapies

The treatment depends on how severe the lesions are. The 5-year reoccurrence rate with conventional therapy is up to 75 percent.

For preinvasive cervical disease

- Conization biopsy
- Cryotherapy
- Laser therapy
- Loop electrical excision procedure (LEEP)

For invasive disease

- Hysterectomy

Precision Medicine Therapies

Precision Medicine therapies address the cause of the problem along with prevention. Precision therapies build the immune system, are anti-inflammatory, hormone-regulating, and antiviral. Treatment of cervical dysplasia requires monitoring and coordination of care between the physician doing the colposcopy and biopsy and the healthcare practitioner doing the precision therapies. Precision Medicine therapies include the following:

- Botanical therapies
- Combination therapy
- Dietary Factors
- Nutritional therapies
- Stress management

Dietary Factors

More than half of patients with cervical cancer have been found to have multiple nutritional deficiencies or other determinants of nutritional inadequacies. A diet containing a lot of fruits and vegetables may help protect against carcinogenesis. A study done in Brazil showed that decreased concentrations of serum lycopene were associated with precancerous lesions of the cervix and cervical cancer. Also, increasing concentrations of dietary intakes of dark green and deep yellow vegetables and fruits were associated with almost a 50 percent reduction in the risk of CIN3. Another study showed that higher levels of vegetable consumption were associated with a 54 percent decreased risk of HPV persistence.

Nutritional Therapies

Numerous nutritional and botanical agents have been shown to be effective treatments for cervical dysplasia. A combination of products works best for most individuals. A medical trial showed multiple vitamins and mineral formulas were associated with a lower viral load and a decreased risk of developing cervical cancer, such as:

- **B_{12} and folate.** A study showed that women with higher levels of serum folate who also had an optimal level of serum B_{12} had a significantly lower risk of getting cervical dysplasia. Therefore, consider supplementing with both B_{12} and folate if you have cervical dysplasia.

- **Copper-zinc ratio and retinol.** A study of over 200 women found an inverse correlation between serum levels of both retinol and zinc and the incidence of cervical dysplasia. Consequently, consider supplementing with a good multivitamin that contains these nutrients.

- **Folic acid.** Low folic acid levels have been shown to be linked to cervical dysplasia. Patients on oral contraceptives may have low folic acid levels. In fact, tissue status as measured by erythrocyte folate is commonly low in patients with cervical dysplasia but may be normal or elevated in blood studies. In addition, low folic acid levels have been shown to also increase the effect of other risk factors for cervical dysplasia. For example, low RBC (red blood cell) folate levels are a major risk factor for HPV infection of the cervix. B_{12} supplementation should also be given with folate to decrease the possibility that a B_{12} deficiency would be masked by treatment with folate.

- **I-3-C/DIM.** Women with precancerous lesions of the cervix may have abnormal estrogen metabolism. Ask your healthcare provider to order an estrogen metabolism urine test. Indole-3-carbinol (I-3-C) is a phytochemical found in cruciferous vegetables which improves estrogen metabolism. Eat more cruciferous vegetables. Two controlled trials have shown I-3-C and/or DIM to be helpful in people with cervical dysplasia. Consider taking I-3-C and or DIM. Dose of I-3-C: 200 to 400 mg a day. Some nutraceutical companies make a combination of I-3-C and DIM.

● **Pyridoxine.** Pyridoxine levels were found to be low in one-third of patients with cervical cancer. Low B_6 levels effect the metabolism of estrogens and tryptophan and may also decrease the immune response. Furthermore, oral contraceptives deplete the body of B_6. Consider supplementing with a B-complex.

● **Selenium.** Individuals with cervical dysplasia may have lower levels of selenium than the general population. Have your healthcare provider measure your selenium level and supplement if needed.

● **Vitamin A and beta-carotene.** People who intake beta-carotene have a decreased risk in development of cervical dysplasia or cancer. A mild association has been shown between low dietary retinoids and the development of cervical cancer or dysplasia. Two other studies showed that lower serum vitamin A and beta-carotene levels were found in patients with cervical dysplasia than in control groups. When patients are treated with vitamin A and/or beta-carotene the response rates have varied. Likewise, supplementation with beta-carotene was found to be more advantageous than with retinoids due to beta-carotene's stronger antioxidant properties.

Moreover, topical vitamin A was used in a study of over 300 women who used either four consecutive 24-hour applications (using a collagen sponge in a cervical cap) of retinoid or placebo; then two more applications at three and six months. The study found that retinoic acid increased the complete regression rate of moderate dysplasia for 43 percent in the treatment group vs. 27 percent in the control group. Women with severe cervical dysplasia did not improve. Furthermore, vitamin A suppositories have also been used along with oral folic acid, vitamin C and carotenes, and herbal vitamin suppositories with good success. Beta-all-trans-retinoic acid as a sponge or cervical cap is also effective.

● **Vitamin C.** Individuals with cervical dysplasia tend to have decreased vitamin C intake and decreased serum vitamin C. Inadequate vitamin C intake has been found to be an independent risk factor for the development of premalignant cervical disease and CIS. Therefore, consider supplementing with vitamin C at 1,000 mg a day.

Botanical Therapies

Botanical therapies have been shown to be effective for cervical dysplasia.

● **Bromelain.** Bromelain is an important therapy in the treatment of cervical dysplasia. It decreases exudation (discharge of certain elements of the blood into tissues) by inhibiting the formation of bradykinin (a peptide that promotes inflammation) at the inflammatory site. Bromelain may also inhibit the arachidonic acid (released when inflammation is involved) pathway. Do not use if you are allergic to pineapple.

HPV

If cervical dysplasia progresses into cervical cancer, most cases are associated with HPV (human papillomavirus), which is the most common STD (sexually transmitted disease). HPV is suggested to be the cause of 99.8 percent of the 320,000 cervical cancer cases that occur throughout the world each year.

HPV is a group of more than 200 related viruses, of which more than 40 are spread through direct sexual contact. Most of them have no harmful effects on the human body. Some can cause warts, but these types are low risk. Some of the high-risk types of HPV cause cell changes that can eventually lead to cancer. Most types of HPV go away after eight to thirteen months, but other forms "hide," making it difficult to diagnose. At least 50 percent of sexually active men and women will contract some form of HPV in their lifetime. Some studies show that up to 80 percent of adults may be infected at some point in their life, with only 10 percent of those studied developing lesions on the cervix.

HPV can lead to many infections including genital warts, cancer of the cervix, anal cancer, various cancers of the vulva, vagina, oropharynx (the middle part of the throat), or head and neck. These infections can progress into diseases or become cancerous. Some people have immune systems that protect against HPV developing into a disease process.

There are a few ways you can lower your risk of developing HPV. There is a vaccine available for women that protects against either two, four, or nine types of HPV. Three vaccines that prevent infection with disease-causing

- **Canendula.** Canendula is used topically for minor inflammation and wound healing. Canendula extracts have been shown to be active against HSV (Herpes Simplex Virus), HIV, and Trichomonas. Canendula is used in other topical applications for cervical dysplasia as suppositories to be used post LEEP (procedure to remove abnormal tissue from the cervix) or biopsy to decrease inflammation and increasing granulation.

- **Goldenseal.** Goldenseal is used topically for cervical dysplasia. It has anti-inflammatory and anti-proliferative actions. It also helps to build the immune system by increasing IgM. No research has been done on Goldenseal for HPV, but it has been found to be active against other organisms such as Chlamydia, Trichomonas, and Giardia. It furthermore has antifungal effects against Candida albicans. Even though

HPV types are licensed for use in the United States: Gardasil®, Gardasil® 9, and Cervarix®. All HPV vaccines protect against at least HPV types 16 and 18 which cause the greatest risk of cervical cancer. Gardasil 9 vaccine is used in girls and women ages 9 through 45 to prevent cervical/vaginal/anal cancers or genital warts caused by certain types of HPV. Gardasil 9 vaccine is also used in boys and men ages 9 through 45 to prevent anal cancer or genital warts caused by certain types of HPV. The Centers for Disease Control and Prevention (CDC) recommends HPV vaccine for all boys and girls ages 11 or 12 years old. The vaccine is also recommended in teenage boys and girls who have not already received the vaccine or have not completed all booster shots. Discuss with your healthcare provider any possible side effects of this vaccine before receiving it.

Using a condom during sexual intercourse also lowers the risk of developing HPV. Forgoing a condom not only increases your risk of developing HPV, but it also increases your risk of developing cervical dysplasia, cervical cancer, and other STDs.

It is possible to catch HPV from examination tables, doorknobs, tanning beds, and other objects, but it is very hard to document. Having other infections, such as chlamydia, herpes simplex, and bacterial vaginosis, may also increase your risk of developing cervical dysplasia or cervical cancer.

Additionally, studies have shown that increased lycopene (a powerful antioxidant) levels in the body are associated with a resolution of HPV for some people. Lycopene isn't made in the body, but you can get it from many dietary sources, including tomatoes and tomato products, like soup, sauce, and ketchup.

Goldenseal has not been specifically studied for use in cervical dysplasia, it helps to decrease inflammation and provides a healthy flora in the vagina. Consider using goldenseal.

- **Green tea.** Components of green tea, polyphenol E and epigallocatechin-3-gallate (EGCG), have been shown to effective against HPV– infected cervical cells and lesions. In studies, the components of green tea were used orally or topically, and all treatment groups improved more than the placebo group. Dose: Green tea extract (>90 percent total polyphenol content): 150 to 300 mg/day for 3 to 12 months. Topical dose: have it compounded.

- **Licorice.** Licorice has been used both topically and orally for cervical dysplasia. It has the following actions in the body: antimicrobial, anti-inflammatory, immunomodulating, antitumorigenic (counteracting the formation of tumors), and inhibits prostaglandin (lipids released to increase inflammatory response) and leukotriene (inflammatory molecules) synthesis. The active component is glycyrrhetinic acid and it has even been shown to be active against HIV. Licorice can be used topically against herpes to reduce the healing time and pain. Do not use if you have high blood pressure.

- **Lomatium.** Lomatium has several properties. It is an antiviral, antibacterial, and antiseptic agent. It may be combined with other herbs to build the immune system. Lomatium has been shown to be effective against HPV and HSV.

- **Marshmallow.** Marshmallow is used to provide a protective, soothing coating to mucosal tissue. It may be helpful for symptoms.

- **Myrrh.** Myrrh can be used as a local anesthetic, antibacterial, and antifungal agent. Vaginal suppositories may have some benefit for cervical dysplasia.

- **Oregano and Thyme.** Oregano and thyme essential oils are used for vaginal infections including HPV. They are also used transdermally (on the skin) against bacteria and fungus. Used undiluted, they can cause irritation to cervical and vaginal tissues. Always dilute.

Stress Management

Stress plays a role in both compromising the immune system along with causing hormonal imbalance. Therefore, it is important that you have normal cortisol levels. See the chapter on cortisol.

It is paramount that individuals with cervical dysplasia be monitored traditionally. It is also important that Precision Medicine therapies be used in conjunction with conventional therapies and not used alone.

See also Cervical Cancer.

CHOLESTEROL ISSUES

See Heart Disease.

CORONARY ARTERY DISEASE

See Heart Disease.

CYSTIC ACNE

Cystic acne is the most painful type of acne. Some people have constant acne, and others experience occasional or frequent breakouts. Women who do not have acne all the time often experience breakouts seven to ten days before their monthly cycle. However, women who suffer from constant acne will notice that it gets worse the week before their cycle.

There are several hormonal imbalances that can cause cystic acne. First, elevated levels of testosterone can cause acne. Consequently, if you have PCOS (see page 299 for more information) you may have an increased risk of developing cystic acne due to elevated testosterone levels. After menopause, you may also have high testosterone levels that predispose you to breakouts. When you are stressed, increased levels of DHEA can also cause skin lesions. Stress may also cause acne through another mechanism—elevated cortisol levels. With high cortisol levels, your body produces excess oil (which clogs the pores and causes acne) and increases the amount of testosterone that you produce.

Existing acne may get worse at perimenopause when estrogen levels start to decline, resulting in testosterone levels becoming out of balance with the amount of estrogen your body is producing even though your testosterone levels may be normal. When your body makes more estrogen it balances sebum production, which lowers your risk of developing acne.

CYSTS

See Fibrocystic Breast Disease; Polycystic Ovarian Disease (PCOS).

DEPRESSION

See Postpartum Depression; Premenstrual Dysphoric Disorder (PMDD); Premenstrual Syndrome (PMS).

DES (DIETHYLSTILBESTROL) BABIES

Diethylstilbestrol (DES) is a synthetic, nonsteroidal estrogenic compound first made in the late 1930s. In the 1940s, the FDA approved it for four uses: gonorrheal vaginitis (vaginal inflammation), atrophic vaginitis (which results from lower estrogen levels after menopause, causing the vaginal tissue to become drier and thinner), menopause symptoms, and postpartum lactation suppression. Additionally, physicians formerly gave it to pregnant women to prevent miscarriages. Women were also given DES to try and treat the nausea and vomiting that can occur during pregnancy. Additionally, DES has also been used as the "morning after pill."

In the 1970s, some health risks associated with DES came into the light. Some of the effects directly affected the women who took DES. A potent endocrine disruptor, prenatal DES exposure has been linked to reproductive tract malformations, adverse pregnancy outcomes, cancer, infertility, and earlier menopause. In addition, side effects concerning the offspring of the women who took DES during pregnancy are now known.

DES DAUGHTERS

Daughters of mothers who used DES (DES daughters) have an increased risk of developing a common type of vaginal cancer called "adenocarcinoma," a cancer that originates in the glandular tissue. Recent studies have shown that DES can also cause abnormalities in the reproductive tract, immune system, and brain. Additionally, DES daughters have an increased risk of tubal pregnancy (when the fertilized egg implants somewhere other than the uterus), infertility, and premature deliveries.

■ Effects of DES on DES Daughters

- Abnormal estrogen production and receptor function

- Abnormal glucose tolerance, which increases your risk of diabetes

- Abnormal progesterone production and receptor function

- Changes in levels of estradiol

- Defects for esophagus, lip or palate, musculoskeletal and circulatory system

- Deformed fallopian tubes and ovaries

- Deformed uteruses that cannot sustain a pregnancy, including uterine defects with both doubling of uterus and bicornuate (heart-shaped uterus) and aplastic uterus (failure of uterus and vagina to develop normally)

- Diminished formation of corpora lutea (eggs)

- Elevated levels of prolactin

- Elevated rates of premature babies

- Higher rates of benign and malignant breast tumors

- Higher rates of uterine tumors, both benign and malignant

- Higher than normal infertility rates

- Immune system dysfunction (changes in the T-helper and natural killer cells)

- Increased frequency of ovarian cysts and abnormal follicles

- Increased rates of ectopic pregnancies (pregnancies when the fertilized egg is implanted outside the uterus) and miscarriages

- Increased rates of endometriosis (tissue similar to the tissue that normally lines the inside of your uterus but grows outside of your uterus)

- Increased rates of prolactinomas (noncancerous tumors of the pituitary)

- Increased risk of obesity

- Variations in concentrations of FSH (follicle-stimulating hormone)

- Variations in concentrations of inhibin B

■ Treatment for DES Daughters

While DES daughters have no control over their exposure to DES, there are some things they can do throughout life to protect their health.

- Conduct a breast self-exam at least once a month.

- Discuss DES with family and especially children. There is not a lot of research on the effects of DES on the children of DES daughters and sons (DES sons will be discussed in the next section), but it is a good idea for them to know about the risks of exposure to DES.

- Schedule regular mammograms and clinical breast examinations. Studies have shown that DES daughters over the age of forty have a greater risk of breast cancer, but younger DES daughters should get checked routinely as well.

- Schedule regular visits to the gynecologist, including Pap smears and pelvic exams. Special precautions during examinations may need to be taken with DES daughters.

- Seek infertility counseling, since many DES daughters have difficulty becoming pregnant.

- Treat all pregnancies as if they are high-risk.

DES SONS

Sons of mothers who took DES (DES sons) can be affected too. According to studies, DES sons are at a higher risk for epididymal cysts, which are sperm-filled cysts in the epididymis, the tube that lies above and behind each testicle. In her book *It's My Ovaries, Stupid,* Dr. Elizabeth Vliet describes these effects.

■ Effects of DES on DES Sons

- Abnormal development of male sexual behavior

- Abnormal glucose tolerance, which increases your risk of diabetes

- Abnormal sperm count and mobility

- Cysts in the epididymis, a part of the male reproductive system

- Defects for esophagus, lip or palate, musculoskeletal and circulatory system

- Higher rate of testicular cancer at earlier than normal ages

- Hypospadias (deformity of the penis)

- Immune system dysfunction

- Increased genital defects

- Low sperm counts

- Reduced fertility

- Stunted testicles and penises

- Undescended testicles (testicles that haven't moved into the proper position)

■ Treatment for DES Sons

There are a few steps DES sons can take to protect their health.

- Discuss DES with family and especially children. There is not a lot of research on the effects of DES on the children of DES daughters and sons, but it is a good idea for them to know about the risks of exposure to DES.

- Perform testicular self-exams monthly.

- There is now an urgent need to find ways to stop the inheritance cycle of DES and prevent adverse effects of DES in the future generations of both daughters and sons. According to a retrospective study conducted in France by Réseau DES France, published in 2016, which included 4,409 DES grandchildren (2,228 girls and 2,181 boys) and about 6,000 controls, about one-quarter of DES grandchildren are born prematurely.

DIABETES

More than 80 percent of the population in the U.S. that are adults have blood glucose levels that are too high. Ten million people in the U.S. have diabetes; another one-half million are believed to be undiagnosed. It is also well known that the incidence of diabetes is higher in postmenopausal women compared with that in premenopausal women. Furthermore, people with hypertension have a two-fold higher prevalence of diabetes and obesity, half are insulin-resistant. Likewise, patients who are obese are twice as likely to have hypertension, hypertriglyceridemia (high triglycerides), or type II diabetes.

■ Disorders Associated With Diabetes

If an individual has diabetes, they have an increased risk in developing the following diseases.

- **Cancer** (particularly breast cancer). Up to 16 percent of patients with breast cancer have diabetes, and two major risk factors for type 2 diabetes—old age and obesity—are also associated with breast cancer. Three mechanisms have been postulated to associate diabetes with breast cancer: activation of the insulin pathway, activation of the insulin-like-growth-factor pathway, and regulation of endogenous sex hormones. Comparative cohort studies and case-control studies suggest that type 2 diabetes may be associated with 10 to 20 percent excess relative risk of breast cancer. In addition, obesity and diabetes are associated with multiple factors that contribute to the increased risk of different cancers, including breast cancer. These factors include hyperinsulinemia, elevated IGFs (insulin-like growth factor), hyperglycemia, dyslipidemia, adipokines (cell signaling proteins secreted by adipose tissue), inflammatory cytokines, and dysfunctional gut microbiome.

- **Cardiovascular disease and stroke.** Having a fasting blood sugar (FBS) high-normal (over 85 mg/dL) the risk of a person dying of cardiovascular disease is increased by 40 percent. Furthermore, having a FBS high normal (over 85 mg/dL) increases your risk of vascular death. People with high after-meal glucose (101 mg/dL) compared to 83 mg/dL) had a 27 percent increased risk of death from stroke in a medical study.

- **Cognitive decline.** Diabetes is associated with an increased risk of developing Alzheimer's disease of 50 percent to 100 percent. A study showed that glucose (blood sugar) at the high end of normal results in significant brain shrinkage. The shrinkage occurs in the hippocampus and amygdala. A study also showed that significant brain shrinkage among participants whose blood sugar levels were high but below 110 mg/dL. In fact, high normal levels of FBS may account for a six percent to 10 percent decrease in the volume of the hippocampus and amygdala.

- **Hypertension.** High levels of insulin correlate with low sodium in the urine. This leads to an increase in water retention which makes it harder for blood to flow through the circulatory system which then leads to an increase in blood pressure. Insulin also elevated blood pressure by affecting the elasticity of arterial walls. Insulin alters the mechanical action of the blood vessel walls by acting on smooth muscle cells, stimulating them and making them larger. As smooth muscle cells grow, they make the arterial walls thicker, stiffer, and less supple. This forces the heart to work harder and exert more pressure to force the blood through the narrowed vessels.

Causes of Diabetes

The following are some of the common causes of diabetes.

- Abuse of alcohol
- Decreased estrogen in females
- Eating processed foods
- Elevated DHEA levels
- Excessive caffeine intake
- Excessive dieting
- Excessive progesterone in females (prescribed)
- Genetic susceptibility (inherited a gene)
- Hypothyroidism
- Increased stress
- Increased testosterone in females
- Insomnia
- Lack of exercise
- Nicotine
- Oral contraceptives

Therapies for Diabetes

Conventional Therapies

Conventional therapies for diabetes are centered around exercise and a healthy eating program. If you are overweight, then weight reduction is very beneficial. If these methods are not successful, then medication may be added, which include one of the following class of drugs:

- Alpha-glucosidase inhibitors
- Biguanides
- Dopamine agonists
- DPP-4 inhibitors
- Glucagon-like peptides
- Meglitinides
- Sodium glucose transporter (SGLT)2 inhibitors
- Sulfonylureas
- Thiazolidinediones

Precision Medicine Therapies

The following are Precision Medicine therapies for diabetes:

Exercise. Lack of exercise is a risk factor for the development of insulin resistance and diabetes in susceptible individuals. Try and exercise four hours a week. If you have not been exercising and you are over the age of 42, see your healthcare provider for a stress test before you begin an exercise program.

Healthy Eating Program. Eat a low glycemic index (GI) diet. The GI ranks carbohydrate-containing foods on a scale from 0 to 100 according to the speed with which they enter the bloodstream and raise glucose levels. Foods high on the list increase blood sugar and cause insulin to be elevated which increases the risk of developing diabetes. The glycemic index is affected by the size of the particles into which the food breaks down into. Therefore, the more processed the food or the longer it is cooked, the higher the glycemic index. Whole versus refined grains have been shown to decrease the incidence of diabetes.

The fat content of a food influences its glycemic index. The fat slows down the absorption and therefore lowers its glycemic index. The right balance of saturated to polyunsaturated to monounsaturated fats is important both for the prevention and treatment of diabetes.

A high fiber (soluble fiber) eating problem helps to control blood sugar. Low fiber intake has been shown to be a risk factor in several studies for the development of diabetes.

Get enough protein in your diet. The protein content of the food also decreases the absorption of sugars and consequently decreases its glycemic load.

Weight loss has been proven to be very beneficial to prevent and control blood sugar.

Good sleep hygiene is very important. If you do not sleep at least six and one-half hours a night and/or do not get restorative sleep, then insulin levels may rise and lead to diabetes.

Nutritional Supplements. Most nutritional supplements can be used with oral hypoglycemic agents (medications that lower blood sugar) provided you have normal liver and kidney function. Check with your compounding pharmacist or healthcare provider if you are unsure of a possible drug-nutrient interaction before using.

- **Alpha lipoic acid (ALA).** Alpha lipoic acid is both fat and water soluble and is a broad-spectrum antioxidant. It also functions as a co-enzyme in carbohydrate metabolism. In addition, it slows the development of diabetic neuropathy and can be an effective therapy for diabetic neuropathy in conjunction with lowering blood sugar and other nutrients. Dose: 300 to 400 mg a day.

- **Biotin.** This important B vitamin is not just for hair and nails. Biotin deficiency results in impaired use of glucose by the body. Biotin is made in your GI tract. Therefore, the best way to have an optimal level is to have optimal gut function. Supplementation may also be helpful. Dose: 1 to 2 mg daily.

- **Chromium.** Chromium is needed for carbohydrate and lipid metabolism. Elevated glucose, insulin, cholesterol, and triglycerides as well as decreased HDL can be improved with chromium. Dose: 600 micrograms to 1,200 micrograms a day with normal kidney function.

- **Conjugated Linoleic Acid (CLA) is the only naturally occurring transfat.** It can improve FBS. Dose: 1,000 mg a day.

- **L-arginine helps insulin work better in the body.** Hence it improves FBS. If you have a heart valve problem, only take under the direction of your doctor. Dose: 1,000 mg a day with normal kidney function.

- **L-carnitine is an antioxidant that influences free fatty acids in glucose oxidation.** It also improves diabetic neuropathy. Dose: 1,000 to 2,000 mg a day with normal kidney function. Have your doctor measure your TMAO level before taking. If it is elevated, you cannot supplement with L-carnitine.

- **L-carnosine is a nutrient that is a combination of two amino acids, beta-alanine and histidine.** It is also an antioxidant and aids the body in preventing glycation, which is more common in diabetes. Carnosine is found in the brain, skeletal muscles, heart, and the lens of the eye. Dose: 1,000 mg a day with normal kidney function.

- **L-taurine is an amino acid.** It requires zinc to help function properly. Taurine has a positive effect on controlling glucose in diabetics. Stress depletes the body of taurine! Dose: 1,000 to 2,000 mg a day with normal renal function.

- **Magnesium.** It functions as an essential cofactor in glucose oxidation, and it also modulates glucose transport across cell membranes. Magnesium deficiency is associated with diabetes. Dose 400 to 600 mg a day of magnesium glycinate or threonate.

- **Omega-3-fatty acids have a positive effect on blood sugar.** Dose: 2,000 mg a day.

- **Vanadium improves insulin sensitivity.** Dose: 10 to 50 micrograms. Do not use doses higher than 50 micrograms since higher doses may exacerbate a bipolar disorder.

- **Vitamin D.** Low levels are associated with diabetes. Studies have shown that supplementing with vitamin D improves insulin sensitivity and blood sugar. Have your healthcare provider measure your vitamin D level.

- **Vitamin E.** If your vitamin E level is low, you are more likely to develop type 2 diabetes. Vitamin E improves glucose tolerance. Dose: 200 to 400 IU a day.

Botanical Supplements. Most botanical supplements can be used with oral hypoglycemic agents (medications) provided you have normal renal and hepatic function. Check with your compounding pharmacists or healthcare provider if you are unsure of a possible drug botanical interaction before using.

- **Aloe vera** in a single-blind, placebo-controlled trial of diabetics over 2 weeks showed improved blood sugar control.

- **Berberine** (*Berberis vulgaris*) has been shown to lower blood sugar. Dose: 200 to 500 mg two to three times a day. It may cause uterine contractions. Therefore, do not use if you are pregnant. Furthermore, it can cause GI upset in some people.

- **Bitter Melon** (*Momordica charantia*) is a tropical fruit widely used in Asia, Africa, and South America. It is also called bitter gourd. The exact mechanism of action is unknown. It has been shown in a medical study to work as well as some medications.

- **Cinnamon, cloves, and bay leaves** have insulin-like or insulin-potentiating action. Possible side effects of all of these include the following: GI upset, stomatitis (inflammation of the mouth and lips), and perioral dermatitis (rash around the mouth).

- **Fenugreek** (*Trigonella foenum graecum*) seeds have a hypoglycemic effect due to its high content of soluble fiber which decreases the rate of gastric emptying and delays the absorption of glucose from the small intestine. There may be a cross-reaction if you are allergic to chickpeas. The possible side effects of this herb include diarrhea, flatulence, and dizziness. Furthermore, fenugreek preparations can contain coumarin derivatives, which may affect clotting. Minerals and medications should be taken separately from fenugreek-containing products since the fiber in the fenugreek may change the absorption rate. If you are taking thyroid medication, fenugreek may interfere with this drug. Consequently, have your healthcare provider measure thyroid levels on a regular basis.

- **Ginseng** species contains triterpenoid glycosides that lower blood sugar by regulating hepatic (liver) glucose uptake, glycogen synthesis, and insulin release. Ginseng (Panax quinquefolius—American ginseng) has been shown to reduce blood sugar levels after eating in both type 2 diabetics and non-diabetics. It has been reported to decrease fasting blood sugar and HgBA1C. Dose: Panax ginseng: 100 to 400 mg of extract standardized to 4 percent ginsenosides.

- **Green coffee bean extract** has been shown to lower blood sugar as well as lower after-meal glucose surges.

- **Green tea** contains epigallocatechin gallate (EGCG) which enhances insulin's activity. It has been also shown to be a possible therapeutic agent for the prevention of diabetes mellitus progression.

- **Gymnema sylvestre** is an herb endemic to India. The common name is gurmar which means "sugar-destroying". It has been shown in clinical trials to lower blood sugar.

- **Ivy Gourd** (*Coccinia indica*) is an herb in the cucumber family. It helps insulin by its effects on several pathways in the body. Two studies have shown that ivy gourd had significant glucose-lowering effects. Dose: dried leaves or extracts at doses equivalent to 15 grams a day with meals. There are no known side effects of ivy gourd.

- **Nopal** (Optunia streptacantha) is also called prickly pear cactus. It is high in fiber and pectin. Studies have shown its hypoglycemic effect.

- **Olive leaf extract** contains oleuropein which has been shown to lower blood sugar. It slows the digestion of starches into simple sugars and slows the absorption of simple sugars from the intestines. Furthermore, it increases the uptake of glucose into tissue from the blood and lowers fasting insulin levels. Dose: 500 mg once or twice a day.

- **Pycnogenol** (*Pinus maritima*) is a standardized extract of French maritime pine bark. A study was conducted on type II diabetics that were given 125 mg of Pycnogenol a day versus a placebo. The people in the treatment group had lower HgA1C, lower blood pressure, and lower LD than before the study began.

Hormones. Many hormones influence blood sugar in women.

- Cortisol levels that are too low or elevated can have a negative impact on blood sugar.

- DHEA has been shown to improve insulin sensitivity and consequently the potential to decrease the risk of a person developing diabetes.

- Estrogen replacement has been shown in several studies to have a positive effect on regulating blood sugar in women.

- Testosterone levels, if they are elevated, are commonly associated with PCOS, which is usually a state of insulin dysregulation that if left untreated, frequently leads to diabetes. Low levels of testosterone in women are associated with an increased risk of developing diabetes.

- Thyroid hormone level is key to glucose regulation. Both hyper- and hypothyroidism have been associated with insulin resistance which has been reported to be the major cause of impaired glucose metabolism in type 2 diabetes. Moreover, type 2 diabetes reduces thyroid-stimulating hormone (TSH) levels and impairs the conversion of T4 to T3 in peripheral tissues.

As you have seen, there are many treatments both conventional and Precision Medicine therapies that have been usefully in helping to regulate blood sugar. Often, a combination of modalities is the most effective.

See also Heart Disease; Polycystic Ovarian Syndrome (PCOS).

DYSMENORRHEA (MENSTRUAL CRAMPS)

Menstrual cramps are dull or throbbing pains throughout the lower abdomen. They affect almost 50 percent of menstruating women just before and during their periods, making them one of the most common symptoms of PMS. The medical term for menstrual cramps is "dysmenorrhea." The pain tends to be intermittent, strongest in the lower part of the abdomen. But it can also radiate to the back and inner thighs. Symptoms may go away after two or three hours, but they can last up to three days.

The severity of symptoms also varies between women. For some, the pain is merely an annoyance, and for others, it can get in the way of daily activities. Worldwide, 45 percent to 95 percent of teens and women have dysmenorrhea and 7 percent to 15 percent of teens and women have dysmenorrhea that interferes with daily activities. Other symptoms of dysmenorrhea include the following: backache, headache, nausea, vomiting, dizziness, or loose stools.

Causes of Dysmenorrhea

Dysmenorrhea can be primary or secondary. Primary dysmenorrhea is pain in the absence of organic pathology. It appears to result from a surge in the level of (PGF2alpha) prostaglandin F2alpha (stimulates the contraction of uterine muscle) around the time of menstruation. This can lead to vasoconstriction (constriction of blood vessels), uterine ischemia, and painful uterine contractions. Women with the disease can produce as much as seven times more PGF2alpha than those who do not have this disease process.

The greatest release of prostaglandin occurs in the first two days of the cycle, which is the time that the symptoms are the most painful. High prostaglandin E2-levels may be associated with lower progesterone levels that occur in your body just before your cycle begins. Painful menstrual cycles occur only in cycles when you have ovulated, because if you have not ovulated during this time, no increase in progesterone occurs in the second part of the cycle.

Secondary dysmenorrhea is associated with underlying pathology such as: endometriosis, infection, or ovarian cysts.

Therapies for Dysmenorrhea

Conventional Treatments

Conventional treatments include the following:

- Prostaglandin synthetase inhibitors such as non-steroidal anti-inflammatory medications. They decrease the synthesis of prostaglandin which reduces uterine hypercontractility, pressure, ischemia, and pain. Other symptoms may also improve with the use of prostaglandin synthetase inhibitors.

- Oral contraceptives. They decrease the production of prostaglandins.

- Pain medications

Precision Medicine Therapies

Precision Medicine therapies include the following:

- Dietary Factors
- Nutritional therapies
- Botanical therapies
- Other therapies

■ Dietary Factors

- It is important to eat breakfast. A study showed that participants that ate breakfast every day had less severe dysmenorrhea than those that ate breakfast less often.

- Food allergies may contribute to dysmenorrhea by causing histamine to be released, which increases inflammation and may cause muscle spasm. Food allergy testing should be considered in individuals with dysmenorrhea, and if you have food allergies, avoid foods you are allergic to. Make sure you see a Precision Medicine practitioner to have your allergy testing done so that both food allergies (IgE) and food sensitivities (IgG) are measured.

- Aspartame intake has been linked to dysmenorrhea in anecdotal cases. Discontinue aspartame if you are using this sweetener.

- Eat a diet high in vegetables which have been shown to help with menstrual pain.

- A study showed that avoiding gluten may be beneficial for dysmenorrhea. Try a gluten-free eating program for 90 days to see if it is of benefit.

■ Nutritional Therapies

- **Calcium.** Two double-blind medical studies have shown that calcium supplementation reduced cyclic uterine pain. Dose: 1,000 to 1,200 mg a day in divided doses.

- **Flavonoids.** In a trial that was not controlled, the patients were given a specific flavonoid preparation (Daflon 1,000 mg daily) that had menorrhagia for 3 menstrual cycles. The Daflon was started 5 days before expected onset of menses and continued until the bleeding stopped. Many of the participants had significant improvement in their symptoms probably due to the inhibition of prostaglandin synthesis by Daflon.

- **Iron.** Iron supplementation in patients that suffer from iron deficiency anemia may be helpful in treating the symptoms of dysmenorrhea.

- **Magnesium.** Magnesium supplementation has been shown to be effective for dysmenorrhea. Magnesium is a cofactor in delta-6 desaturase which is involved in anti-inflammatory prostaglandins (PGE1), and it also has a relaxing effect on the skeletal and smooth muscles. In one of the trials, magnesium was used with vitamin B_6 since B_6 enhances cellular uptake of magnesium. Magnesium was given continuously in some studies and around the menstrual cycle in other studies. Continuous use would provide a more stable magnesium level. Dose: 300 to 600 mg a day of magnesium glycinate to bowel tolerance. Magnesium use is contraindicated in heart block and severe kidney disease.

- **Niacin.** In an uncontrolled study, niacin (100 to 200 mg twice a day and increased every 2 to 3 hours during cramps) was given to women with dysmenorrhea. Niacin was beneficial for most of the patients. Use the niacin 7 to 10 days before the onset of your menstrual cycle and continue for 4 to 5 days after the cycle begins. Taking vitamin C (300 mg) and rutin (60 mg) may help the efficacy of the niacin. You may experience a niacin flush. If this occurs, then take an aspirin 30 to 60 minutes before taking niacin.

- **Omega-3-fatty acids.** Omega-3-fatty acids inhibit the synthesis of inflammatory prostaglandins that play a role in the development of dysmenorrhea. A medical trial showed an inverse relationship between the intake of omega-3-fatty acids and severity of menstrual pain.

Studies have also shown omega-3-fatty acid supplementation was a very effective therapy for dysmenorrhea. Dose: 2,000 mg to 6,000 mg a day. In doses above 3,000 mg a day, omega-3-fatty acids have blood thinning qualities. Therefore, do not use high dose omega-3-fatty acids if you are taking a blood thinner.

- **Thiamine.** In a double-blind study, patients were given 100 mg a day of thiamine for 3 months. Most of the people were symptom free by the end of the trial. The mechanism of action is unknown, but it may be due to thiamine possibly improving inflammation of pelvic sympathetic nerves. When taking any B vitamin, it is important that you take all B vitamins. B vitamins are water soluble and should be taken twice a day.

- **Vitamin D.** Vitamin D was shown to be helpful in two medical trials in women with dysmenorrhea. Have your healthcare provider measure your vitamin D level and take the dose according to your lab results.

- **Vitamin E.** Vitamin E is an inhibitor of prostaglandin synthesis and can also increase endorphin levels which may decrease pain levels. Studies have shown that vitamin E decreased the severity of the dysmenorrhea in many of the participants. Dose: 150 to 500 IU starting ten days before the menstrual cycle begins and continuing through day four of bleeding. Vitamin E is a blood thinner, therefore use with caution if you are on a medication or nutrient that thins the blood.

- **Zinc.** One double-blind study revealed that zinc supplementation may be an effective therapy for dysmenorrhea. Suggested dose and the length of therapy were not discussed in the article. With long-term use of zinc, take copper in a ratio: 10 to 15 mg zinc to 1 mg copper.

■ Botanical Therapies

- **Black cohosh.** Black cohosh (Actaea racemosa) is a spasmolytic and anti-inflammatory to the smooth and skeletal muscles. The salicylates and gallic acid in black cohosh are analgesic and anti-inflammatory, which may reduce prostaglandin excess if it is given before menses (when your cycle starts). Black cohosh contains ferulic and isoferulic acids which inhibit leukotriene production. Black cohosh is approved by German Commission E for the treatment of dysmenorrhea and premenstrual complaints. Dose: 20 to 40 mg twice a day of standardized extract. Black cohosh may interact with medications processed by the liver, including but not limited to acetaminophen, atorvastatin, carbamazepine, isoniazid, and methotrexate.

- **Blue cohosh.** Blue cohosh is used when there is dysmenorrhea that is due to uterine atony in which the uterus fails to contract after birth. It promotes uterine contractions and relieves spasticity when used with uterine spasmolytics (muscle relaxant). It is an emmenagogue (herbs which stimulate blood flow in the area) and utero-tonic. It is not used as frequently as other herbal therapies since it may increase blood pressure.

- **Chamomile.** Chamomile is an antispasmodic and anti-inflammatory due to the flavonoids that it contains, and it also has sedative qualities. Chamomile works very well for dysmenorrhea with diarrhea, bloating, and gas, as well as irritability and anxiety. Research recommends chamomile tea be sipped hot for a rapid decrease in menstrual cramps.

- **Corydalis.** Corydalis is an effective analgesic. The analgesic effect is 1 percent to 10 percent that of opium. It may be useful for acute spasms and for associated headache and musculoskeletal discomfort.

- **Cramp bark.** Cramp bark (Viburnum opulus) is taken as a tea. It is used with caution in patients who take diuretics or lithium. It acts as a uterine antispasmodic and tonic and is used for pain, dysmenorrhea, and amenorrhea—absence of menstruation. The mechanism of action is unknown. Clinical trials need to be done.

- **Dong quai.** Dong quai has been used for dysmenorrhea since the 16th century. It relaxes smooth muscle due to its volatile oil-containing fraction, and the aqueous extract contains ferulic acid and acts as both a muscle relaxant and stimulant. Dong quai likewise has an analgesic and anti-inflammatory effect. It also contains nicotinic acid which has blood vessel relaxing and/or vasodilating action. Regular use may make the menstrual flow heavier. Some herbalists suggest stopping Dong quai during the cycle in patients that tend to have heavy cycles. It is usually used in conjunction with other herbs.

- **Fennel.** Fennel essential oil (FEO) has an antispasmodic effect and therefore helps with the symptoms of dysmenorrhea. Studies have confirmed its efficacy.

- **Ginger.** Ginger root (Zingiber officinale) is used both internally and transdermally (on the skin) as a warming circulatory stimulant and anti-inflammatory agent in the treatment of dysmenorrhea. The anti-inflammatory effects are on the prostaglandin synthesis pathway. Also, ginger is a thromboxane synthetase inhibitor (antiplatelet drug) and a prostacyclin agonist (inhibits platelet activation), so it has analgesic effects in dysmenorrhea and also helps with nausea. Dose: 250 mg four times a day starting two days before the cycle begins and continuing for three days after the cycle begins. Two medical trials have shown ginger to be helpful, including one that revealed it to be as effective as a NSAID for relieving pain.

- **Jamaican dogwood.** Jamaican dogwood is a strong uterine antispasmodic and analgesic for the treatment of acute and severe dysmenorrhea. Recommended doses should not be exceeded. Possible side effects include nausea, vomiting, and headache.

- **Licorice.** Licorice inhibits prostaglandins. Studies have shown that the traditional Chinese Medicine formula shakuyaku-kanzo-to which is one-half licorice and one-half peony inhibits prostaglandins and improves dysmenorrhea. Do not take if you have high blood pressure. If you develop hypertension while taking it then discontinue using it.

- **Motherwort.** Motherwort has uterine spasmolytic and sedative effects. It also is a uterine tonic and improves atony due to pelvic floor congestion. It also improves circulation and relieves vascular congestion. Likewise, motherwort may reduce pain due to a decrease in endogenous inflammatory mediators and an increase in the synthesis of prostaglandins. It furthermore contains substances which inhibit platelet aggregation. Moreover, it is a hypotensive nervine that helps headaches, insomnia, and vertigo. Motherwort works for pelvic pain with concomitant heart palpitations, anxiety attacks, and stress in patients with dysmenorrhea. Motherwort contains the following:

  - Flavonol and iridoid glycosides
  - Lectins
  - Leonurin
  - Leonurine, an alkaloid which restores uteine tone
  - Phytosterols
  - Tannins
  - Vitamin C
  - Volatile oils

- **Peony.** Peony is used to treat dysmenorrhea and muscle cramping. It is employed commonly with licorice root and has been shown to lower testosterone in women with PCOS. It also has been shown to reduce the size of fibroids in a trial of 100 women using P. suffructicosa, Poria cocos, Cinnamomum cassia, and Prunus persica.

- **Pulsatilla.** Pulsatilla is helpful for painful or inflammatory reproductive conditions including dysmenorrhea. Pulsatilla's sedative action works for nervous tension that may be associated with dysmenorrhea and it also helps with uterine pain. It should not be used during pregnancy. Pulsatilla should also not be used in high doses.

- **Yarrow.** Yarrow contains sesquiterpene lactones which have antiphlogistic activity (acting against inflammation or fever) and flavonoids which have spasmolytic action—relieves spasms. Research has shown that yarrow has antispasmodic and anti-inflammatory action that is therapeutic for dysmenorrhea.

■ Other Therapies

Yoga, exercise, and massage have been found to be helpful for the pain of dysmenorrhea.

Acupuncture and acupressure both have been found to be beneficial, according to clinical trials, for individuals with dysmenorrhea.

See also Endometriosis; Premenstrual Syndrome (PMS).

DYSPAREUNIA

See Endometriosis.

ELEVATED C-REACTIVE PROTEIN (CRP)

See Heart Disease.

ENDOMETRIOSIS

In endometriosis, the cells that form the endometrium—mucous membrane lining the uterus—grow outside of the uterus, usually in the abdomen, pelvis fallopian tubes, or ovaries. However, the endometrial tissue can grow anywhere including the eyes and can also migrate to the spinal cord and cause severe lower back pain.

The areas of tissue growing outside of the uterus are called implants. The tissue thickens, breaks down, and bleeds every month. The implants produce their own estrogen by aromatization—conversion of testosterone to estrogen. Consequently, even if you are prescribed medications to lower estrogen, the implants still produce their own estrogen and cause the surrounding areas to grow. Implants can also go into the muscle wall of the uterus which is called adenomyosis. This can cause bleeding into the uterine muscle during the menstrual cycle and cause pain. Endometriosis affects 1 percent to 15 percent of women that are menstruating between the ages of 24 and 40. In addition, endometriosis is linked to 25 percent of the cases of infertility.

The pain and the symptoms the patient experiences with endometriosis may not correlate with the extent of the disease. The amount of pain seems to be related to the depth of the lesions and not the number of lesions. Signs and symptoms include excessive bleeding during or between cycles, infertility, dyspareunia (pain that occurs when engaging in sexual intercourse), dysmenorrhea (painful menstrual cycles), and pelvic pain. Less common symptoms of endometriosis include the following:

- Back pain that radiates down the legs
- Blood in the bowels, nose, or eyes
- Diarrhea
- Fainting
- Fatigue
- Pain during urination
- Painful bowel movements
- Vomiting

Therapies for Endometriosis

Conventional Therapies

The following are conventional treatment for endometriosis.

- Danazol
- Gonadotropin-releasing hormone agonists
- Oral contraceptives
- Progestins
- Surgical removal of affected tissue

Risk Factors for Endometriosis

The cause has yet to be determined of endometriosis. The following are risk factors for this disease process:

- D&C history

- Diet low in fruit

- Diet low in green vegetables

- Environmental toxins may also play a role. The patient may have a genetic predisposition (SNP) which increases their risk of developing the disease when exposed to any of the following toxins: bisphenol-A, parabens, phthalates, pesticides, dioxins, PCBs, and formaldehyde.

- Estrogen dominance

- Genetic influences are likely involved in the etiology of endometriosis. Endometriosis occurs more commonly in family groups including twin studies. Furthermore, abnormalities in detoxification enzymes, tumor suppressor genes, and other genetic actors may be involved in the development and also the progression of endometriosis.

- High fat diet

- High intake of red meat

- History of abuse

- History of repeated uterine and vaginal infections

- Immune dysfunction can occur in severe ways to promote endometriosis. There may be a lack of good immune surveillance in the pelvic area. Patients with endometriosis have suppressed natural killer (NK) cell activity in their peritoneal fluid. High levels of IgG and IgM are also seen in patients with endometriosis. They also have high levels of autoantibodies against ovary and endometrial cells, which occur in this disease process. Both types of immunity, cell-mediated and humoral, have been implicated in endometriosis with immunologic defects present in all forms of the disease. In addition, macrophages are found in greater numbers in the early stages of endometriosis. Cytokines, macrophages, T lymphocytes, and TNF are increased in the peritoneal fluid and their increase is related to the severity of the disease. Growth factors, angiogenic factors, and lipid peroxidation—oxidative degradation of lipids—in the peritoneal fluid may also stimulate endometrial cell growth.

- Intense stress

- Lack of exercise from an early age

- Menstrual cycles that occur more frequently than every 28 days, with menstrual bleeding lasting more than seven days

- Naturally red hair

- Use of intrauterine devices

Other possible risk factors for the development of endometriosis:

- Exposure to environmental estrogens or estrogen disruptors (weed killers, plastics, detergents, household cleaners, and tin can liners)

- Liver dysfunction

- Poor estrogen metabolism

- Prenatal exposure to high levels of estrogen

None of the above treatments is preferred over the other. All can have significant side effects. Likewise, all are associated with a high recurrence rate (20 percent to 50 percent) when the treatment is discontinued except for total abdominal hysterectomy with bilateral salpingo-oophorectomy (ovaries also taken out).

Precision Medicine Therapies

The following are Precision Medicine therapies for endometriosis.

Dietary factors. These are very important if you have endometriosis. Decreasing your caffeine intake has been shown to be beneficial. A study revealed that women that drank more than 5 to 7 grams a month of caffeine had a higher risk of developing endometriosis; consequently, consider lowering your caffeine intake.

Try and decrease your intake of trans-fats. One study showed that women that ate the most trans-fats were almost 50 percent more likely to develop endometriosis than women that did not intake a lot of trans-fats. Other researchers have suggested that avoiding gluten, dairy, refined sugar, and alcohol may also be helpful for patients with endometriosis. Therefore, try and avoid these foods and drinks.

Increase consumption of foods that contain sulfur, such as onions, garlic, and leeks, which elevate the body's ability to detoxify and also builds the immune system. These foods also contain quercetin which stimulates the immune system, blocks the inflammatory response, protects against oxidation, and helps inhibit tumor growth.

Furthermore, increase vegetable intake that contain indole-3-carbinol so that the body will break down estrogen into more desirous forms, such as: broccoli, Brussels sprouts, cauliflower, cabbage, and kale. As much as possible, consume foods and drinks that are organic.

Furthermore, increase foods that are high in fiber in your diet. Decrease your intake of red meat. Eat foods that cleanse the liver: carrots, lemons, artichokes, beets, watercress, and dandelion greens.

Nutrients. There are also nutrients that have been shown to be beneficial for individuals with endometriosis. They have the following functions in the body:

- **B vitamins.** B vitamins may help detoxify estrogen in the body by improving methylation. Take a B complex vitamin twice a day.

- **Beta-carotene.** Beta-carotene can moderately affect IL-6 which is implicated in endometriosis. Beta-carotene, in addition, helps enhance immunity and promotes phagocytosis (process where immune cells ingest and destroy microbes and cellular debris). A large dose is required. Therefore, beta-carotene is not the best option for treatment.

- **Essential fatty acids.** Essential fatty acids play a major role in decreasing inflammation.
  - Omega-3-fatty acids. Dose: 1,000 mg a day.
  - Gamma-linoleic acids. Dose: 1,000 mg daily of one of the following: borage oil or evening primrose oil.
  - Alpha-linolenic acid. It is found in foods such as flaxseed, pumpkin, or walnuts.

- **Lipotropic factors.** Lipotropic factors aid in enhancing liver function and detoxification. They also promote the flow of fat and bile containing estrogen metabolites from the liver to the colon. Lipotropic factors include choline, methionine, and cysteine. Before supplementing with choline, have your doctor measure TMAO (trimethylamine N-oxide) levels in your body. This is a blood study. If you have high TMAO you cannot take choline as a nutrient.

- **Selenium.** Selenium aids in the synthesis of antioxidant enzymes that are responsible for detoxification of the liver, stimulates WBCs, and stimulates thymic function. If you have a low selenium level, you may have sub-optimal cell-mediated immunity and decreased T cells. Low selenium levels increase inflammation in the body. Dose: 200 to 400 micrograms a day. You can become toxic when using selenium, therefore have your healthcare provider measure levels in the body before supplementing.

- **Vitamin C** is helpful to decrease autoimmune progression, fatigue, capillary fragility, and decrease tumor growth. It also enhances general immunity and increases cellular immunity. Dose: 6 to 10 grams a day to bowel tolerance.

- **Vitamin E.** Vitamin E helps to inhibit the arachidonic acid pathway which aids in the prevention of the release of chemicals that can cause edema (swelling), inflammation, and contraction of the smooth muscle. Moreover, free radical production may contribute to the inflammation and excessive growth of the tissue of the endometrium. Vitamin E is an excellent free radical scavenger and when used with n-acetyl cysteine (NAC) has been shown to decrease tissue replication. Long-term use of NAC depletes the body of zinc and copper. Therefore, make sure you also take a multivitamin. Long-term use of NAC also can increase the risk of developing cysteine kidney stones. If you are predisposed to this condition, then take 1,000 mg a day of vitamin C. Dose 400 to 800 IU a day of natural vitamin E. Vitamin E is a blood thinner, therefore use with caution if you are taking a medication that is a blood thinner.

Botanicals

- **Blue Vervain.** Blue vervain stimulates LH and FSH (stimulates follicular growth and ovulation) and is immunomodulatory by inhibiting phagocytosis by granulocytes—a type of white blood cell. It is used for endometriosis, irregular cycles, nervous conditions, exhaustion, and sluggish liver.

- **Cotton Root.** Cotton root has short-term efficacy of up to 90 percent in treating endometriosis. Long-term effectiveness of treating endometriosis after 1 and 3 years is 54 percent to 63 percent. Individuals that are treated with cotton root generally have amenorrhea (no menstrual cycle) for up to 6 months in 80 percent of women. Gossypol is the active component in the roots and seeds of cotton, and it antagonizes the actions of estrogen and progesterone. Cotton root may mimic pseudo-menopause. It is not available in Western countries. You may need to take a potassium supplement if you are taking cotton root since it may cause low potassium levels. High dosages may cause any of the following symptoms:

- Edema
- Elevated liver enzymes
- Fatigue
- Nausea
- Possible decrease in mitochondrial energy metabolism

- Palpitations
- Possible inhibition of thyroid function
- Rash
- Reduced appetite

- **Dandelion root (*Taraxacum officinale*).** Dandelion root helps to detoxify the liver and gall bladder. It contains vitamins A, C, and K and also contains calcium and choline.

- **Dong quai.** Dong quai may be helpful for individuals with endometriosis since it is an antispasmodic, analgesic, anti-inflammatory, and has tonic effects. It also functions as an antioxidant and free radical scavenger. Likewise, Dong quai has immunomodulatory effects since it stimulates phagocytic activity (ability to engulf and destroy). It increases the production of IL-2. IL-2, which promotes the growth and invasion of endometriotic stromal cells that cause endometriosis.

- **Chaste tree (*Vitex agnus castus*).** Chaste tree increases progesterone by increasing LH and makes estrogen less available to stimulate the tissues of the endometrium.

- **Echinacea.** Echinacea is an herbal therapy that enhances phagocytosis and stimulates cytokine production. It increases immunoglobulin production and is anti-inflammatory. Echinacea is furthermore an antioxidant and free radical scavenger. Echinacea should not be used on a daily basis.

- **Motherwort.** Motherwort (*Leonorus cardiac*) decreases spasms and helps with the pain that occurs with endometriosis. It also soothes nerves.

- **Pine bark (Pycnogenol).** Pycnogenol is the trademarked name for a mixture of forty different antioxidants from the bark of the maritime pine tree (Pinus maritime). It is an oligomeric proanthocyanidin (OPC). It inhibits inflammatory cells. A randomized medical trial of women with endometriosis were given pycnogenol 30 mg versus leuprorelin acetate IM every 4 to 6 weeks for 24 weeks. The pycnogenol group had a 1/3 reduction in symptoms but maintained cycles and normal estrogen levels during therapy. The leuprorelin group had a greater response during treatment but relapsed after the medication was stopped. They also had low estrogen levels during treatment. Dose of pycnogenol was 60 to 150 mg a day.

- **Prickly ash (*Xanthoxylum americanum*).** Prickly ash stimulates blood flow and increases transport of oxygen and nutrients. It removes waste products and helps with circulation of the pelvis.

- **Turska's formula.** Turska's formula may interfere with the placement of the endometrial implants—tissue growing outside of the uterus—and it also enhances the immune system. Turska's formula contains the following:

  - Aconite napelus (Monkshood)
  - Bryonia alba (Bryony)
  - Gelsemium sempervirens (Yellow jasmine)
  - Phytolacca americana (Poke root)

Yeast Infections *(Candidiasis).* Anecdotally some patients have done better with symptoms of endometriosis on a diet that decreases yeast-containing foods and treatment with an antifungal medication. Have your doctor order a GI health test and treat yeast if present.

Hormones

- **Melatonin.** Melatonin has many functions in the body including but not limited to being an antioxidant, analgesic, and anti-inflammatory agent. A double-blind, randomized, placebo-controlled study gave women with endometriosis 10 mg of melatonin at bedtime for two months. Melatonin improved pain, dysmenorrhea, dyspareunia, dysuria, and pain during defecation in a statistically significant number of people. Have your healthcare provider measure melatonin levels by saliva testing.

- **Progesterone.** Progesterone modifies the action of estradiol, which decreases the amount of time estrogen stays on the receptor sites and decreases the number of uterine contractions which can cause pain. Have your healthcare provider order a 28-day salivary test to determine if your progesterone level is low.

FATIGUE

See Endometriosis; Postpartum Depression; Premenstrual Dysphoric Disorder (PMDD); Premenstrual Syndrome (PMS).

FIBROCYSTIC BREAST DISEASE

Fibrocystic breast disease is a benign condition where an individual has lumps in her breast. The lumps may be tender. Less commonly the patient may have pain severe enough to interfere with daily activities. This condition is called mastalgia. The lumps may occur at around the same time of the menstrual cycle each month or may not be related to the time of the cycle. Fibrocystic breast disease is common, occurring in about 50 percent of all women. Cysts are benign conditions and are not associated with an increased risk of breast cancer. However, they must be distinguished from a cancerous mass. Mammography, ultrasound, MRI, and needle aspirations or biopsies are modalities that are used to evaluate breast lumps.

Therapies for Fibrocystic Breast Disease

Conventional Treatments

- Danazol
- Diuretics (water pills) prior to menstruation to decrease breast swelling
- Oral contraceptives
- Stop smoking
- Wear support bras

Precision Medicine Therapies

Dietary changes. Studies have shown that limiting the intake of coffee, tea, cola, chocolate, and caffeinated medications (methylxanthines) in the diet resulted in improvement in fibrocystic breast disease in almost all

Causes of Fibrocystic Breast Disease

Studies have shown a strong association between fibrocystic breast disease and the intake of caffeine. Caffeine, the medications theophylline, and theobromine, all inhibit the action of cyclic adenosine monophosphate (cAMP)—involved in the regulation of glycogen, sugar, and lipid metabolism—and cyclic guanosine monophosphate phosphodiesterase and elevate their levels in the tissues of the breast. High levels of these nucleotides stimulate protein-kinase activity which increases the production of fibrous tissue and cystic fluid. In adults, ingestion of 1,000 mg or more of caffeine can cause symptoms such as nausea, vomiting, diarrhea, reflex, peptic ulcers, tremors, increased heart rate, high blood pressure, and rarely death. Large amounts of caffeine intake can also lead to premature aging. Caffeine is metabolized in the body at different rates by individuals. In adults, the elimination half-life of caffeine is between three to seven and one-half hours. However, some studies do not show an association between caffeine intake and fibrocystic breast disease.

Stress has been shown to also play a role in fibrocystic breast disease since fibrocystic breast respond more to epinephrine (adrenaline) which increases cAMP production. A study found a correlation between fat intake and the risk of severity of fibrocystic breast disease. The association was positive for all forms of fat but particularly for saturated fat.

Iodine deficiency may furthermore be a contributing factor to fibrocystic breast disease.

Fibrocystic changes in the female breast may be the end result of a series of biochemical events initiated by the mast cell degranulation products histamine and heparin. Two mechanisms are proposed which could lead to mast cell degranulation in breast tissue. First, low progesterone levels lead to decreased intracellular cAMP levels in mast cells, which enhance mast cell degranulation. Second, low progesterone levels lead to increased solubilization of breast collagen during tissue turnover. Susceptible patients may undergo an allergic reaction to soluble collagen resulting in further mast cell degranulation. The degranulation products histamine and heparin may stimulate increased stromal proliferation (growth of cells in supporting tissue) and vascularization (excessive formation of blood vessels) respectively.

Likewise, estrogen dominance has been associated with an increased risk of developing fibrocystic breast disease. A study showed an inverse correlation between the intake of fiber and the rate risk of developing benign disorders of the breast.

women who did not use these products. There are other dietary considerations that affect fibrocystic breast disease. Since low fiber intake has been
associated with an increased risk of developing benign breast disease,
intake more fiber in your diet.

Furthermore, a study showed that supplementation with a good soy
protein has revealed a reduction in breast tenderness and fibrocystic
breast disease. The study found a decrease in variability of tissue activity
after one year of soy use.

Likewise, in a trial that was uncontrolled, the patients that ate a low-
fat diet had less mastalgia (breast pain) and improvement in their fibrocystic breast changes. A healthy eating pattern contain good fats, such as
avocados and lamb.

Nutritional Supplements. The following supplements have been shown
to be helpful in individuals with fibrocystic breast disease: evening primrose oil, iodine, vitamin A, vitamin E, and thiamine.

- **Evening Primrose Oil (EPO).** Evening primrose oil has been shown to
  be effective for both fibrocystic breast disease and mastalgia. Evening
  primrose oil is made from the seeds of the flowers of the plant and
  is very rich in the omega-6 fatty acid known as gamma-linolenic acid
  (GLA).

The dosage has varied in medical studies. The common suggested
dose is 2,000 to 3,000 mg a day. Evening primrose oil can act as a blood
thinner. If you have a bleeding disorder or are taking a medication or supplement that may thin your blood, do not take this herb. If you are planning to have surgery, discontinue this herbal therapy two weeks before
the procedure. Speak to your healthcare provider or pharmacist to learn if
any drugs you are taking might make it unwise to take evening primrose
oil. Do not use if you have a seizure disorder, since its use can precipitate
a seizure. This supplement can also cause some mild side effects, including the following: bloating, diarrhea, headaches, indigestion, nausea, and
vomiting.

- **Iodine.** Iodine is a micromineral best known for its role in making
  thyroid hormone which controls the body's metabolism. Studies have
  shown that women with fibrocystic breast disease obtain substantial
  relief from oral administration of iodine. According to the World Health
  Organization, up to 72 percent of the world's population is affected by

an iodine deficiency disorder. It is worth noting that sea salt contains little iodine unless you purchase an iodized product.

There are many causes of iodine deficiency including any medication that contains fluoride or bromide, diets containing food grown in iodine-depleted soil, diets high in pasta, and sodas that contain brominated vegetable oil, which is an emulsifier that can affect iodine metabolism. Also diets low in fish or sea vegetables, fluoride use in toothpaste and other products, and the use of sucralose which contains chlorinated table sugar.

If you are a vegan or vegetarian, you may also have low iodine levels. Always have your healthcare provider measure iodine levels, which is a urine test before supplementing. Individuals have an increased risk of developing thyroiditis or thyroid cancer if supplemented with iodine when it is not needed. Other possible side effects of iodine use include the following: acne, nausea, diarrhea, hair thinning, skin rash, headache, or hyperthyroidism (over functioning of your thyroid gland).

The dose of iodine for fibrocystic breast disease is 3 to 6 mg a day. This is a high dose since most people take 150 micrograms daily. Have your doctor remeasure iodine levels in 3 months. Many people no longer need to supplement with iodine after this time frame.

- **Thiamine.** In a case report, a woman who was deficient in thiamine due to alcohol intake had fibrocystic breast disease. She was given thiamine and had a resolution of small and large cysts in both breasts within three weeks of treatment with the thiamine. Thiamine is a B vitamin. It is best to always take all of the B vitamins instead of just one of them. Also, B vitamins are water soluble and therefore need to be taken twice a day to be effective.

- **Vitamin A.** There are retinoid receptors in breast tissue which may affect breast changes. A small clinical trial, 12 women, with fibrocystic breast disease were given a large dose of vitamin A (150,000 IU daily for 3 months). More than half who finished the study had significant improvement. Some people had to drop out of the study due to symptoms. Beta-carotene would be a better retinol to use in most people that do not have a genetic variation that impedes the conversion of beta-carotene to vitamin A.

If you are a smoker do not supplement with more than 8,000 IU of vitamin A in a day. There is an increased risk of developing lung cancer in smokers that use doses of vitamin A above 8,000 IU. This therapy is a high dose of vitamin A and therefore is not the best suggested treatment for fibrocystic breast disease.

- **Vitamin E.** Alpha-tocopherol has been shown to relieve symptoms of fibrocystic breast disease in double-blind trials. In uncontrolled trials, vitamin E was effective in many of the women studied with fibrocystic changes. Studies used between 200 IU and 600 IU of vitamin E. It is preferable to use vitamin E as the mixed tocopherol form. Vitamin E is a blood thinner. Use with caution if you are taking a blood thinning medication.

Medications

Thyroid Hormone Replacement. In human trials, thyroid hormone replacement resulted in clinical improvement of fibrocystic breast disease. One of the studies found that treatment with desiccated (porcine) thyroid resulted in improvement in over 200 women with fibrocystic breast disease who had hypothyroidism. Have your healthcare provider measure your complete thyroid studies. If you are hypothyroid, discuss thyroid replacement with your doctor.

Likewise, it is best to measure iodine levels first and replace iodine if levels are low before starting on thyroid medication. Your thyroid may not be functioning optimally due to iodine deficiency. If that is the case, taking iodine may decrease the need for thyroid medication, particularly if your thyroid function is borderline low.

Progesterone Replacement. Fibrocystic breast disease is commonly an estrogen dominant state where progesterone levels are low in relationship to estrogen levels. Have your healthcare provider measure hormone levels with saliva testing. If your progesterone level is low, your doctor or other healthcare provider can prescribe you compounded progesterone medication to balance the estrogen your body is producing.

Other Therapies

If you are estrogen dominant, then your body's ability to break down estrogen may be decreased. A formal liver cleanse may be beneficial to improve estrogen metabolism. Likewise, some of the estrogen your body makes is broken down in the GI tract (gut).

A study revealed that women who had fewer than three bowel movements per week had a risk of fibrocystic disease that was 4.5 times greater than women who had at least one bowel movement a day. Microorganisms in the GI tract can make estrogens as well as metabolize them. This may result in the absorption of estrogens made from bacteria along with reabsorption of estrogens that were previously conjugated. See your doctor or compounding pharmacist to start a gut restoration program. Most people would benefit from at least a good pharmaceutic grade probiotic.

GOITER

See Hyperthyroidism.

GRAVES' DISEASE

Graves' disease is the most common form of hyperthyroidism. It is also known as diffuse toxic goiter and Flajani-Basedow-Graves' disease. It represents 85 percent of all hyperthyroid cases. It is considered an auto-immune disease because of the way in which the body's immune system works against itself. The pituitary gland produces thyroid stimulating hormone (TSH). TSH in turn triggers the thyroid gland into producing enough T3 and T4 hormones that the body requires. For any number of reasons, the body's immune system produces thyrotropin receptor anti-body (TRAb) that acts in the same way TSH does, simulating the thyroid tissue to overproduce T3 and T4. In some cases, the symptoms may be mild, while in other cases, the symptoms can be serious. Normally in Graves' disease, the entire thyroid gland becomes enlarged.

Unlike other forms of hyperthyroidism, Graves' disease can also affect the tissues and muscles surrounding the eyes and the eye socket inducing swelling and inflammation. This condition is called thyroid eye disease (TED) or ophthalmopathy. Only 30 percent of Graves' patients show signs of TED. For those who do, the symptoms can range from mild, to moderate, to severe. While there are a number of therapies designed to reverse the overproduction of hormones brought about by Graves' disease, because TED involves the eyes, it may require other specialized treatments.

Risk Factors for Graves' Disease

The flare-up of antibodies that are at the root cause of Graves' disease can be initiated by any number of reasons. The following factors may indicate if an individual is at a higher risk.

- **Age.** The signs of Graves' disease usually present between the ages of 20 and 40.

- **Gender.** For every single male patient with Graves' disease, there are eight females. However, the ratio of patients that develop eye complications is equal in both men and women. Women with normal hormone levels of the estrogen but with an increased sensitivity to the estrogen have a higher prevalence of antibodies that may affect the thyroid.

- **Genetics.** Statistics strongly indicate that genetics plays a role in a person's predisposition to develop Graves' disease. While there is no evidence that only one gene is to blame, it is more likely that the presence of several specific genes increases the incidence of Graves' disease. Research has shown that Graves' disease is passed on from one generation to another as well as showing up in identical twins. However, it may require one or more triggers, as listed below, to initiate this condition.

- **Left-Handedness.** Oddly enough, a study done by Wood and Cooper showed a statistically significant trend for left-handed people to be affected by Graves' disease.

■ Causes

Although Graves' disease has been studied for years, its causes remain unclear. There are, however, some conditions that are thought to be likely triggers.

Emotional and Physical Stress. Recent stress may be a precipitating factor in the development of Graves' disease. The most common precipitating factor is the actual or threatened separation from an individual upon whom the patient is emotionally dependent. Furthermore, studies now support the idea that Graves' disease often follows an emotional shock.

Existing Autoimmune Diseases. Graves' disease is caused by a breakdown in the body's disease-fighting immune system. For those people with preexisting immune system disorders, such as type 1 diabetes or rheumatoid arthritis, studies have shown that there is an increased risk of developing Graves' disease.

Infections. Viral and bacterial infections have been reported in a large percentage of patients with Graves' disease. Studies indicate that a number of these pathogens can trigger the body's immune system to create antibodies; and it is in the body's natural response that a specific antibody may attach itself to the thyroid cells to overproduce hormones.

Studies have reported an increase in the frequency of anti-influenza B virus antibodies found in patients with thyrotoxicosis. A large prevalence of circulating antibodies against the bacteria *Yersinia enterocolitica*, strain 0:3 have been seen in patients with Graves' disease. Also, *Yersinia* antibodies have been found to interact with thyroid structures. Low-affinity binding sites for TSH have been found in other bacteria—*Leishmania* and *Mycoplasma*. Retroviral sequences or proteins have also been found in the thyroid gland of patients with Graves' disease. This may be due to a secondary infection.

Pregnancy and Recent Childbirth. For women going through pregnancy, there are a number of hormonal changes that their bodies experience. This includes increases in progesterone, estrogen, oxytocin, prolactin, and relaxin—any one of these or a combination of these hormones could trigger the development of Graves' disease.

Smoking. Studies showed a relatively small correlation between smoking and Graves' thyroid eye disease. There also appears to be an increase in symptoms when smoking is combined with drugs designed to stop the overproduction of thyroid hormones.

■ Signs and Symptoms

The following are the common signs and symptoms of Graves' disease. The progression of these, however, may also differ from one individual to another. It is also important to keep in mind that many of these symptoms can be caused by other underlying problems.

❑ Anxiety, nervousness, and irritability

❑ Breast enlargement in men (rare)

❑ Bulging eyes (exophthalmia)

❑ Chest pains and/or rapid or irregular heartbeat (palpitations)

- Difficulty in managing diabetes
- Erectile dysfunction or reduced sexual urges
- Eyelid retraction, puffy eyelids, reddening around the eyes, pressure on the eyes, and irritation of the eyes as well as double vision (Graves' thyroid eye disease)
- Goiter (enlargement of the thyroid gland)
- Heat intolerance
- Increase in bowel movements and/or diarrhea

- Lumpy thickening and reddening of the skin, usually on the shins or tops of the feet (Graves' dermopathy)
- Personality or psychological changes
- Perspiring profusely (diaphoresis)
- Shortness of breath
- Slight trembling of the hands or fingers
- Thinning hair
- Weight change (weight loss or gain)

◼ Testing for Graves' Disease

There are several tests available to determine whether you have Graves' disease or another potential form of hyperthyroidism.

Physical Examination. Normally, a physician can see some of the more pronounced signs, such as irritated or bulging eyes, thyroid enlargement, or signs of tremors which can indicate Graves' disease.

Blood Tests. In a standard blood test, there would be an increase in the level of thyroid hormones (T3 and T4) as would be expected with hyperthyroidism and there would be a decrease in the level of the thyroid-stimulating hormone (TSH). Because the thyroid is now being stimulated by an antibody, TSH production would naturally drop. In another specialized blood test, the level of the thyroid peroxidase antibody (TPO) is measured. This may indicate that there is an autoimmune disorder present. However, since 5 percent to 10 percent of healthy individuals test positive for TPO, the results of this antibody test may not be conclusive. If the tests all come back within a normal range, these blood tests can at least rule out Graves' disease.

Radioactive Iodine Uptake (RAIU). A radioactive iodine uptake test (RAIU) is designed to measure the amount of iodine your thyroid absorbs and determine whether all or only part of the thyroid is overactive. The amount of radioactive tracer your thyroid absorbs determines if your thyroid function is normal or abnormal. A high uptake of iodine tracer may mean you have hyperthyroidism or Graves' disease.

Scan of the Area Around Your Eyes. If the patient is showing either irritation around the eye and eye socket, or there is a bulging of the eyes several scans can be ordered. Ultrasound, magnetic resonance imaging (MRI), or computed tomography (CT) scan may be performed to determine the extent of impact the irritation has caused.

Based upon the patient's family history, risk factors, symptoms, and test results, the doctor will determine if the problem is Graves' disease.

■ Treatment of Graves' Disease

There are a number of the medical options available to combat Graves' disease. Each option should be considered in light of how far the Graves' disease has progressed.

■ Beta Blockers (B-Adrenergic Antagonist Drugs)

Beta blockers were originally designed to reduce blood pressure by blocking the effects of the hormone epinephrine, also called adrenaline. It does this by slowing down the number of heart beats per minute as well opening blocked vessels. This, in turn, reduces tachycardia, palpitations, tremor, and anxiety. The effects of beta blockers are fast, so it is important for use early in the treatment of Graves' disease. These drugs do not affect thyroid function, release, or synthesis. Beta blockers are not usually used alone for treatment of Grave's disease except for short time frames before and/or after radioactive therapy. Beta blockers should not be used if you have asthma, emphysema, congestive heart failure, bradycardia (slow heartbeat), hypotension (low blood pressure), COPD (chronic obstructive pulmonary disease), or Raynaud's phenomenon.

■ Anti-Thyroid Medication

One of the first options offered is anti-thyroid medications. Anti-thyroid drugs are designed to interfere with the thyroid gland's ability to produce hormones, thereby decreasing hormone production. Unlike other treatments, once they are discontinued, they allow the thyroid to function as usual. Side effects many vary with each drug. These may include nausea, vomiting, heartburn, headache, rash, joint pain, loss of taste, liver failure, or a decrease in disease-fighting white blood cells. Pregnant women should always check with their doctor regarding when they can start on such medications. These drugs can usually be discontinued once a stable normal thyroid balance has been achieved with other therapies. These medications include the following:

- **Glucocorticoids.** Glucocorticoids in high doses inhibit the peripheral conversion of T4 to T3. In the treatment of Grave's disease, glucocorticoids decrease T4 secretion by the thyroid gland. How effective this response is or how long it lasts is not known. Use of glucocorticoids is usually not suggested for Graves' disease unless there is major eye or skin involvement or if the patient is in thyroid storm. Short-term use only for these conditions is suggested.

- **Iodine and iodine-containing compounds.** Pharmacologic doses of iodine such as Lugol's solution or saturated solution of potassium iodide (SSKI) work by the following mechanisms:
  - Decreases iodine transport into the thyroid
  - Decreases the vascularity of the thyroid in Graves' disease
  - Inhibits iodine organification and blocks the release of T4 and T3 from the thyroid gland

The effects are only transient, lasting only a few days to weeks. Thyrotoxicosis may return and even worsen. Consequently, iodine therapy is used only short term in preparation for surgery after a normal state has been achieved and maintained with the use of thionamides. Iodine is also used to treat thyroid storm since it can inhibit thyroid hormone immediately. Use iodine only under your doctor's direction.

- **Oral cholecystographic agents.** Oral cholecystographic agents (iodine containing radiocontrast agents), such as iopanoic acid and sodium ipodate, produce a rapid fall in thyroid hormones. They act by inhibition of the peripheral conversion of T4 to T3 and by prevention of thyroid hormone secretion because of the inorganic iodine that is released from the drug. Both iopanoic acid and sodium ipodate because of their rapid onset of action are very effective treatments for Graves' disease.

They are not effective for long-term treatment because of the escape of thyroid hormone synthesis from the blocking action of iodine. Furthermore, iopanoic acid and sodium ipodate provide a load of iodine to the thyroid which makes the using of radioactive iodine not feasible for weeks. Therefore, these drugs are best used for emergency situations for a rapid decrease in thyroid hormone production or prior to surgery.

● **Perchlorate.** Perchlorate works by inhibiting the transport of iodine into the thyroid. Possible side effects include stomach irritation and aplastic anemia. These side effects are somewhat common; therefore, it stops the use of perchlorate as treatment for Graves' disease long-term. Used in conjunction with thionamides, perchlorate has been used successfully for depleting the thyroidal iodine overload in amiodarone-induced hyperthyroidism.

● **Thionamades.** There are three thionamides drugs, methimazole (MMI), carbimazole, and propylthiouracil (PTU) which are effective in their treatment of Graves'. Thionamides do not block the release of pre-formed thyroid hormone. Consequently, it takes 1 to 6 weeks for the thyroid hormones that are already stored and the iodine that is stored to be depleted and the patient to have total relief of symptoms and normalization of thyroid studies. Large goiters with large deposits of thyroid hormone may show a delayed response to thionamides.

The main problem with the use of thionamides is that there is a high relapse rate when the medications are stopped. Recurrence rate is 50 to 80 percent depending on the length of follow-up. Most relapses occur within 3 to 6 months but can occur much later. Remission rates have decreased over the last decade, perhaps due to an increased iodine supply in the diet of the average American. Relapse after treatment suggests that another form of treatment may be necessary. Some patients become hypothyroid after therapy.

Mild side effects have been reported in 1 to 15 percent of patients that take thionamides, such as:

● Hives (urticaria)

● Itching (pruritus)

● Joint pain (arthralgias)

● Slightly elevated liver enzymes

● Skin rash

Severe side effects of thionamides are rare and require prompt discontinuation of the medication. These side effects include:

- Cholestatic necrotic hepatitis

- Decrease of white blood cells (agranulocytosis)

- Inflammation of blood vessels (vasculitis)

- Lupus-like syndrome

- Toxic hepatitis

Thionamides can be used prior to thyroid surgery, with radioactive iodine, or as primary treatment. Treatment is usually for 1 to 2 years and then stopped.

■ Radioactive Iodine Therapy

As discussed earlier, in order to function, the thyroid gland needs to absorb iodine on a daily basis. With this therapy, a radioactive form of iodine is orally taken by the patient. As the reactive iodine is absorbed, the low-level radiation is enough to destroy the overactive thyroid cells causing the thyroid to shrink and produce less hormones. The treatment is taken over several weeks. With the decrease in thyroid hormones, the symptoms of Graves' disease are lessened.

Unfortunately, in cases where there is eye muscle irritation, the outcome is more complicated. For patients with mild inflammation of the eye muscles, the results may be mild and temporary, however in cases that are moderate to severe this therapy is not recommended, nor is it recommended for women who are pregnant or nursing.

Because this treatment involves destroying thyroid cells, it will likely have an effect on the amount of thyroid hormones produced in the future. For that reason, an individual's thyroid hormone levels must be checked regularly, and that patient may require taking thyroid medication to make up for a drop in thyroid hormone production.

■ Surgery

In serious cases, surgically removing part or the whole thyroid gland may be considered. With the partial or whole removal of your thyroid gland, a patient's levels of thyroid hormones must be carefully monitored. If the entire or partial gland is removed, individuals will normally be required to take thyroid medication for the remainder of their lives.

■ Thyroid Eye Disease (TED) Treatments

For mild symptoms of TED, patients can use over-the-counter artificial tears during the day and lubricating gels at night to avoid corneal damage caused by exposure and for relief. For moderate to severe symptoms, your doctor may recommend the following treatments:

- **Corrective lens.** In cases of double vision because of Graves' disease, or as a side effect of surgery for Graves', glasses containing prism lens may be prescribed to normalize vision. The outcome of vision improvement may vary from patient to patient.

- **Corticosteroids.** Treatment with corticosteroids, such as prednisone, will help reduce swelling behind your eyeballs. Side effects may include fluid retention, weight gain, elevated blood sugar levels, increased blood pressure, and mood swings.

- **Dry eyes.** As soon as you begin to experience dry eyes or a sensation of grit or irritation in the eye, start to use artificial tears or eye drops to prevent any scratching of the cornea. Check with your doctor for a brand recommendation. You can also use eye covers at night to keep the eyes shut and prevent them from becoming dry.

- **Eyelid surgery.** This procedure may be performed to restore the eyelid to an appropriate position allowing a patient to either close their eyes or to reduce sagging eyelid tissue to improve appearance.

- **Orbital decompression surgery.** In this operation, the surgeon removes the bone between the eye socket and your sinuses, providing more room for the eyes to move back to their original position. This treatment should be considered when the pressure on the optic nerve may lead to blindness. Possible complications include double vision.

- **Teprotumumab** (the brand name is Tepezza) is the new medication that can help people with thyroid eye disease. The way it works is by binding to the IGF-1 receptor which causes degradation of the antibody-receptor complex I. This in turn has been shown in trials to decrease proptosis (abnormal protrusion or displacement of the eye), double vision, and other symptoms associated with moderate to severe cases of thyroid eye disease. Unlike other non-surgical options for thyroid eye disease (for example, corticosteroids), teprotumumab can stop the progression of thyroid eye disease.

■ Natural Treatments

While there are no natural short-cuts for treating Graves' disease, there are a number of natural treatment options to consider. These should be used in conjunction with standard medical treatment. Before starting each natural option, they should be discussed with your healthcare provider.

■ Acupuncture

Acupuncture, the use of small needles strategically placed in the skin, has been used as a treatment in China for thousands of years. Studies in China have shown it effective in treating Graves' disease.

■ Cold Packs

By placing ice packs over the thyroid gland, found at the base of your neck, three times a day you can reduce swelling. The cold will also help slow down the function of the thyroid gland.

■ Diet

Eat foods that are good for you. Whole fruits, vegetables, and nuts head the list. In addition, a high protein diet has been shown to be mildly effective against mild Graves' disease. Moreover, these foods contain goitrogens, a naturally occurring chemical, which has been shown to prevent or make it more difficult for utilization of iodine. In so doing, they block thyroid synthesis. These goitrogenic foods include:

- Almonds
- Broccoli
- Brussels sprouts
- Cabbage
- Cassava root
- Cauliflower
- Kohlrabi
- Millet
- Mustard
- Peaches
- Peanuts
- Pine nuts
- Rapeseeds
- Rutabagas
- Soybeans
- Sweet potatoes
- Turnip

However, it is important to understand these foods cannot be reliably used in place of medications in the treatment of Graves' disease since their goitrogen content is low. Furthermore, cooking inactivates the goitrogens. Likewise, no substantial documentation is available to show that dietary goitrogens interfere with thyroid function if the patient has adequate levels of iodine. Also, foods that are high in iodine content, such as seaweeds, should be avoided.

Studies have shown that people should eat foods that contain flavonoids since they decrease serum T4 and inhibit both the conversion of T4 to T3 and 5′deiodinase activity. For example, fruits and vegetables of yellow, orange, red, and purple color, such as blueberries, purple grapes, and cherries, contain flavonoids.

■ Exercise and Light-Weight Training

While exercise is good for so many healthful reasons, when it comes to Graves' disease it can help in two ways. When the issue is weight gain, burning carbs through exercise can help keep pounds off. Secondly, with Graves' there is a tendency to have brittle bones. Light-weight training can strengthen bones as well as strengthen leg muscles for better balance and to prevent falls from occurring.

■ Limiting Your Food Choices

When treating Graves' disease, you should avoid consuming any foods that will interfere with normal thyroid function.

- **Avoid all gluten permanently.** Since Graves' disease is an autoimmune process, avoiding all gluten and gluten-containing products is imperative.

- **Avoid caffeine.** Caffeine can increase the severity of many Graves' disease symptoms, such as rapid heart rate, anxiety, and tremors. By eliminating products such as soda, coffee, tea, and chocolate from your diet, you can control some of these persistent issues.

- **Avoid foods that you are allergic to.** While it may be easy to identify foods and avoid the foods you are allergic to, there are people who have hidden food allergies that they may not be aware of—from dairy (containing lactose) to soy, to wheat (containing gluten) products. Many of these food allergies can aggravate Graves' symptoms. Make sure you are aware of all the foods you may be allergic to.

- **Avoid foods with high iodine content.** It is wise to avoid foods containing a high level of iodine, such as sea vegetables, iodized salt, and some fish and seafood, since iodine can affect the overproduction of the thyroid hormones. In addition, betadine washes, and iodine containing medications, such as amiodarone and radiographic dyes, should be avoided if possible. Do not discontinue any medication without working with your physician. Iodine excess may be a problem particularly in people that take iodine without having their levels measured. The use of iodine in patients that have Graves' disease is unpredictable and it is not suggested for usage.

- **Avoid heavily processed foods.** Cut down or stop consuming foods that are heavily processed, salted, and/or sugared. Also, make sure to consume foods low in iodine. Find a healthful diet that you can stick to.

■ Reducing Stress

Studies have shown that stress may trigger or worsen Graves' disease symptoms. By learning how to control stress in your life, you can avoid those stress-related hormones that may interfere in your healing process. Find the activity you enjoy most that you can relax doing—from taking long walks and hot baths to learning yoga exercises. This simple change in your life can make a difference.

■ Stop Smoking

Research has shown that smoking can increase the symptoms associated with Graves' disease—especially those who suffer from Graves' thyroid eye disease. In addition, it can affect the outcome of various thyroid treatments. Giving up smoking may not be easy, but it may be a lot easier to do knowing it's something that can help you beat the disease.

■ Medication

Since Graves' disease is an autoimmune process, discuss with your health-care provider starting on a compounded low-dose naltrexone (LDN) to decrease the inflammatory component of this disease. It has been shown that LDN reduces inflammation by reducing multiple pro-inflammatory cytokines. These effects are unique to low dosages of naltrexone and appear to be entirely independent from naltrexone's better-known activity on opioid receptors. As a daily oral therapy, LDN is inexpensive and well-tolerated, and most people have no side effects or few side effects. Possible side effects include insomnia, fatigue, hair-thinning, nausea, vivid dreams, loss of appetite, mood swings, and mild disorientation.

Contraindications are acute hepatitis, liver failure, and recent or current opioid ingestion or history of alcohol abuse.

■ Nutritional Supplements

Another option for people with Graves' is taking nutritional supplements. However, taking nutritional supplements alone may not be enough to overcome this thyroid disease. There are several factors that should be considered when trying to improve your thyroid health and taking certain nutritional supplements can be beneficial.

Calcium citrate. Calcium metabolism may be changed in hyperthyroidism where patients with Graves' disease have an increased risk of developing osteoporosis. Supplementing with calcium may be beneficial.

Coenzyme Q-10. Similar to a vitamin, this substance is a cofactor in the electron-transport chain which is the energy producing cycle in the body. Q-10 levels have been shown to be low in adults and children with hyperthyroidism. Studies have also shown that coenzyme Q-10 levels may return to normal after treatment of hyperthyroidism with conventional therapies. It may be helpful to supplement with Q-10 in people with Graves' disease that have cardiac disease and also in individuals with long-standing uncorrected hyperthyroidism.

L-carnitine. This amino acid is used for the transport of long-chain fatty acids into the mitochondria. L-carnitine is an antagonist of thyroid hormone in peripheral tissues by inhibiting thyroid hormone entry into the nucleus of the cells. One study conducted over 6 months used carnitine in patients with hyperthyroidism. Patients taking L-carnitine improved their symptoms and liver profiles, but the patients that did not take L-carnitine were worse. The form of L-carnitine used should be L-carnitine alone or the acetic or propionic acid form and not the D-form. Also, L-carnitine is cleared through the kidneys so it should only be considered in individuals with normal kidney function. A contraindication to the use of carnitine is if you have an elevated TMAO level. Therefore, ask your healthcare provider to measure TMAO. It is a blood study. If you have high TMAO levels and you supplement with any form of L-carnitine, it increases your risk of developing heart disease.

Selenium. People with Graves' commonly have low selenium (a trace mineral) levels. In fact, selenium deficiency alters the conversion of T4 to T3 in peripheral tissues such as the kidney and liver. One study found men fed high selenium diets had their serum T3 levels increase. Selenium is one of the supplements that should be considered as a therapy for mild hyperthyroidism in people that are not high in selenium or selenium toxic. Eating Brazil nuts and other foods that are high in selenium is also helpful.

In several studies, it was found that a deficiency of selenium was found in a number of patients suffering from Graves' thyroid eye disease. When put on a daily dosage of 100 micrograms of selenium selenite twice daily for 6 months, there was an observable improvement of symptoms associated with mild TED. Additionally, the same amount of selenium taken by Graves' patients showed a significant decrease in their thyroid peroxidase antibody levels—one of the culprits that trigger the thyroid's overproduction of hormones.

Vitamin A. Given in large doses this antioxidant has an inhibitory effect on the thyroid gland. Vitamin A supplementation has been shown to decrease the symptoms of Graves' disease. The exact mechanism by which vitamin A works is unknown. If you smoke, then do not consider this therapy since large doses of vitamin A in smokers may be linked to an increased risk of developing lung cancer.

Vitamin C (Ascorbic acid). Animal studies have shown that thyroid hormone in excess can reduce ascorbic acid levels in the serum, blood, liver, adrenal glands, thymus, and kidney. Studies in human trials in patients with hyperthyroidism have also shown an increase in excretion of ascorbic acid. Furthermore, trials have shown that the medications thiourea and thiouracil also lower ascorbic acid levels. Consequently, supplementation with vitamin C is suggested in patients with hyperthyroidism. Supplementation does not affect the course of the disease, but it may decrease the symptoms and metabolic effects.

Vitamin E. This vitamin may be protective against oxidative damage caused by Graves' disease. In an animal study, animals with hyperthyroidism were given vitamin E which helped to prevent the lipid peroxidation that is associated with hyperthyroidism. Human studies have shown that individuals with hyperthyroidism have low vitamin E levels. Consequently, supplementation with vitamin E is suggested.

Zinc. Red blood cell (RBC) zinc levels are lower in patients with Graves' disease since zinc needs are increased because of greater urinary zinc excretion in this disease process. Therapy with anti-thyroid medications has been shown to normalize RBC zinc levels 2 months after free T3 and free T4 were normalized.

■ Herbs

There are botanical supplements that may be helpful in some patients with Graves' disease. It is always advisable to work with a trained professional when using these herbal supplementation.

Bugleweed. In fact, the German Commission E, Germany's equivalent to the FDA, recognizes the use of bugleweed for mild hyperthyroid conditions associated with the dysfunction of the nervous system based on pharmacologic studies. Activity is mediated by a reduction in TSH, T4, and inhibition of the conversion of T4 to T3. Bugleweed also inhibits the receptor-binding and biological activity of Graves' immunoglobulins. However, be aware that in rare situations high dosages have resulted in thyroid enlargement and sudden discontinuation has increased disease symptoms.

Club moss. This herb has a long history of use for hyperthyroidism like bugleweed. Animal studies using club moss have shown its ability to block TSH activity at the receptor level, block the release of TSH from the thyroid, and suppress the iodine pump. It can also inhibit the peripheral T4-deiodination and conversion to T3.

Emblica officinalis. Animal studies using Emblica officinalis are promising. It was shown to reduce T3 and T4 concentrations by a significant amount. Human trials need to be done.

Ginger. It has been found that ginger has a positive effect on thyroid function. Ginger contains magnesium which has been proven to be a key factor in controlling thyroid disease. Since it aids in regulating inflammation, it is considered to also protect against thyroid conditions that are caused by inflammation. Ginger can be used in various ways. Fresh ginger root can be added when cooking or baking in the diced or powder form. In pill form, start with one capsule twice a day.

Lemon balm. Lemon balm has calming effects on the nervous system and has been used since ancient times for this issue. In vitro studies have confirmed lemon balm's ability to block TSH receptors and inhibit both binding of bovine TSH to human thyroid tissue and binding of autoantibodies in Graves' disease. It is usually combined with bugleweed to treat Graves' disease. Studies show that this herb is helpful in lowering the production of thyroid hormones when given in injection form. More studies need to be done on the oral form.

Milk thistle. Milk thistle is another natural therapy for the treatment of Graves' disease and is usually taken in supplement form for this purpose. It contains a flavonoid called silymarin that contains powerful antioxidant properties that are beneficial in the treatment of this disorder. It also may be helpful for treating eye problems caused by Graves' disease.

Motherwort. This is used traditionally to treat anxiety, depression, heart palpitations, and tachycardia. Therefore, it may be good for the relief of symptoms of Graves' disease. It can be used with bugleweed. The German Commission E supports the use of motherwort for the treatment of cardiac disorders associated with anxiety and for the symptomatic relief of mild hyperthyroidism.

Turmeric. Turmeric is an herb that has been used for thousands of years. Like ginger, it can be beneficial in treating inflammation. It has anti-inflammatory properties which help to treat thyroid dysfunctions such as Graves' disease. You can add turmeric when cooking or it can be taken in capsule form. Follow dosage directions on the package.

There are also botanical medicines that contain flavonoids, such as Hawthorne berry, astragalus, ginkgo biloba, licorice, and chamomile that may be helpful therapies in Graves' disease.

See also Hyperthyroidism.

HASHIMOTO'S THYROIDITIS

Hashimoto's thyroiditis also called Hashimoto's disease, chronic lymphocytic thyroiditis, and autoimmune thyroiditis is an autoimmune condition. Normally our immune system is designed to attack disease-causing invaders such as bacteria and virus, however, under certain conditions, it can attack the thyroid gland which can result in an inflammation of the thyroid called Hashimoto's thyroiditis. As the tissues of the gland become inflamed, the thyroid produces less hormones interfering with the body's normal metabolism. The disease begins slowly and may go undetected for months or even years.

Hashimoto's thyroiditis is the most common cause of hypothyroidism. It can result from inherited genetic and environment factors which often lead to a low functioning thyroid. It most often affects middle-aged women, although it can also affect men and teenagers. Generally, the symptoms and signs resemble those of hypothyroidism. However, some individuals with Hashimoto's thyroiditis have normal thyroid function, particularly early in the course of the disease.

Risk Factors for Hashimoto's Thyroiditis

The flare-up of antibodies that are at the root cause of Hashimoto's thyroiditis can be initiated for any number of reasons. The following factors may indicate if an individual is at a higher risk:

- **Age.** The signs of this disease usually present between the ages of 30 and 50, the disease can occur in children, teens, and young women.

- **Gender.** As with most thyroid related diseases, women are more prone to develop Hashimoto's thyroiditis than men.

- **Genetics.** Recent research has shown a significant role of heredity in the development of autoimmune thyroid disease for Hashimoto's thyroiditis. In addition, other autoimmune-prone genes may trigger this condition as well. However, it may require one or more environmental factors, as listed below, to initiate this condition.

■ Causes of Hashimoto's Thyroiditis

There are several conditions that may trigger Hashimoto's thyroiditis. These include the following:

- **Environmental Exposure.** There are several chemicals that can lead to Hashimoto's thyroiditis as well as other forms of autoimmune diseases. These include perchlorate, fluoride, lithium, mercury, bisphenol A, and Teflon.

- **Excessive Iodine.** A diet heavy in foods containing iodine, taking iodine supplements, and/or taking drugs containing large amounts of iodine can trigger Hashimoto's thyroiditis.

- **Pregnancy.** Pregnancy creates great hormonal changes in a woman's body. Sometimes this can result in some form of thyroid dysfunction during or after pregnancy. Statistics indicated that approximately 20 percent of these women who have thyroid issues during pregnancy will develop this disorder in later years.

- **Radiation Exposure.** While less common, research has shown that being exposed to large amounts of radiation can bring on autoimmune thyroid diseases.

■ Signs and Symptoms

The signs and symptoms of Hashimoto's thyroiditis are the same as those for hypothyroidism if you have Hashimoto's thyroiditis with low thyroid function. (See page 253.) However, if you have Hashimoto's thyroiditis and have normal thyroid function, you may not initially have any symptoms of hypothyroidism.

■ Diagnosis

Early diagnosis of Hashimoto's thyroiditis isn't always easy. Many people with normal thyroid function or with an underactive thyroid aren't aware that they have this condition. There are several tests that can be performed to indicate whether there is an autoimmune process affecting your thyroid gland.

■ Consult With Your Doctor

If you feel a problem does exist, it is very important that you see your healthcare provider for an evaluation of your thyroid gland; and, that you have a complete workup done and not a partial workup.

Clinical Evaluation. Your physician will perform a complete physical exam of the gland, where he palpates your thyroid to determine if there are any lumps, nodules, growths (goiters), or masses. In addition, he/she will be checking the thyroid's size, and if it is solid and firmly fixed in place.

Blood Tests. The blood test is the most common test and plays an important role in diagnosing thyroid disease and treating thyroid conditions. A
number of blood tests will be done in order to determine if you are suffering from hypothyroidism. Your physician will be evaluating your TSH,
free T4, free T3, rt3 (reverse T3), and thyroid antibodies (see page 75).

Thyroid binding globulin (TBG) can also be measured, see page 82.
This is the amount of stored hormone. It is produced by the liver and
is affected by illness, liver disease, and some medications. Sometimes
estrogens can raise TBG, so this is another test that you doctor may order.
Your healthcare provide may also order thyroid releasing hormone (TRH)
also called thyrotropin-releasing factor (TRF) which is a hormone that
stimulates the release of thyroid stimulating hormone (TSH) and prolactin
from the pituitary, see page 82.

In addition, with Hashimoto's thyroiditis, the individual's high antibody level compared to a lowered level of thyroid hormones will indicate
the presence of autoimmune problem. Likewise, it is not as common, but
you can have normal levels of TSH, free T3 and free T4 with positive
antibodies and you would still have Hashimoto's thyroiditis but without
hypothyroidism, as mentioned earlier.

Fine Needle Aspiration (FNA). Fine needle aspiration is a type of biopsy
procedure that is commonly performed to detect or rule out cancer cells
in the thyroid. It is performed on swellings or lumps found in the thyroid.
The fine needle aspiration can identify the type of cells contained in the
abnormal tissue or fluid.

Imaging Tests. Laboratory tests may not be enough to diagnosis thyroid
dysfunction. Sometimes more tests are ordered. Imaging tests are administered to help determine a diagnosis of various thyroid disorders. The
following are some other tests that may be performed:

- Iodine Uptake Scan: to measure the absorption of iodine in the thyroid.

- Thyroid Scan: a radioisotope is administered, usually given with
  the iodine uptake. Cells that do not absorb iodine will appear "cold
  (lighter on the scan);" a cell absorbing too much iodine will appear
  "hot (darker)."

- Thyroid Ultrasound: high frequency sound waves provide an image of
  the thyroid gland. It aids in performing fine need biopsies.

■ Treatment Of Hashimoto's Thyroiditis

Once a diagnosis of Hashimoto's thyroiditis has been confirmed there are several therapies available to treat the condition (detailed on page 252) if you have low thyroid function. Moreover, with Hashimoto's thyroiditis, the goal is to reduce the level of the body's autoimmune response. Consider going on a detox diet that pulls out inflammatory foods which may alleviate thyroid symptoms. Also avoiding all gluten, foods you are allergic to, and having optimal gastrointestinal function may decrease or resolve your symptoms. In fact, a recent study revealed that a gluten-free diet reduced thyroid antibody titers.

Furthermore, nutritional therapies have also been shown to be beneficial. Studies have revealed that supplementing with selenium at a dose of 200 micrograms decreased TPO antibodies and normalized the levels in some of the patients. Please check with your healthcare provider before starting selenium since this is a nutrient that you can develop symptoms of toxicity if you take too much. Individuals with Hashimoto's thyroiditis are frequently iron deficient as well. Have your healthcare provider measure your ferritin and TIBC level to see if your iron levels are decreased.

In addition, lower vitamin D status has been found in Hashimoto's thyroiditis individuals than in controls. The low vitamin D status may be the result of autoimmune disease processes that includes vitamin D receptor dysfunction. Moreover, vitamin D levels must be measured since you can become vitamin D toxic. Your doctor will frequently also start you on low dose naltrexone (LDN) which is a compounded medication to decrease the inflammatory response that occurs in Hashimoto's thyroiditis. See page 177 for more information on LDN. Last, if you are hypothyroid, then your healthcare provider will start you on thyroid medication.

See also Hypothyroidism.

HEADACHES

See Migraine Headaches: Hormonally Related; Premenstrual Dysphoric Disorder (PMDD); Premenstrual Syndrome (PMS).

HEART ATTACK

See Heart Disease.

HEART DISEASE

Heart disease is not a specific disease, but rather a broad term used to describe several diseases that can affect your heart and, in some cases, your blood vessels. Heart disease is also called cardiovascular disease, and can include coronary artery disease, arrhythmias, blocked vessels that can lead to heart attacks or stroke, heart infections, and heart defects you are born with. Women experiencing an acute cardiac event often do not recognize the symptoms. In fact, you may be misdiagnosed by your healthcare provider because you may have atypical symptoms. This can lead to a significant delay in treatment. Most women when they are having a heart attack do not get chest pain or they may have right sided chest pain. Women may have extreme fatigue, nausea, vomiting, or muscle aches and pains.

Even with a great deal of news coverage, most people do not realize that heart disease is the number one killer of women worldwide. Therefore, it is important to do all you can to prevent and treat heart disease before it affects you and your loved ones. To do this, you need to know what the risk factors for heart disease are. Many people think that if they watch their cholesterol, they will drastically reduce their risk of developing heart disease. However, cholesterol is only part of the picture—one-half of women who die of heart disease have normal cholesterol levels. There are quite a few other risk factors that have to do with hormones and menopause that women should pay attention to.

Let's begin a look at heart disease with high cholesterol and elevated triglyceride levels and then progress onto other risk factors for heart disease.

■ Hypercholesterolemia (High Cholesterol)

Cholesterol is a wax-like fatty substance (lipid) found in the cell membranes of all body tissues. About 75 percent of it is synthesized by the body with the remainder being of dietary origin. High-density lipoproteins (HDL) carry cholesterol from the blood to the liver. Low-density

Primary Risk Factors for Heart Disease

Along with elevated cholesterol, some common risk factors for heart disease are:

- **Age.** The older you are, the higher your risk of developing heart disease.

- **Blood pressure.** High blood pressure (hypertension) increases your chance of developing heart disease.

- **Diabetes.** Diabetics have a greater risk of developing heart disease.

- **Diet.** A diet high in fat, salt, or cholesterol can increase your chances of getting heart disease.

- **Gender.** Men are usually at a higher risk of developing heart disease than women, until after menopause when women have as high or higher risk of developing the disease.

- **Genetics.** Having heart disease in your family increases your chances of developing the disease.

- **Hygiene.** Poor oral hygiene can lead to infections, which can worsen your risk of developing heart disease.

- **Lack of exercise.** Not exercising increases your risk of developing heart disease.

- **Obesity.** Excess weight increases your chances of developing the disease.

- **Smoking.** Smoking increases your chances of developing the disease.

- **Stress.** Unresolved stress can damage arteries and worsen other risk factors.

lipoproteins (LDL) carry cholesterol from the liver to the remainder of the body. LDL cholesterol particles have more triglycerides and less protein than HDL cholesterol particles. Because they are less dense, LDL particles are also larger than HDL particles. Very low-density lipoprotein (VLDL) particles have the highest ratio of triglycerides to protein and are the largest of the three types of cholesterol.

Cholesterol is important for many biological functions in the body including making pregnenolone and other hormones, helping the body produce vitamin D from the sun, aiding the body in digesting fat, enhancing cell structure since some of the cell membranes are made of cholesterol, along with other functions. However, high cholesterol levels, particularly LDL is associated with an increased risk in developing heart disease. Excess triglycerides are also detrimental to your healthy and increase your risk of heart disease. After you eat, and especially if you consume a high-sugar meal, any excess blood sugar that goes unused turns into triglycerides that are then deposited in fat storage areas throughout the body.

What the Cholesterol Ratio?

Sometimes, heart disease risk is assessed using cholesterol ratios. Your healthcare provider will determine a cholesterol ratio by taking your total cholesterol count and dividing it by your HDL cholesterol count. This cholesterol ratio should ideally fall between 1 and 3.5, which signifies that HDL cholesterol comprises a significant portion of your total cholesterol. If your level is above 3.5 you are at a higher risk of developing heart disease.

Therapies to Lower Cholesterol

Conventional Therapies

The following are conventional therapies to lower cholesterol:

- Exercise
- High fiber diet
- Medications:
  - Bile acid binding resins
  - Cholesterol absorption inhibitors (Ezetimibe)
- Niacin
- Omega-3-fatty acids
- PCSK9 (injectable) inhibitors: Evolocumab, Alirocumab
- Statin drugs

Precision Medicine Therapies

The following are Precision Medicine therapies to lower cholesterol:

Amino acids. Testing amino acids and balancing them according to lab results will help optimize your cholesterol level. Research shows that getting optimal ratios of essential amino acids may play an important role in lowering LDL cholesterol levels and triglycerides. A study found that supplementing with a combination of essential amino acids and phytosterols promoted lower levels of total cholesterol, LDL cholesterol, and triglycerides. Have your doctor order an amino acid test.

Balance hormones. See a Precision Medicine specialist or pharmacist to order salivary testing to test your sex hormones and have them replaced with natural hormones if you are a candidate for hormone replacement. On the salivary test will also be DHEA and cortisol levels. Elevation of

Causes of High Cholesterol

The following are some of the etiologies of hypercholesterolemia:

- Alcoholism
- Amino acid deficiency
- Biotin deficiency
- Carnitine deficiency
- Deficiency of natural antioxidants (such as vitamin E, selenium, and beta-carotene)
- Essential fatty acid deficiency
- Excess dietary starch
- Excess dietary sugar
- Excess hydrogenated or processed fats (such as lard, shortening, cotton-seed oil, palm oil, margarine)
- Fiber deficiency
- Food allergies
- Hormone deficiencies (DHEA, estrogen, pregnenolone)
- Hypothyroidism (low thyroid level)
- Increased tissue damage due to infection, radiation, or oxidative activity (free radical production)
- Liver dysfunction
- Medications: cyclosporine, cimetidine, antiepileptic drugs, tamoxifen, thiazides, alpha blockers, retinoids
- Vitamin C deficiency

either of these hormones can also raise your cholesterol. Make sure that complete thyroid studies have been done since high cholesterol levels may be a manifestation of hypothyroidism.

Nutrition. Have your healthcare provider order a comprehensive nutritional test to coordinate your nutritional therapy to help lower your cholesterol.

Diet. Eating a diet that is high in soluble fiber will help lower cholesterol. Decrease your intake of trans fats. Add nuts to your diet, such as almonds, walnuts, pecans, pistachios, hazelnuts, and macadamia nuts. Adding sesame seeds to your diet may be beneficial. Also add beans to your meal, such as lentils, chickpeas, pinto beans, and navy beans. If you have a normal TAMO (Trimethylamine N-oxide) level (see section on risk factors for heart disease, page 183), most studies have shown that eating up to 28 eggs a week does not raise your cholesterol.

Evaluate for infection. Have your doctor evaluate you for infection. There are two different methods that bacterial and viral infections can raise your cholesterol. One is by altering lipid metabolism which causes your LDL level to rise. Secondly, recent evidence suggests that LDL has antimicrobial properties and LDL is elevated as the body tries to inactivate the pathogens.

Exercise. Exercise helps to lower cholesterol. Exercising three to four times a week for 20 minutes not only lowers cholesterol, but it will help lower blood sugar and cause weight loss if you are overweight. If you are over 45 and have not been exercising, then see your healthcare provider before you begin an exercise program.

Fatty acids. Fatty acid testing is also an important examination to have your doctor perform to help lower your cholesterol level. Both omega-6 fatty acids, such as safflower oil, soybean oil, and sunflower oil, can help decrease cholesterol as can omega-3-fatty acids.

GI health. Have your healthcare provider order a gut health test. GI infections, such as H. pylori, parasitic infections, and small intestinal small overgrowth (SIBO), can raise your cholesterol level. Leaky gut is when the gut barrier becomes more permeable to endotoxins such as lipopolysaccharides (LPS). These toxins enter the bloodstream and create an immune response. As part of the body's defense against these toxins, it releases a protein called LPS binding protein which circulates with the LDL, this leads to an up regulation of your LDL levels. Addressing gut bacterial infections and dysbiosis (too much bad bacteria and not enough good bacteria) can decrease cholesterol levels by 30 to 40 points.

Nutrients. The following are nutrients found to be effective in lowering cholesterol.

- **Artichoke** (Cynara scolymus, Cynara cardunculus) decreases LDL, total cholesterol, and triglycerides. Its components luteolin and chlorogenic acid play a key role.

- **Berberine** induces LDL excretion. It works very effectively. Some individuals may get nausea and loose stools with berberine use. Dose: 200 mg to 500 mg three times a day. Do not use this supplement during pregnancy since it can cause uterine contractions.

- **Bergamot** (Citrus bergamia) inhibits cholesterol synthesis. It has been shown to be one of the most effective natural ways to lower cholesterol. Dose: 500 mg twice a day.

- **Beta-sitosterol** is a plant sterol. It works by inhibiting intestinal absorption of cholesterol and is usually taken twice a day.

- **Carnitine** lowers total cholesterol and triglycerides. It also causes a significant reduction of Lp(a) level. In addition, carnitine aids in fat metabolism enhancing the transport of fatty acids into the mitochondria. It likewise raises HDL-C. Ask your doctor to measure your TMAO level before supplementing with carnitine. If your TMAO level is elevated, you cannot take carnitine. Dose: 1,000 to 3,000 mg a day if you have normal kidney function.

- **Chitosan** inhibits cholesterol absorption.

- **Chromium** has been shown to lower total cholesterol and raise HDL-C in some studies. Not all trials show any benefit of this mineral.

- **Fiber,** the soluble form, as a supplement inhibits cholesterol absorption. Soluble fiber includes pectin, guar gum, mucilage, oats, and psyllium. Dose: 20 to 30 grams a day.

- **Garlic** is one of the best methods to lower your cholesterol since it inhibits cholesterol synthesis. Dose: 10 mg allicin or a total allicin potential of 4,000 micrograms (equal to one clove of garlic) once a day. Garlic is a blood thinner. Do not use if you are taking any kind of blood-thinning medication or supplement.

- **Green tea.** Drinking green tea or taking it as a supplement (EGCG) lowers total cholesterol and LDL-C. Green tea extract can interact with a number of drugs. Check with your healthcare provider before taking this supplement. Dose: 200 to 400 mg twice a day.

- **Gugulipid** lowers cholesterol. Do not take if you are taking a blood thinning medication or a nutrient that causes your blood to thin, since gugulipid has anticoagulant activity. Dose: 50 mg twice a day.

- **Magnesium glycinate** increase HDL-C. It also has many other functions in the body. Dose: 400 to 500 mg a day.

- **Niacin** works by lowering total cholesterol, LDL-C, and triglycerides. It also raises HDL-C. Do not use if you are taking a statin drug. This nutrient in large doses may also raise your blood sugar and can increase your liver enzymes. Dose: 1.5 to 3 grams a day.

- **Pantethine** inhibits cholesterol synthesis and lowers total cholesterol and triglycerides. It also raises HDL-C. Dose: 900 mg a day.

- **Policosanol** (from sugar cane) inhibits the making of cholesterol by the body. Dose: 10 mg twice a day.

- **Red yeast rice** lowers cholesterol very effectively. It works by inhibiting cholesterol synthesis and improving endothelial (thin membrane inside of heart and blood vessels) function. It lowers both total cholesterol and LDL-C. In addition, it decreases C-reactive protein (CRP). Like statin drugs, it can deplete the body of the important nutrient coenzyme Q-10. Therefore, supplement with coenzyme Q-10: 100 mg a day. Do not take red yeast rice with a statin drug. Dose: 600 mg twice a day.

- **Tocotrienols** are natural analogs of vitamin E. Taken twice a day they have been shown to reduce cholesterol levels.

- **Targeted probiotics** inhibit cholesterol absorption. In addition, keep alcohol intake to a minimum.

Conventional medications may be mixed with Precision Medicine therapies to effectively help you lower cholesterol, except for statin drugs, niacin, and red yeast rice.

■ Hypertriglyceridemia (High Triglycerides)

Triglycerides are the form that fat takes when it is being stored for energy in the body. High triglyceride levels increase the person's risk of developing heart disease and pancreatitis. Furthermore, elevated triglyceride levels are the second most common dyslipidemic (blood lipid levels that are too high or too low) change in individuals with hypertension after an increase in LDL-C. In addition, hypertriglyceridemia influences the metabolism of other lipoproteins, transport of proteins, enzymes, on coagulation, and endothelial dysfunction (damage to the vascular tissue).

Causes of High Triglycerides

High triglycerides tend to show up along with other problems, like high blood pressure, diabetes, obesity, high levels of "bad" LDL cholesterol. It's not uncommon for people with high triglycerides to have more than one etiology factoring into their condition. The following can cause or contribute to the rise of triglyceride levels:

- Alcohol
- Caffeine
- Diuretics
- Family inheritance
- Fruit juice
- High fat diet
- Insulin resistance
- Lack of physical activity
- Nephrotic syndrome
- Nicotine

- Oral contraceptives
- Skipping breakfast and/or lunch and making up for it at supper
- Soft drinks
- Stress
- Too much fruit
- White bread, cakes, cookies, candies
- White flour
- White sugar

■ Ways to Lower Triglyceride Levels

There are many ways to lower high triglyceride levels. Decreasing your intake of fruits to two serving a day and eliminating fruit juices has been shown to be beneficial. Also eating a good fat diet, low glycemic index (low sugar) eating program has been shown to be helpful. Of course, like many things that can help us be healthier, exercise will lower triglycerides. There are many nutrients that can also lower your triglyceride level. EPA/ DHA (fish oil) has been shown to be the most effective, as well as the nutrients in the table of supplements below.

SUPPLEMENTS THAT DECREASE TRIGLYCERIDES		
Supplements	**Dosage**	**Considerations**
Alpha-ketoglutarate	500 to 1,000 mg once a day	Use with caution if you get cold sores.
Arginine	2 to 4 g once a day	If you have kidney disease, liver disease, or herpes, only take under a doctor's supervision.
Chromium	300 mcg once a day	Combining with the protein picolinate allows your body to absorb chromium more efficiently. However, some chromium picolinate supplements contain more chromium than necessary. Ask your healthcare provider for a recommendation on chromium consumption.
Coenzyme Q-10	60 to 120 mg once a day	May reduce the effects of blood thinners. May cause diarrhea in dosages above 100 mg once a day.
EPA/DHA (fish oil)	2,000 to 4,000 mg once a day	Choose a source that contains vitamin E to prevent oxidation. Doses of 4,000 mg a day or more act as a blood thinner. Do not take more than 3,000 mg a day if you are taking a prescription blood thinning drug.
Gugulipid	500 to 1,000 mg once a day	
Lysine	1,000 to 3,000 mg once a day	Taking for more than six months can cause an imbalance of arginine. Do not take if you have diabetes or are allergic to eggs, milk, or wheat.
Magnesium	600 mg once a day	Consult healthcare provider for dosage if you have kidney disease. Discontinue use and see your doctor if you experience abdominal pain. Take a lower dose if it causes diarrhea.
Methionine	250 to 500 mg once a day	Take with vitamins B_6 and B_9 to prevent a build-up of homocysteine. May counter the effects of levodopa (a drug used to treat Parkinson's disease).
Niacin	1 to 2 g once a day	Do not take the suggested dosage without first consulting your doctor. Large dosages can cause a "flush" feeling, which can be eliminated by taking an aspirin one hour before the niacin. Do not drink alcohol or hot drinks within one hour of taking niacin.

Supplements	Dosage	Considerations
Policosanol	10 to 20 mg once a day	
Vitamin B5 (pantothenic acid)	100 mg once a day	High doses can deplete your body of other vitamins in the B complex.
Vitamin B9 (folic acid)	1 mg twice a day	High doses can deplete your body of other vitamins in the B complex.
Vitamin E	400 IU once a day	Take tocotrienols, the most active type of vitamin E.
Zinc	25 mg once a day	The best zinc supplements are zinc picolinate and zinc citrate. If you are taking zinc and iron supplements, take one in the morning and one in the evening. (Taking them together reduces the efficiency of both.)

In addition, natural hormone replacement has been shown to lower your triglyceride level.

Since lipids, such as cholesterol and triglycerides, are insoluble in water these lipids must be transported in association with proteins (lipoproteins) in the circulation. Large quantities of fatty acids from meals must be transported as triglycerides to avoid toxicity. These lipoproteins play a key role in the absorption and transport of dietary lipids by the small intestine; in the transport of lipids from the liver to peripheral tissues, and the transport of lipids from peripheral tissues to the liver and intestine (reverse cholesterol transport). A secondary function is to transport toxic foreign hydrophobic (doesn't dissolve easily in water) and amphipathic (contains both water-soluble and not water-soluble) compounds, such as bacterial endotoxin (found in outer membrane of bacteria), from areas of invasion and infection.

To be more specific, cholesterol and triglycerides are insoluble in water and therefore these lipids must be transported in association with proteins. Lipoproteins are complex particles with a central core containing cholesterol esters—chemical compound derived from an acid—and triglycerides surrounded by free cholesterol. These help with the formation and function of substances (lipoprotein) made of protein and fat that carry cholesterol through the bloodstream. Plasma lipoproteins can be divided into seven classes based on size, lipid composition, and if elevated they can increase your risk of heart disease. HDL decreases your risk.

■ Lipoprotein Particles

Chylomicrons. These are large triglyceride rich particles made by the intestine, which are involved in the transport of dietary triglycerides and cholesterol to peripheral tissues and liver. These particles contain apolipoproteins—proteins that bind lipids. The size of chylomicrons varies depending on the amount of fat ingested. A high fat meal leads to the formation of large chylomicron particles due to the increased amount of triglyceride being transported; whereas in the fasting state the chylomicron particles are small carrying decreased quantities of triglyceride.

Chylomicron Remnants. The removal of triglyceride from chylomicrons by peripheral tissues results in smaller particles called chylomicron remnants. Compared to chylomicrons, these particles are enriched in cholesterol and are pro-atherogenic (cause heart disease).

Very Low-Density Lipoproteins (VLDL). These particles are produced by the liver and are triglyceride rich. They contain apolipoprotein. Similar to chylomicrons the size of the VLDL particles can vary depending on the quantity of triglyceride carried in the particle. When triglyceride production in the liver is increased, the secreted VLDL particles are large. However, VLDL particles are smaller than chylomicrons.

Intermediate-Density Lipoproteins (IDL; VLDL Remnants). The removal of triglycerides from VLDL by muscle and adipose tissue—body fat— results in the formation of IDL particles which are enriched in cholesterol. These particles contain apolipoprotein B-100 and E. These IDL particles if elevated increase your risk of heart disease.

Low-Density Lipoproteins (LDL). These particles are derived from VLDL and IDL particles and they are even further enriched in cholesterol. LDL carries the majority of the cholesterol that is in the circulation. LDL consists of a spectrum of particles varying in size and density. An abundance of small dense LDL particles are seen in association with hypertriglyceridemia (high triglycerides), low HDL levels, obesity, type 2 diabetes, infectious, and inflammatory states. These small dense LDL particles are considered to be more pro-atherogenic (promoting fatty deposits in the arterial walls) than large LDL particles for a number of reasons. Small dense LDL particles have a decreased affinity for the LDL receptor resulting in a prolonged retention time in the circulation. In addition, they more easily enter the arterial wall and bind more avidly to intra-arterial proteo-glycans (compounds containing carbohydrate linked to protein), which traps them in the arterial wall. Finally, small dense LDL particles are more susceptible to oxidation, which could result in an enhanced uptake by macrophages—a type of white blood cell.

High-Density Lipoproteins (HDL). These particles play an important role in reverse cholesterol transport from peripheral tissues to the liver, which is one potential mechanism by which HDL may be anti-athero-genic. In addition, HDL particles have antioxidant, anti-inflammatory, anti-thrombotic, and anti-apoptotic (cause cell destruction) properties, which may also contribute to their ability to inhibit atherosclerosis. HDL particles are enriched in cholesterol and phospholipids. Apolipoproteins are associated with these particles. Apo A-I is the core structural protein, and each HDL particle may contain multiple Apo A-I molecules. HDL particles are very heterogeneous and can be classified based on density, size, charge, or apolipoprotein composition.

Apolipoprotein (a). Apo (a) is synthesized in the liver. High levels of Apo (a) are associated with an increased risk of atherosclerosis. Apo (a) is an inhibitor of fibrinolysis (prevents blood clots from growing) and can also enhance the uptake of lipoproteins by macrophages, both of which could increase the risk of atherosclerosis. The physiologic function of Apo (a) is unknown.

■ Advanced Cholesterol Profile

It is important that as a woman you also have the lipoprotein subgroups of cholesterol measured, not just the basic panel, to evaluate new risk factors, which is crucial for an accurate assessment of cardiovascular risk.

   This test is called NMR® LipoProfile test. This is a more accurate way of measuring LDL (bad cholesterol) since it is a direct measure of LDL circulating in your body. A typical cholesterol panel gives you a calculated measurement instead. The test also allows for measurement of the lipo-protein subclasses of HDL and LDL.

   The NMR® LipoProfile contains the following tests:

- LDL particle number (LDL-P)
- HDL particle number (HDL-P)
- Small LDL particle number (small LDL-P)
- LDL particle size

- A standard cholesterol test
  (LDL-C, HDL-C, triglycerides,
  and total cholesterol)

- LP-IR

These subclasses examine particle size and number. If the particle size of cholesterol is small, it is more of a risk factor for heart disease than if the particle size is large. For example, you can have a high HDL (good cholesterol) level but if the particle size of HDL is mostly small, then your risk for developing heart disease is still increased.

Apolipoprotein (a). Apo (a) is synthesized in the liver. High levels of Apo (a) are associated with an increased risk of atherosclerosis. Apo (a) is an inhibitor of fibrinolysis (prevents blood clots from growing) and can also enhance the uptake of lipoproteins by macrophages, both of which could increase the risk of atherosclerosis, as previously discussed. The physiologic function of Apo (a) is unknown.

Secondary Risk Factors for Heart Disease

It is also important that as a woman, you also have your secondary risk factors for heart disease measured. The risk factors you need to look out for are elevated levels of homocysteine, iron (ferritin), lipoprotein A, fibrinogen, c-reactive protein, and Interleukin 6 (IL-6).

■ Homocysteine

Homocysteine is an amino acid not supplied by the diet that can be converted into cysteine or recycled into methionine, an essential amino acid, with the aid of specific B vitamins. High levels promote free radical production. Free radicals are molecules that lack an electron. They will search through your body for an electron until they find a healthy cell, and then they steal the healthy cell's electron. This process kills the cell. If enough cells die, it leads to death.

This process is also one of the causes of oxidative stress, which can lead to vascular disease, a condition that affects your circulatory system. Oxidative stress is a term used to describe internal inflammation and the free radicals produced as a result of this inflammation. It is caused by an imbalance between the production of reactive oxygen and the body's ability to detoxify it.

In addition, studies have indicated that elevated homocysteine levels are directly related to strokes, peripheral vascular disease, cardiovascular disease, cognitive decline, osteoporosis, diabetes, polycystic ovary syndrome (PCOS), and depression.

Elevated homocysteine levels have also been associated with several other disease processes, including multiple sclerosis (MS), spina bifida/neural tube defects, spontaneous abortion, placental abruption, renal failure, and rheumatoid arthritis. Additionally, elevated homocysteine levels have been associated with an increase in breast cancer risk. When homocysteine levels are greater than normal limits, it signifies a disruption in the metabolism of homocysteine.

Causes of Excess Homocysteine

- Drugs
- Genetic mutations and enzyme deficiencies
- Hypothyroidism
- Menopause
- Renal failure
- Rich diet
- Smoking
- Toxins

In instances where high homocysteine levels are hereditary, it is commonly due to the lack of the enzyme methylenetetrahydrofolate reductase, which breaks down homocysteine. A deficiency of this enzyme increases the need for folate in order to prevent high homocysteine levels. This occurs in 12 percent of the population.

Elevated homocysteine levels have also been associated with several other disease processes, including depression, osteoporosis, multiple sclerosis (MS), spina bifida/neural tube defects, spontaneous abortion, placental abruption, type-2 diabetes, renal failure, and rheumatoid arthritis. Additionally, elevated homocysteine levels have recently been associated with the risk of memory loss later in life and an increase in breast cancer risk.

As mentioned, your homocysteine levels are lower before menopause. As you go through menopause, your homocysteine levels will rise because your lowering estrogen status is associated with elevated homocysteine concentrations. Optimal homocysteine level is 6 to 8 micromol/L.

Your homocysteine levels may naturally increase with menopause. Likewise, as you have seen in the section on PCOS, women with polycystic ovarian disease also may have elevated homocysteine levels. Therefore, it's good to get your levels checked regularly at that age.

High homocysteine levels can damage the arterial lining of the heart, making it narrow and inelastic (a condition also known as "hardening" of the arteries, or arteriosclerosis). When levels are elevated, homocysteine can reduce nitric oxide production, which can lead to high blood pressure, a risk factor for heart disease. High homocysteine levels also elevate triglyceride and cholesterol synthesis.

Studies suggest that 42 percent of strokes, 28 percent of peripheral vascular disease (which causes leg pain, cramping, and loss of circulation), and approximately 30 percent of cardiovascular disease (heart attacks, chest pain) are directly related to elevated homocysteine levels. Furthermore, a study published in the *New England Journal of Medicine* in July 1997 showed that people with homocysteine levels below nine were much less likely to die. Optimal levels of homocysteine are six to eight. Another study showed that women with a history of high blood pressure and elevated homocysteine levels were 25 times more likely to have a heart attack or stroke than women whose blood pressure and homocysteine levels were closer to normal.

Ways to Lower Homocysteine Levels

- Exercise

- Hormone replacement therapy that includes natural estrogen if you are deficient and a candidate for hormone replacement.

- Stress reduction

- Quit smoking if you smoke cigarettes

- If you are hypothyroid, optimizing thyroid function can lower homocysteine levels.

- Improve methylation

Supplementation with vitamins B_6, B_{12}, and folate. As previously stated, your body needs adequate amounts of B_6, B_{12}, and folate to break down homocysteine. B vitamins are water soluble and excessive ingestion of caffeine products, alcohol, or diuretics (water pills) will wash B vitamins out of your system. Some people may still have elevated homocysteine levels after supplementing with B_6, B_{12}, and folate. These people will need to take the active form of vitamin B$_{12}$ (methylcobalamin) and/or folic acid (L-5-MTHF).

Researchers have suggested that folate supplementation could save 20,000 to 50,000 lives from heart disease every year. In addition to supplementation, folate can be found in dark green leafy vegetables, beans, legumes, and oranges.

Consuming broccoli, spinach, and beets also increase the conversion of homocysteine in your body. Likewise, SAM-e (s-adenosylmethionine) will help break down homocysteine. The suggested dosage is 200 to 400 mg a day.

Garlic at the dosage of 1,000 mg a day and trimethylglycine (TMG) at 500 to 1,000 mg a day have also been found to lower homocysteine levels.

Consult your doctor to discontinue medications that can raise homocysteine levels, such as prescription niacin (high dose), some diuretics (water pills), and oral contraceptives.

If your testosterone level is elevated, then work with your healthcare provider to use the techniques suggested in this book to lower your testosterone level.

■ Iron (Ferritin)

When women menstruate, many of them are instructed by medical professionals to take iron supplementation, because blood loss sometimes results in low iron levels, or in some cases, anemia. Consequently, when you go through menopause, you are no longer menstruating, so there is a good chance that if you once needed iron supplementation, you will no longer need it after menopause.

In many cases, if you continue with iron supplementation after menopause, your iron levels will become too high. Studies have shown that too much iron can increase your risk of heart disease. Every 1 percent increase in ferritin (serum iron) causes a 4 percent elevation in risk of heart attack. Thus, continuing iron supplementation if you do not need it may elevate your ferritin level and predispose you to a heart attack. Also, your levels of iron increase naturally after menopause since you are no longer bleeding every month, so it is a good idea to have your ferritin (iron) levels measured.

Elevated iron is seen often in individuals with hemochromatosis or hemosiderosis but also in people that have a chronic inflammatory condition. The following are inflammatory conditions associated with iron overload besides heart disease:

- Cancer, such as leukemia, lymphoma, breast
- Hyperthyroidism
- Iron poisoning
- Liver disease

- Metabolic syndrome
- Recent blood transfusion
- Rheumatoid arthritis
- Type 2 diabetes

How to Lower Ferritin Levels

- Donate blood
- Eat egg yolks (Have your healthcare provider measure TMAO levels first. If you have an elevated TMAO level, you should not eat egg yolks.)
- Exercise
- Fiber
- Polyphenolic-containing beverages:

  - Black tea
  - Chamomile
  - Cocoa
  - Lime flower
  - Pennyroyal
  - Peppermint tea
  - Vervain

- Reduce alcohol intake
- Stop cigarette smoking

In addition, if your iron level is elevated do not eat foods that are high in iron until your levels are optimized.

■ Foods Sources of Iron

The following list is reprinted with permission from Jeffrey Bland's *Clinical Nutrition: A Functional Approach*. Foods that contain the most iron are listed first, followed by foods that contain progressively less iron. The listed number describes how many milligrams of iron are in 100 grams (3.5 ounces) of food.

Iron in meat is more bioavailable than iron found in vegetables. Additionally, your body will absorb more iron from vegetables if they are eaten *with* meat than if they were eaten alone.

100	Kelp	11.2	Pumpkin and squash seeds
17.3	Brewer's yeast	9.4	Wheat germ
16.1	Blackstrap molasses	8.8	Beef liver
14.9	Wheat bran	7.1	Sunflower seeds

6.8	Millet	1.1	Currants
6.2	Parsley	1.1	Whole wheat bread
6.1	Clams	1.1	Cauliflower
4.7	Almonds	1.0	Cheddar cheese
3.9	Dried prunes	1.0	Strawberries
3.8	Cashews	1.0	Asparagus
3.7	Lean beef	0.9	Blackberries
3.5	Raisins	0.8	Red cabbage
3.4	Jerusalem artichoke	0.8	Pumpkin
3.4	Brazil nuts	0.8	Mushrooms
3.3	Beet greens	0.7	Banana
3.2	Swiss chard	0.7	Beets
3.1	Dandelion greens	0.7	Carrot
3.1	English walnut	0.7	Eggplant
3.0	Dates	0.7	Sweet potato
2.9	Pork	0.6	Avocado
2.7	Cooked dry beans	0.6	Figs
2.4	Sesame seeds, hulled	0.6	Potato
2.4	Pecans	0.6	Corn
2.3	Eggs	0.5	Pineapple
2.1	Lentils	0.5	Nectarine
2.1	Peanuts	0.5	Watermelon
1.9	Lamb	0.5	Winter squash
1.9	Tofu	0.5	Brown rice, cooked
1.8	Green peas	0.5	Tomato
1.6	Brown rice	0.4	Orange
1.6	Ripe olives	0.4	Cherries
1.5	Chicken	0.4	Summer squash
1.3	Artichoke	0.3	Papaya
1.3	Mung bean sprouts	0.3	Celery
1.2	Salmon	0.3	Cottage cheese
1.1	Broccoli	0.3	Apple

■ Lipoprotein (a)

Lipoprotein (a) Lp(a) is a small cholesterol particle that causes inflammation and can clog blood vessels. Research has shown that patients with high lipoprotein (a) have a 70 percent higher risk of developing heart disease over 10 years. High levels of lipoprotein (a) are due to an inherited trait, declining estrogen levels in women at menopause, and statin drug use.

According to the National Lipid Association website lipoprotein (a) is considered elevated at levels greater than 50 mg/DL or 125 nmol/L. There are factors that can affect your test results such as fever, infection, recent and considerable weight loss, and pregnancy. Therefore, do not have your Lipoprotein (a) level measured if you are running temperature, are infected, or are pregnant.

There are many ways you can lower your lipoprotein (a) level. If you plan to use any of these methods to reduce your levels, be sure to take them daily. You should work with a physician who is familiar with treating high lipoprotein (a) levels to determine which treatment is right for you. Therapies that accelerate LDL clearance and lower LDL levels do not lower lipoprotein (a) levels (for example statin therapy). The kidney appears to play an important role in Lp (a) clearance as kidney disease is associated with delayed clearance and elevated levels.

Ways to Lower Lipoprotein (a)

● Aged garlic: 1,200 mg twice a day

● Bergamot (Citrus bergamia) inhibits cholesterol synthesis. It has been shown to be one of the most effective natural ways to also lower cholesterol. Dose: 500 mg twice a day.

● Bio-identical estrogen replacement in women that are candidates for hormone replacement

● Coenzyme Q-10: 200 to 300 mg once to twice a day

● Curcumin: 500 mg a day

● EPA/DHA: 1 to 2 grams

● Flaxseed

● Ginkgo biloba: 120 mg twice a day

- L-carnitine: 1 to 2 grams in individuals with normal kidney function and normal TMAO levels. L-carnitine should not be taken as a supplement if your TMAO levels are elevated. Therefore, have your healthcare provider measure your TMAO levels before taking this important amino acid.

- L-lysine: 500 to 1,000 mg

- L-proline: 500 to 1,000 mg

- N-acetyl cysteine (NAC): 500 mg to 1,000 mg twice a day. NAC depletes the body of zinc and copper. Therefore, if you are taking NAC long-term, make sure you also take a multivitamin. Also take vitamin C 1,000 mg a day to prevent precipitation of cysteine kidney stones if you are supplementing with NAC.

- Niacin: 1 to 2 grams

- Red yeast rice: 600 mg twice a day. Red yeast rice depletes the body of coenzyme Q-10. Therefore, take 100 mg of coenzyme Q-10 once or twice a day in addition to the red yeast rice.

- Resveratrol: 500 mg a day

- Tocotrienols: 400 IU a day

- Vitamin C: 2 to 4 grams

Exercise also effectively lowers high lipoprotein levels.

For some individuals it is difficult to lower their lipoprotein (a) level. If that occurs, your doctor may start you on vitamin C 2,000 mg a day and nattokinase 50 mg twice a day. Nattokinase is a blood thinner and, therefore, should not be taken if you are on a blood thinner or if you have another reason for increased bleeding.

■ Fibrinogen

Fibrinogen is a clot promoting substance that if elevated is a marker for an increased risk of developing heart disease. Fibrinogen concentrations vary widely among populations and increase with age. Levels are higher in women than men and rise after menopause. People with diabetes, hypertension, and high cholesterol have a higher risk of having elevated fibrinogen levels, as do sedentary and obese individuals.

During menopause, estrogen levels decline. Fibrinogen increases as estrogen decreases, so when you become menopausal, your fibrinogen levels can elevate. Additionally, fibrinogen elevates if you are a smoker.

Research has shown that estrogen replacement therapy can decrease fibrinogen. Nutritional support includes garlic, cold water fish, vitamin E, ginkgo, and bromelain. In addition, fish oil (EPA/DHA) 2,000 mg a day has been shown to be effective, as has green tea and ginger. Also, if you smoke cigarettes, discontinuing smoking is helpful. One of the best ways to lower fibrinogen levels is targeted probiotics. A study showed that L. reuteri as a supplement lowered fibrinogen by 14 percent. All of these substances can offset the clotting effects of elevated fibrinogen.

■ C-Reactive Protein

C-reactive protein (hs-CRP) is a marker of inflammation. It is part of the non-specific acute phase response to most forms of inflammation, infection, and tissue damage by activating the complement system and increasing phagocytosis—ingestion of bacteria. It stimulates monocytes to release pro-inflammatory cytokines: IL-1, IL-6, TNF-alpha. Furthermore, CRP stimulates endothelial cells (cells lining the inside of the heart and blood vessels) to express intracellular adhesion molecule (ICAM)-1 and vascular adhesion molecule (VCAM)-1. Decreasing hs-CRP reduces vascular events independent of LDL reduction.

Scientists believe that some infections can cause heart disease. Chlamydia, herpes, and cytomegalovirus, an infection in the herpes group, can cause inflammation in your blood vessels and cause plaque formation, eventually leading to heart disease. Chronic gum disease and an H. pylori infection in your stomach are also causes of inflammation. Elevated levels of C-reactive protein occur when there is inflammation in the body. High levels are a risk factor for heart disease, diabetes, hypertension, depression, peripheral artery disease, congestive heart failure, stroke, atrial fibrillation, and sudden cardiac death.

Since CRP levels can be elevated due to many causes of inflammation, your doctor will want to get a high-sensitivity CRP test (hs-CRP), which is designed for greater accuracy in measuring risk factors for cardiovascular disease. Studies have shown that C-reactive protein can be predictive of future heart attacks, even if you have a normal cholesterol level. Many physicians believe that an elevated CRP level is the most important risk factor for heart disease.

Ways to Lower CRP

- Aged garlic

- Berberine

- Bromelain (do not use of patient is allergic to pineapple)

- Curcumin

- EPA/DHA

- Estrogen replacement in women who are candidates for estrogen replacement

- Exercise

- Ginger

- Natural Cox-2 inhibitors: grapeseed extract (100 to 200 mg/day), curcumin (300 to 600 mg/day), green tea (3 cups or 3 capsules/day)

- Quercetin

- Red yeast rice (supplement with Q-10)

- Statin drugs (supplement with Q-10)

- Targeted probiotics. L. reuteri has been shown to lower CRP in a clinical trial. In this study, hs-CRP was decreased by 62 percent.

■ Interleukin-6 (IL-6)

Interleukin-6 (IL-6) is a polypeptide product of monocytes and macrophages. Adipocytes (cells storing fat) also produce IL-6. It is one of more than 30 members of the interleukin family and IL-6 induces the synthesis of C-reactive protein and fibrinogen, which you have seen are risk factors for heart disease.

Ways to Lower IL-6

- Antidepressants: Imipramine, Venlafaxine

- Botanicals: Astragalus, cat's claw, reishi mushroom, red clover, bitter melon, tart cherry, ashwagandha, berberine, Hawthorne

- Eating a Mediterranean diet

- Exercise three to four times a week (If you have not been exercising and you are over the age of 42, then see your healthcare provider to have an ECG done before starting an exercise program.)

- Good sleep hygiene

Causes of Elevated IL-6

The following are causes of elevated IL-6:

- Aging process
- Cigarette smoking
- Excessive alcohol consumption
- Excessive exercising
- Infection
- Insomnia
- Nutrient deficiencies: Vitamin D, zinc, magnesium, calcium, choline
- Poor sleep hygiene
- Stress
- Weight gain

IL-6 stimulates the inflammatory processes in many diseases for example: diabetes, depression, heart disease, Alzheimer's disease, systemic lupus erythematosus (SLE), multiple myeloma, breast cancer, prostate cancer, rheumatoid arthritis, COVID-19, and Behcet's disease.

- Medications: tocilzumab, metformin, low-dose naltrexone (LDN)

- Optimizing hormone function: leptin, thyroid, melatonin, angiotensin II, cortisol

- Replacing nutritional deficiencies

- Spices: Oregano

- Stop smoking cigarettes

- Supplements: Curcumin, EGCG, grape seed extract, phosphatidylcholine (do not take if you have an elevated TMAO level—therefore, have your healthcare provider measure levels before starting), quercetin, MSM, omega-3-fatty acids, Schisandra

- Treating infection if present

- Weight loss

As you have seen, there are many risk factors for heart disease. The good news is that most of them can be mitigated using many of the methods described in this chapter. It may also surprise you to discover that hormones also help prevent and treat heart disease. See Part III of this book for a discussion of the beneficial effects that hormone replacement has on women in relationship to heart disease.

HEAVY PERIODS

See Endometriosis; Metrorrhagia.

HIGH BLOOD PRESSURE

See Heart Disease; Hypertension (High Blood Pressure); Polycystic Ovarian Syndrome (PCOS).

HOT FLASHES AND NIGHT SWEATS

Hot flashes, defined as transient sensations of heat, sweating, flushing, anxiety, and chills lasting for 1 to 5 minutes, constitute one of the most common symptoms of menopause among women. About 75 percent of women in the U.S. have hot flashes and/or night sweats during perimenopause or menopause. This may persist for up to 5 years after menopause and rarely as long as 15 years. A study showed that 72 percent to 80 percent of women view hot flashes as one of the worst symptoms of menopause.

Causes of Hot Flashes and Night Sweats

Hot flashes and night sweats occur as a result of decreased or changing estrogen. This leads to inappropriate peripheral vasodilation and the feeling of heat, followed by perspiration which leads to rapid heat loss and cooling of the core temperature of the body to lower than normal. Hot flashes and night sweats can also be a symptom of adrenal dysfunction. Have your healthcare provider order a salivary test to examine your female hormone levels as well as your cortisol level.

Therapies for Hot Flashes and Night Sweats

Conventional Therapies

Conventional therapies for hot flashes include the following:

- Clonidine has been shown to be effect for hot flashes. A study showed that clonidine reduced hot flashes by 15 percent to 20 percent but may have significant side effects.

  - Edema

  - Hypotension in normotensive patients

  - Rebound hypertension upon discontinuation

  - Weight gain

- Gabapentin: Shown to be more effective when combined with SSRIs than when used alone. The possible usual side effects may occur with this drug.

- SSRIs: A study showed that it reduced hot flashes by 19 percent to 65 percent. It may have the usual side effects of SSRIs.

- Venlafaxine (SNRI) has been found to be effective for hot flashes.

Precision Medicine Therapies

Precision Medicine therapies are used commonly by women for hot flashes and night sweats. The estimates are that 50 percent to 75 percent of women use alternative therapies for menopausal symptoms. The rate may be higher in patients with breast cancer. Seventy-two percent of women found Precision Medicine therapies effective. They include the following:

- Acupuncture

- Botanicals are plant compounds. Some of them bind naturally to human estrogen receptors and are effective for hot flashes and night sweats. They are classified in three categories.

  - Isoflavones: alfalfa, chickpeas, lentils, lima beans, pinto beans, soy

  - Phytosterols: bean sprouts, red clover, sunflower seeds

  - Lignins: flaxseeds, fruits, genistein, vegetables, whole grains

- Hypnosis

- If symptoms are due to adrenal dysfunction, treat the case of the problem. See the chapter on cortisol for therapies.

- Natural prescription hormone replacement if hormone levels are low in individuals and they are a candidate for natural hormone replacement.

- Regular aerobic exercise

- Vitamin E 1,200 IU. Vitamin E is a blood thinner so do not use if you are taking a blood thinner.

See also Menopause and Perimenopause.

HUMAN PAPILLOMAVIRUS (HPV)

See Cervical Dysplasia (Abnormal Pap Smear).

HYPERCHOLESTEROLEMIA (HIGH CHOLESTEROL)

See Heart Disease.

HYPERPARATHYROIDISM

Hyperparathyroidism occurs when the parathyroid glands create too much parathyroid hormone in the bloodstream. Hyperparathyroidism is characterized as primary, secondary, or tertiary dysfunction.

■ Primary Hyperparathyroidism

Primary hyperparathyroidism (PHPT), the most common cause of hypercalcemia (high calcium), is most often identified in postmenopausal women with hypercalcemia and parathyroid hormone (PTH) levels that are either elevated or inappropriately normal. Most people have no symptoms, and primary hyperparathyroidism usually is diagnosed after an elevated serum calcium level is found incidentally on a basic chemistry panel testing. If symptoms are present, they are attributable to hypercalcemia and may include muscle weakness, bone pain (resulting in the risk of developing osteoporosis), abdominal pain, easy fatigability, anorexia, or anxiety.

Primary hyperparathyroidism refers to an abnormality to the parathyroid gland itself, such as an adenoma or hyperplasia causing the gland to oversecrete. This is characterized by lab values that show elevated PTH levels, hypercalcemia (high calcium), and hypophosphatemia (low phosphate). These are the diagnostic criteria for primary hyperparathyroidism. Primary hyperparathyroidism is customarily due to an adenoma, hyperplasia, or even more rare, a carcinoma. Adenomas are very sporadic and can be surgically resected.

Although in most of the cases hyperparathyroidism is a sporadic disease, it can also present as a manifestation of a familial syndrome. Many benign and malignant sporadic parathyroid neoplasms are caused by loss-of-function mutations in tumor suppressor genes. These were initially identified by the study of genomic DNA from patients who developed hyperparathyroidism as a manifestation of an inherited syndrome. Somatic and inherited mutations in certain proto-oncogenes can also result in the development of parathyroid tumors.

The clinical presentation of PHPT includes three phenotypes: target organ involvement of the renal and skeletal systems; mild asymptomatic hypercalcemia; and high PTH levels in the setting of persistently normal albumin-corrected and ionized serum calcium values. Interestingly, the factors that determine which of these three clinical presentations is more likely to occur include the extent to which biochemical screening is employed, the prevalence of vitamin D deficiency, and whether a medical center or practitioner tends to routinely measure PTH levels in the evaluation of low bone density or frank osteoporosis. When screening is common, asymptomatic primary hyperparathyroidism is the most likely form of the disease. In places where vitamin D deficiency is prevalent and biochemical screening is not frequently done, symptomatic disease with skeletal abnormalities is likely to be most common.

Higher PTH concentrations are associated with an increased mortality risk among older populations. Parathyroidectomy (removal of one or more of the parathyroid glands) is the definitive treatment for primary hyperparathyroidism. When performed by experienced endocrine surgeons, the procedure has success rates of 90 to 95 percent and a low rate of complications. Asymptomatic individuals who decline surgery and meet criteria for medical management must commit to long-term monitoring. Any unexplained elevation of the serum calcium level should be evaluated promptly to prevent complications from hypercalcemia.

◼ Secondary Hyperparathyroidism

Secondary hyperparathyroidism (SHPT) is an increased secretion of PTH due to parathyroid hyperplasia (abnormal cells in the parathyroid glands) caused by triggers such as hypocalcemia (low calcium level), hyperphosphatemia (high phosphate level in the blood), or decreased active vitamin

D. The increased PTH secretion, in turn, causes increased calcium in the blood by acting on bones, intestines, and kidneys. Prolonged SHPT is often associated with disturbances of bone turnover, as well as visceral and vascular calcifications, which are responsible for cardiovascular morbidity and mortality. Despite improvements in medical treatment, surgical treatment of secondary hyperparathyroidism is often necessary, especially in refractory cases. Renal transplantation is a therapeutic alternative but is frequently followed by the persistence of hyperparathyroidism.

In secondary and tertiary hyperparathyroidism, the kidney cannot convert vitamin D into the physiologically active 1,25-cholecalciferol. Reduced intestinal absorption of calcium results in low serum calcium and elevated phosphate due to the kidney's failure to excrete phosphate which increases secretion of parathyroid hormone. Prolonged stimulation results in parathyroid hyperplasia. This manifestation also occurs in vitamin D-deficient rickets, malabsorption, and pseudohypoparathyroidism—a disorder in which the body fails to respond to the parathyroid hormone.

Lab values differ according to the underlying cause. In chronic kidney failure, there will be elevated PTH, but with decreased calcium and elevated phosphate. In the setting of malabsorption and vitamin D deficiency, there will be elevated PTH but decreased calcium and phosphate.

■ Tertiary Hyperparathyroidism

Tertiary hyperparathyroidism occurs when an excess of parathyroid hormone is secreted by the parathyroid glands, usually after longstanding secondary hyperparathyroidism. This occurs when the parathyroid glands are producing high levels of parathyroid hormone for such a long time that they become overgrown and permanently overactive leading to high level blood calcium.

Some scientists reserve the term for secondary hyperparathyroidism that persists after successful renal transplantation. Long-standing chronic kidney disease (CKD) is associated with several metabolic disturbances that lead to increased secretion of PTH, including hyperphosphatemia (high phosphate levels), calcitriol deficiency, and hypocalcemia. Hyperphosphatemia has a direct stimulatory effect on the parathyroid gland cell, resulting in nodular hyperplasia and increased PTH secretion. Prolonged hypocalcemia also causes parathyroid chief cell hyperplasia and excess PTH. After correction of the primary disorder chronic kidney disease by renal transplant, the hypertrophied parathyroid tissue fails to resolute and continues to over secrete PTH, despite serum calcium levels that are within the reference range or even elevated.

■ Disorders Associated With Hyperparathyroidism

In individuals with hyperparathyroidism, there is often an interplay between bone disorders, renal (kidney) dysfunction, and cardiovascular disorders. Calcium balance regulates the interplay between these organ systems.

Let's begin by looking at hyperparathyroidism and heart disease. Hyperparathyroidism affects the cardiovascular system in several ways: vascular inflammation, hypertension, vascular/valvular calcification, cardiac hypertrophy (thickening of the heart muscle), and metabolic syndrome. Moreover, parathyroid hormone is a principal regulator of calcium balance in physiological and pathological conditions associated with cardiovascular disorders and plays a major physiological role in bone homeostasis.

Accumulating evidence suggests that higher PTH levels may be associated with low-grade inflammation. Dietary-induced hyperparathyroidism in lab animals led to increased serum proinflammatory cytokine production. This study indicates that serum PTH levels are independently associated with several inflammatory markers in the U.S. population including CRP and IL-6. PTH stimulates interleukin-6 (IL-6) production by osteoblasts and liver cells. In turn, IL-6 may modulate acute-phase protein synthesis in the liver. It has been proposed to supplement with vitamin D in the elderly to reduce serum levels of IL-6 and C-reactive protein (CRP) and, possibly, to decrease the risk of thromboembolic vascular (blood clots in the vessels) events. It is important to always measure levels of vitamin D and frequently repeat vitamin D levels.

Clinically, patients with primary hyperparathyroidism have a higher risk of cardiovascular mortality and suffer from a broad spectrum of adverse cardiovascular disorders, such as coronary microvascular dysfunction, subclinical aortic valve calcification, increased aortic stiffness, endothelial dysfunction, and hypertension. Moreover, cardiovascular disease is the most common cause of death in patients with CKD. A PTH level greater than 70 pg/mL is independently associated with cardiovascular disease events in patients with CKD stages 3 and 4. No association was observed between serum phosphorus or calcium level and CVD events. These findings provide support for intact PTH testing, along with testing for other indicators of CKD mineral and bone disorders, at earlier CKD stages.

Furthermore, secondary hyperparathyroidism, the most significant complication in patients with chronic kidney disease (CKD), causes abnormal bone disorders as well as extra-skeletal calcification, such as vascular and valvular calcification, and increased risk of cardiovascular mortality. In addition, hyperparathyroidism is associated with increased risk of cardiovascular events in patients with stage 3/4 CKD independent of calcium-phosphate levels. Furthermore, the association between long-term exposure of high PTH and valvular calcification has been demonstrated mainly in individuals with renal (kidney) dysfunction.

Vitamin D deficiency has been associated with cardiovascular disease (CVD), suggesting a role for bioregulators (naturally occurring organic compounds needed to regulate diverse cellular processes) of bone and mineral metabolism in heart health. Vitamin D deficiency can lead to secondary hyperparathyroidism, and both primary and secondary hyperparathyroidism are associated with cardiovascular pathology. Elevated PTH is associated with a greater prevalence and incidence of cardiovascular risk factors and predicts a greater likelihood of disease, including mortality. Likewise, risk persists when adjusted for vitamin D, renal function, and standard risk factors. Consequently, parathyroid hormone represents an important new cardiovascular risk factor that adds complementary and independent predictive value for heart disease and mortality.

Furthermore, the presence of PTH receptors within the cardiovascular system, including vasculature (smooth muscle cells, endothelial cells) and heart (cardiomyocytes), suggests that secreted PTH may play a role in the pathophysiology of cardiovascular diseases beyond its role in mineral and bone metabolism. In addition, hyperparathyroidism is considered to be a complementary biomarker in heart failure. A study found that in a racially/ethnically diverse population without prevalent cardiovascular disease, higher serum PTH concentration was associated with increased left ventricular mass and increased risk of incident heart failure. Further studies should be performed to determine whether PTH excess may be a modifiable risk factor for heart failure.

Inappropriate aldosterone and parathyroid hormone secretion are strongly linked with development and progression of cardiovascular disease. Aldosterone is a hormone produced by the adrenal gland that is essential for sodium conservation in the kidney, salivary glands, sweat glands, and colon. It plays a major role in the regulation of blood pressure, sodium, and potassium levels. Accumulating evidence suggests a bidirectional interplay between parathyroid hormone and aldosterone. This interaction may lead to a disproportionally increased risk of cardiovascular damage and metabolic and bone diseases.

Calcium is essential to heart, kidney, bone, and nervous system functioning, making PTH's functioning crucial. Calcium plays an integral part in cardiac contractions. The contractility of the heart is predicated on the availability and role of calcium inside myocardial cells. When there is an excess amount of calcium within cardiac cells, contractility will increase, and similarly, when there is a lower calcium level within the cardiac cells, contractility will decrease. This can potentially lead to prolonged QT intervals seen on ECG. QT prolongation occurs when the heart muscle takes a longer time to contract and relax than usual. QT prolongation may increase the risk of developing abnormal heart rhythms and may lead to sudden cardiac arrest.

Extreme hypercalcemia's effect on the myocardium can be manifested in ECG changes, causing very short QT intervals which could potentially precipitate the onset of fatal arrhythmias such as ventricular tachycardia or even ventricular fibrillation if not treated.

Also, serum concentrations of 25(OH)D (active form of vitamin D) and PTH were found to be independently associated with blood pressure and the presence of hypertension or prehypertension among United States adults. The "Multi-Ethnic Study of Atherosclerosis (MESA)" demonstrated the association among PTH and hypertension, and an association between parathyroid hormone, carotid stiffness, and systolic blood pressure, thus providing supplementary evidence for the role of PTH in cardiovascular diseases. Serum 25(OH)D was not associated with the presence of hypertension, whereas serum PTH was positively associated, suggesting that serum PTH may be an independent risk factor for high blood pressure as well.

Last, the parathyroid level, but not the vitamin D level, was found to be an independent predictor of metabolic syndrome in yet another trial.

As you have seen, the parathyroid gland is a very interesting organ in the body. In the blood, the sensitive process of calcium and phosphate balance is maintained primarily by optimally functioning parathyroid glands. Hyperparathyroidism, if not recognized and treated, can have significant consequences to your health.

HYPERTENSION (HIGH BLOOD PRESSURE)

According to data from the National Health and Nutrition Examination Survey, overall hypertension prevalence decreased from 47 percent in 1999–2000 to 41.7 percent in 2013–2014 and then increased to 45.4 percent in 2017–2018. In addition, hypertension increased with age: 22.4 percent (aged 18 to 39), 54.5 percent (40 to 59), and 74.5 percent (60 and over).

Systemic arterial hypertension is characterized by persistently high blood pressure in the systemic arteries—branches directly or indirectly from the aorta. Hypertension is commonly expressed as the ratio of the systolic blood pressure (BP) which is the pressure that the blood exerts on the arterial walls when the heart contracts and the diastolic BP which is the pressure when the heart relaxes.

The new American College of Cardiology/American Heart Association guidelines eliminate the classification of prehypertension and divides it into two levels: (1) elevated BP, with a systolic pressure (SBP) between 120 mm Hg and 129 mm Hg and diastolic pressure (DBP) less than 80 mm Hg, and (2) stage 1 hypertension, with an systolic blood pressure of 130 to 139 mm Hg or a diastolic blood pressure of 80 to 89 mm Hg.

Fewer than half of those with hypertension are aware of their condition, and many others are aware but not treated or inadequately treated. High blood pressure is a major risk factor for coronary heart disease, cerebrovascular disease, kidney disease, and congestive heart failure.

Conventional Therapies

Lifestyle Changes

- Weight loss if the patient is overweight. Up to 60 percent of all individuals with hypertension are more than 20 percent overweight.

- Exercise is very important to prevent and treat hypertension. Regular aerobic physical activity can facilitate weight loss, decrease BP, and reduce the overall risk of cardiovascular disease. In fact, your blood pressure may be lowered by 4 to 9 mm Hg with moderately intensive physical activity.

- Limiting salt intake is key for some people. The American Heart Association recommends that the average daily consumption of sodium chloride not to exceed 6 grams. This may lower blood pressure by 2 to 8 mm Hg.

Causes of Hypertension

There are many contributing factors to hypertension, some of which include the following:

- Diet
- Genetics
- Lack of exercise
- Lead and/or cadmium exposure
- Other disease processes, such as:
  - Diabetes
  - Hypercalcemia
- Hypothyroidism
- Pheochromocytoma
- Polyarteritis nodosa
- Primary hyperaldosteronism
- Renal diseases
- Toxemia of pregnancy
- Overweight/obesity
- Poor sleep hygiene
- Stress

However, 90 percent of patients with hypertension have essential hypertension where no known cause is present. Individuals with essential hypertension are divided into three categories based on renin activity—measure of the plasma enzyme renin. Renin plays a critical role in vascular reactivity due to its effects in producing the peptide angiotensin II which is vasoconstricting (narrows blood vessels). The secretion of renin is influenced mainly by the person's salt intake and volume status. The categories are:

- Patients with **low** renin have low renin activity. Aldosterone—steroid hormone which regulates salt and water in the body—production in these individuals is not being suppressed. This leads to a mild form of hyperaldosteronism (overproduction of aldosterone) resulting in elevated blood pressure. The elevation in blood pressure is due to the retention of sodium being increased along with an increase in fluid volume and blood pressure.

- Patients with **normal** renin hypertension are commonly insulin resistant and have abdominal obesity. However, hypertension can occur in people that have a normal body weight and do not have non-insulin-dependent diabetes. This suggests that there is a relationship between insulin sensitivity and blood pressure. People with normal renin essential hypertension do not commonly respond to sodium restriction.

- **High** renin essential hypertension is less common than other forms of essential hypertension. In this form of high blood pressure high renin levels are associated with hypertension and it is believed to be due to a secondary increase in sympathetic nervous system activation.

  In addition, if the individual is categorized by renin production, the production of renin may not stay constant.

- A healthy eating program is also important. The DASH eating plan encompasses a diet rich in fruits, vegetables, and low-fat dairy products and may lower blood pressure by 8 to 14 mm Hg.

- Limiting alcohol intake is also paramount. The consumption of three or more drinks per day is associated with an elevation in blood pressure. Daily alcohol intake should be decreased to less than one ounce of ethanol in man and 0.5 ounces in women. The 2011 ADA standard supports limiting alcohol consumption in patients with diabetes and hypertension.

- Nutrients have also been shown in clinical trials to improve blood pressure. Potassium and magnesium are particularly important. However, you can have side effects if you take too much of either of these nutrients. Have your doctor measure your potassium level which is part of your electrolyte studies. Magnesium is best measured as RBC magnesium which is the amount of magnesium in your red blood cells.

Medications

- Ace inhibitors (ACE)
- Alpha-adrenergic blockers
- Angiotensin receptor blockers (ARBs)
- Beta-adrenergic blockers
  - Beta-adrenergic blockers with alpha-blocking properties
- Beta-adrenergic blockers with intrinsic sympathomimetic activity
- Beta-adrenergic blockers with nitric oxide-mediated vasodilating activity
- Traditional beta-adrenergic blockers
- Calcium channel blockers
  - Dihydropyridines

- Non-dihydropyridines
- Central alpha-adrenergic agonists
- Combination drugs
- Direct renin inhibitor
- Direct vasodilators

- Diuretics
  - Aldosterone antagonists
  - Loop diuretics
  - Potassium-sparing
  - Thiazide and thiazide-like

The updated Eighth Joint National Committee (JNC 8) guidelines no longer recommend only thiazide-type diuretics as the initial therapy in most patients. According to the JNC 8 guidelines, angiotensin-converting enzyme inhibitors (ACEIs /angiotensin receptor blockers (ARBs), calcium channel blockers (CCBs), and thiazide diuretics are equally effective in hypertensive non-black patients, whereas CCBs and thiazide diuretics are favored in black patients with hypertension.

■ Precision Medicine Therapies

The following are Precision Medicine therapies for hypertension.

Lifestyle Changes

- Weight loss if you are overweight will help lower blood pressure in almost everyone. One study showed that weight loss was as effective as metoprolol (BP medication) in controlling blood pressure.

- Exercise is beneficial to help control blood pressure. One study revealed that approximately 75 percent of people with hypertension were able to lower their blood pressure with a regular exercise program.

- Limiting salt intake is also productive. Avoid high salt foods and try not to add additional salt to your diet.

- A healthy eating program is very important to help regulate your blood pressure. The following are some important ways to change your diet to help with blood pressure control.
  - The DASH diet has been shown to lower BP.
  - The Mediterranean diet has also been shown to lower BP.
  - Adding extra virgin olive oil to the diet is also beneficial.

- A raw food diet also aids in lowering blood pressure.
- Crude onion extract has been shown to decrease blood pressure.
- Garlic: raw, powdered, aqueous extract, or other preparations have been shown to lower blood pressure. Garlic is a direct vasodilator, calcium channel blocker, ACE inhibitor, angiotensin II receptor blocker, and central alpha agonist. All of these mechanisms help to lower your blood pressure. Dose: 10,000 micrograms of allicin per day which is equal to four cloves of garlic (4 grams).
- Whole oats added to the diet lowers blood pressure.
- Milled flaxseed effectively reduces blood pressure.
- Pomegranate juice, 6 to 8 ounces a day, is beneficial.
- Increasing dietary fiber has been shown to lower blood pressure.
- A small amount of dark chocolate lowers blood pressure. White and milk chocolate do not.
- Avoid foods you are allergic to. Studies have shown that food allergy contributes to hypertension.
- Limiting caffeine intake is beneficial.
- Limiting sugar intake helps to control blood pressure.
- Celery has been shown to lower blood pressure since it contains apigenin. Celery is a diuretic (increase the excretion of water from your body), angiotensin II receptor blocker, central alpha agonist, and calcium channel blocker. All of these methods help lower blood pressure. Dose: 4 stalks of celery a day, or 8 tsp. of celery juice three times a day, or 1,000 mg of celery seed extract twice a day, or ½ to 1 tsp. of celery oil three times a day in tincture form.
- Stress reduction lowers blood pressure. Have your healthcare provider measure your cortisol levels and treat according to lab. See chapter on cortisol.
- Smoking cessation lowers blood pressure in many patients.

Nutrients and Herbal Therapies

- **Alpha lipoic acid** has been shown to lower blood pressure since it is a natural calcium channel blocker and direct vasodilator. It also lowers BP through several other mechanisms including reducing oxidative stress and improving mitochondrial function. Dose: 100 to 200 mg a day.

- B vitamins such as riboflavin also have a positive effect on blood pressure. Dose: 500 to 750 mg a day. Folic acid is another B vitamin that studies have shown lowers blood pressure. In addition, vitamin B_6 is effect to lower BP by acting as a diuretic, calcium channel blocker, angiotensin II receptor blocker, and central alpha agonist. Dose: 50 mg twice a day.

- **Calcium** lowers BP by acting as a diuretic, calcium channel blocker, and direct vasodilator. Some studies show that taking calcium does not have an influence on blood pressure.

- **Coenzyme** Q-10 supplementation lowers blood pressure by acting as a diuretic, angiotensin II receptor blocker, central alpha agonist, and direct vasodilator. Patients with essential hypertension have been shown to have lower Q-10 levels than controls. Dose is 100 to 200 mg a day.

- **Flavonoids**, such as quercetin, have been shown to lower blood pressure by functioning as an angiotensin II blocker and vasodilator. Dose: 150 to 750 mg a day. Hesperidin has also been shown to lower BP. Dose: 250 to 500 mg three times a day.

- **Guizhi decoction** (GZD) contains 112 active ingredients. It is a classical Chinese herbal formula to treat hypertension and is now being evaluated in clinical animal trials. The potential mechanisms and therapeutic effects of GZD on hypertension may be attributed to the regulation of cardiac inflammation and fibrosis.

- Hawthorne berry lowers blood pressure since it functions as an ace inhibitor, diuretic, and calcium channel blocker. Dose: 160 to 900 mg a day.

- **Hibiscus sabdariffa.** Medical studies have shown that hibiscus tea and hibiscus extracts have anti-hypertensive affects. Dose: 250 mg of total anthocyanins a day or a tea preparation three times a day.

- **L-arginine** is an amino acid and is a precursor to nitric oxide which is a vasodilator. Dose: 2,000 mg three times a day up to 6,000 mg three times a day. Do not use if you have heart valve abnormalities without seeing your cardiologist.

- **L-carnitine** has been shown to lower BP by acting as a diuretic. Dose:

1,000 mg twice a day. Do not supplement with L-carnitine without seeing your healthcare provider to have your TMO level measured. If you have an elevated TMAO level, then you are not a candidate to take carnitine.

- **Magnesium** has been shown in medical studies to lower blood pressure by acting as a diuretic, calcium channel blocker, and direct vasodilator. Magnesium glycinate or threonate are the best forms to use. Dose: 400 to 600 mg a day. Not all studies reveal a blood pressure lower effect with the use of magnesium.

- **N-acetyl cysteine (NAC)** lowers blood pressure by decreasing arterial resistance and functioning as a natural calcium channel blocker. Dose: 500 mg twice a day. Long-term use of NAC depletes the body of zinc and copper. Therefore, make sure you also take a multivitamin. If you are prone to cysteine kidney stones, then take 1,000 a day of vitamin C to help prevent stone formation.

- **Olive leaf extract** lowers blood pressure by functioning as an ACE inhibitor. It contains compounds called secoiridoid glycosides. Dose: 1,000 mg a day standardized to 16 percent oleuropein.

- **Omega-3-fatty acids** are one of the best document nutrients that have an anti-hypertensive effect. Many studies have shown that supplementing with fish oil lowers blood pressure by functioning as a direct vasodilator, ACE inhibitor, central alpha agonist, and calcium channel blocker. Omega-3-fatty acids also decrease blood viscosity.

- Omega-6-fatty acids, in the form of gamma alpha linoleic acid (GLA), lower blood pressure by promoting the blood vessels to dilate. It also functions as a diuretic, central alpha agonists, and angiotensin II receptor blocker. Safflower oil or sunflower oil are the most common forms of GLA used to control hypertension.

- **Potassium** has been shown to lower both systolic and diastolic blood pressure. It also aids in balancing the hypertensive effects of sodium. Potassium functions as a diuretic, direct vasodilator, central alpha agonist, and angiotensin II receptor blocker. All these mechanisms aid in reducing hypertension. Have your healthcare provider measure your potassium level since you can have side effects if you take too much potassium.

- **Taurine** has been shown to lower blood pressure by functioning as a diuretic, direct vasodilator, and central alpha agonist. Dose: 1,000 to 2,000 mg twice a day.

- **Tomato extract** contains lycopene which is a therapy for hypertension. Dose: 250 mg a day of tomato extract that contains 15 mg of lycopene.

- **Vitamin C** has been shown to decrease blood pressure by lowering oxidative stress and arterial stiffness. It also functions as a diuretic, direct vasodilator, angiotensin II receptor blocker, central alpha agonist, and calcium channel blocker. Dose: 400 to 1,000 mg a day.

- **Vitamin D** has a positive effect on blood pressure according to most clinical trials. Some studies did not show any effect. Have your doctor measure your vitamin D level so that you know the best dose for you.

- **Zinc** has been shown to lower blood pressure by inhibiting the expression of unfavorable genes, improving insulin resistance, and inhibiting the renin-angiotensin-aldosterone system. Dose: 25 mg a day. Zinc and copper need to balance in the body: 10 to 15 mg of zinc to 1 mg of copper.

Hormones

- **Female hormones.** Optimizing and balancing estrogen, progesterone, and testosterone aids in lowering blood pressure in women. Menopause is accompanied by a dramatic rise in the prevalence of hypertension in women, suggesting a protective role of endogenous estradiol on blood pressure. Both animal experimental and human clinical investigations suggest that estrogen engages several mechanisms that protect against hypertension, such as activation of the vasodilator pathway mediated by nitric oxide and prostacyclin and inhibition of the vasoconstrictor pathway mediated by the sympathetic nervous system and angiotensin. However, oral estrogen raises blood pressure. Transdermal delivery of estrogen, which avoids the first-pass hepatic metabolism of estradiol, has a blood pressure lowering effect in postmenopausal women. Consequently, this is another reason that estrogen should always be applied to the skin and not taken by mouth.

- **Thyroid hormones** must be functioning optimally in order to control your blood pressure. One of the symptoms of hypothyroidism (low thyroid function) is hypertension. See the chapter on thyroid hormones.

In fact, one study even showed that patients with subclinical hypothyroidism are at a higher risk of developing high blood pressure and dyslipidemia—high level of lipids—compared to controls. Have your doctor measure all the thyroid studies discussed in the chapter on thyroid hormones.

- **Cortisol.** An optimized cortisol level has been shown to lower blood pressure.

- **Insulin** is the hormone that regulates your blood sugar. Insulin also increases the retention of sodium in the body which increases blood volume and drives up blood pressure if insulin levels are elevated. Normalizing blood sugar and insulin levels aids in controlling your blood pressure. See the chapter on insulin.

- **Melatonin** is the hormone that helps you sleep. However, it also has been shown to lower night-time blood pressure by dilating blood vessels and inhibiting signals from the sympathetic nervous system. In addition, melatonin has proven to lower the high blood pressure that is caused by poor diet choices. It has been shown to protect the kidneys and other organs from long-term consequences of elevated blood pressure. Likewise, controlled release melatonin has been shown to lower both systolic and diastolic blood pressure.

Other Therapies

- **Stevioside** is a constituent of Stevia rebaudiana (Stevia). It has been shown to lower blood pressure since it is a natural calcium channel blocker. Dose: 750 to 1,500 mg a day.

See also Heart Disease.

HYPERTHYROIDISM

As a general definition hyperthyroidism usually refers to the overproduction of thyroid hormones in the body. However, when you read medical texts there are two terms that are associated with the over production of thyroid hormones. They are hyperthyroidism and thyrotoxicosis, and while they both refer to the production of too much thyroid hormone in your body, they are distinctly two different conditions.

The term hyperthyroidism refers to disorders that result from long-term overproduction and release of hormones by the thyroid gland. For individuals with hyperthyroidism the greater number of symptoms can be very subtle and take several weeks to months to be noticed. This occurs because the slight elevation in thyroid hormones is so small that the patient may not notice or put off going to the doctor. Hyperthyroidism is a long-term condition.

On the other hand, thyrotoxicosis refers to excessive thyroid hormone production that is caused by a physiologically based change in the gland. It can be caused by an inflamed or damaged thyroid gland, or by taking or stopping certain drugs. People that have thyrotoxicosis can usually pinpoint the date that their symptoms began and seek medical attention immediately.

With a normally functioning thyroid gland, hormones are released into the blood stream over a 30- to 60-day period. In the case of thyrotoxicosis,

Risk Factors

There are several risks that can increase the possibility of developing hyperthyroidism. The following factors may indicate if an individual is at increased risk:

- **Age.** Hyperthyroidism can occur at any age; it is more common in people 60 years old or older. On the other hand, Graves' disease usually occurs between the ages of 20 and 40.

- **Gender.** In general, women are more likely to develop hyperthyroidism than men. Regarding Graves' disease, there are eight females for every one male with this specific disease.

- **Genetics.** Statistics strongly indicate that genetics plays a role in a person's predisposition to develop hyperthyroidism. While there is no evidence that only one gene is to blame, it is more likely that the presence of several specific genes increases the incidence of hyperthyroidism. However, in order to turn these genes on, it may require one or more triggers or causes, as listed on page 223, to initiate this condition.

- **Ethnicity.** Statistically, the Japanese appear to be at greater risk for hyperthyroidism than other people. This may be attributed to either genetics or a diet high in iodine rich foods.

hormones are released over a shorter period of time, such as a few days or a couple of weeks. This is referred to as a transient hormones excess state. Should thyrotoxicosis occur within an even shorter time frame, this condition is referred to as a thyroid storm or thyroid crisis. It should be considered an emergency and be treated immediately. If left untreated, it can lead to death.

Because hyperthyroidism is sometimes used as an overall term for the overproduction of thyroid hormones, thyrotoxicosis may be considered a category of hyperthyroidism. This can be confusing because the treatments for thyrotoxicosis may be very different from those offered for other hyperthyroid-related disorders. There are a number of disorders caused by, or associated with, hyperthyroidism and/or thyrotoxicosis. These include the following:

- Exogenous causes

- Factitious hyperthyroidism (seen in patients trying to lose weight)

- Iatrogenic hyperthyroidism

- Iodine-induced hyperthyroidism (Jod-Basdow disease)

- Grave's disease (an autoimmune process)

- Hashimoto's thyroiditis in the early stages

- Painless thyroiditis

- Radiation thyroiditis

- Subacute thyroiditis

- Thyroiditis

- Toxic goiters

- Multinodular goiter

- Toxic adenomas

As we see, there are several forms hyperthyroidism can take. To establish if it is hyperthyroidism, we need to be able to identify the condition and know what the options are.

■ Causes of Hyperthyroidism

When the thyroid is diseased, it may produce and release too much thyroid hormone. Various conditions may be the cause for the overproduction of the thyroid hormone, including:

- **Emotional and physical stress.** Recent stress may be a precipitating factor in the development of hyperthyroidism, especially in the class of Graves' disease. The most common precipitating factor is the "actual or threatened" separation from an individual upon whom the patient is emotionally dependent.

- **Environmental toxic exposure.** Studies performed on lab animals showed that exposure to toxic levels of cadmium and/or mercury increased the risk of developing hyperthyroidism.

- **Excess dietary iodine supplementation.** Iodine excess may be a problem particularly in people that take iodine without having their iodine levels measured. Common sources of iodine are iodized salt, betadine washes, and iodine-containing medications, such as amiodarone and radiographic dyes.

A large study looked at the rate of Graves' disease in a population that was required to consume iodized salt. The rate of thyrotoxicosis and Graves' disease was higher throughout the entire study time. The increase in rate included both nodular and diffuse goiters. The conclusion of the study was that iodine supplementation in a group of people that were iodine-sufficient can increase the risk of developing thyrotoxicosis in susceptible people. However, it is important to point out that not having enough iodine can also lead to additional thyroid issues. Make sure to talk to your healthcare provider regarding your own situation, and keep track of your iodine levels when your test results come in. Iodine levels are best measured in the urine.

- **Existing autoimmune diseases.** For those people with pre-existing immune system disorders, such as type 1 diabetes or rheumatoid arthritis, studies have shown that there is an increased risk of developing an overactive thyroid.

- **Foods.** Certain foods can suppress thyroid function, such as cruciferous vegetables, which include broccoli, Brussels sprouts, cabbage, cauliflower, kale, leafy greens, peaches, pears, and soybeans.

- **Infections.** Viral and bacterial infections have been reported in a large percentage of patients with Graves' disease. Studies indicate that a number of these pathogens can trigger the body's immune system to create antibodies; and it is in the body's natural response that a specific antibody may attach itself to the thyroid cells to overproduce hormones.

- **Medications.** Some medications, such as amiodarone, lithium, interferon-alpha, IL-2, and GM-CSF (granulocyte-macrophage colony-stimulating factor), can cause an inflammation of the thyroid gland which in turn can cause an overproduction of thyroid hormones. In addition, taking excessive synthetic thyroid hormone can lead to hyperthyroidism.

- **Pregnancy and recent childbirth.** For women going through pregnancy, there are a number of hormonal changes that their bodies experience. This includes increases in progesterone, estrogen, oxytocin, prolactin, and relaxin—any of these hormones could trigger the development of Graves' disease.

- **Smoking.** Smoking has a significant impact on thyroid function, interfering with the thyroid's ability to absorb iodine. Oddly enough, in some individuals it can result in an excess amount of thyroid hormone production, and in others, a reduction.

- **Thyroid nodules** (Toxic Adenoma, Toxic Multinodular Goiter, Plummer's Disease). A benign growth or nodule that has walled itself off from the rest of the gland may cause an enlargement of the thyroid. When this happens the gland may produce an excess amount of the hormone T4 which will then enter the bloodstream.

- **Thyroiditis (inflamed thyroid gland).** The thyroid gland can become inflamed for a variety of reasons. This inflammation can cause the gland to increase in size and to produce excess amounts of thyroid hormone which will then enter the bloodstream.

■ Signs and Symptoms

The following are the most common signs and symptoms of hyperthyroidism and/or thyrotoxicosis. The progression of these individual symptoms, however, may also differ from one individual to another. It is also important to keep in mind that many of these symptoms can be caused by other underlying problems.

Early Symptoms

- ❑ Anxiety, nervousness, and irritability
- ❑ Brittle fingernails
- ❑ Breast enlargement in men (rare)
- ❑ Bulging eyes (exophthalmia)
- ❑ Constipation
- ❑ Diarrhea and/or an increase in bowel movements

❑ Difficulty in managing diabetes

❑ Elevated heart rate (tachycardia) and/or chest pain

❑ Erectile dysfunction or reduced sexual urges

❑ Eyelid retraction, puffy eyelids, reddening around the eyes, pressure on the eyes, and irritation of the eyes as well as double vision (Graves' thyroid eye disease)

❑ Goiter (enlargement of the thyroid gland)

❑ Heart palpitations (sensation heart is pounding)

❑ Heat or cold intolerance

❑ Muscle weakness

❑ Personality or psychological changes

❑ Perspiring profusely (diaphoresis)

❑ Separation of nail from the nail bed (onycholysis)

❑ Shortness of breath

❑ Skin changes

❑ Slight trembling of the hands or fingers

❑ Weight change (weight loss and gain)

Late Symptoms

❑ Decreased ability to hear

❑ Hoarseness

❑ Lumpy thickening and reddening of the skin, usually on the shins or tops of the feet (Graves' dermopathy)

❑ Menstrual disorders

❑ Puffy face, hands, and feet

❑ Slow speech

❑ Thinning eyebrow hair

Most commonly, younger patients tend to show symptoms of sympathetic activation—that is, the fight or flight response—which brings on anxiety, hyperactivity, and tremors. With patients over 60, the symptoms may more frequently involve cardiovascular related issues which need to be carefully monitored.

■ Testing for Hyperthyroidism

If you are experiencing any of the symptoms associated with

hyperthyroidism, there are a number of tests available to determine whether you have hyperthyroidism or thyrotoxicosis.

- **Physical examination.** Normally, a physician can see some of the more pronounced signs, such as a goiter, high blood pressure, or signs of tremors which can indicate hyperthyroidism.

- **Blood tests.** In a standard blood test, there is usually an increase in the level of thyroid hormones (T3 and T4). There is also a compensatory decrease in the level of the thyroid-stimulating hormone (TSH) since the thyroid is now being stimulated by an antibody, TSH production would naturally drop. In another specialized blood test, the level of the thyroid peroxidase antibody (TPO) is measured. This may indicate that there is an autoimmune disorder present. However, since 5 percent to 10 percent of healthy individuals test positive for TPO, the results of this antibody test may not be conclusive. If the tests all come back within a normal range, these blood tests can at least rule out hyperthyroidism.

- **Fine-needle aspiration (FNA).** If a node is found, a fine-needle aspiration is done. The skin above the node is numbed, and a thin needle is inserted into the node to remove cells and fluid for review. These samples are then sent to a laboratory where a pathologist examines them under a microscope to determine the exact nature of the cells. The pathologist writes up a report on the findings and sends back the report to the ordering physician. While the FNA is designed to determine if the cells are benign or cancerous, up to 30 percent of the FNA biopsies may be inconclusive. When this happens a blood test may be able to provide an answer. However, should it not, traditionally, surgery is the next step to determine if the node is benign or cancerous. Recently, however, a new precision genetic test has been developed to provide an answer based on the initial FNA biopsy which can help prevent unnecessary surgeries.

- **Genetic tests.** Beyond testing for inherited thyroid cancer-prone genes, there are new customized genetic tests available which may be able to rule out whether the cells taken from a FNA procedure are benign or malignant. The tests may also be able to determine how aggressive a cancerous thyroid cell may be. These tests are based upon molecular identification. The results of such tests can enable a surgeon to determine how extensive a surgery is needed or if one is required at all.

- **Radioactive iodine uptake (RAIU).** A radioactive iodine uptake test (RAIU) is designed to measure the amount of iodine your thyroid absorbs and determine whether all or only part of the thyroid is overactive. The amount of radioactive tracer your thyroid absorbs determines if your thyroid function is normal or abnormal. A high uptake of iodine tracer may mean you have hyperthyroidism.

- **Scan of your eye area.** In the case of Graves' disease, if the patient is showing either irritation around the eye and socket, or there is a bulging of the eyes, an ultrasound, magnetic resonance imaging (MRI), or computed tomography (CT) scan may be taken to determine the extent of impact the irritation has caused.

- **Thyroid scan.** A radioactive iodine tracer is injected into the vein in the arm or hand. You then lie on a table with a scanner that produces an image of your thyroid on a computer screen. The image can show whether parts of the thyroid gland are absorbing too much or too little of the radioactive iodine. This test may be given as part of a radioactive iodine uptake test. In that case, orally administered radioactive iodine is normally used to image the thyroid gland.

Based upon the patient's family history, risk factors, symptoms, and test results, the doctor will determine if the diagnosis is hyperthyroidism.

■ Treatment of Hyperthyroidism

The treatment of choice for hyperthyroidism is governed by many factors. It depends on age, goiter size and association with nodular disease, existence of Grave's eye disease, standard of care in the area in which one lives, the personal preference of the treating physician, any other disease processes one may have, and of course the patient's choice. Treatment of thyroid storm is a medical emergency and must be implemented immediately.

The goal of these treatments is to correct the overproduction of thyroid hormone. The following is a summary of common treatments for hyperthyroidism and thyrotoxicosis.

- **Anti-thyroid medication.** One of the first options offered is anti-thyroid medications. Anti-thyroid drugs are designed to interfere with the thyroid glands ability to produce hormones thereby decreasing hormone production. Unlike other treatments, once they are discontinued, they allow the thyroid to function as it previously did. Side effects many vary with each drug. These may include nausea, vomiting, heartburn, headache, rash, joint pain, loss of taste, liver failure, or a decrease in disease-fighting white blood cells. Pregnant women should always check with their doctor regarding when they can start on such medications. These drugs can usually be discontinued once a stable normal thyroid balance has been achieved with other therapies. These medications include the following:

- **Glucocorticoids.** Glucocorticoids in high doses inhibit the peripheral conversion of T4 to T3. In the treatment of Grave's disease, glucocorticoids decrease T4 secretion by the thyroid gland. How effective this response is or how long it lasts is not known. Use of glucocorticoids is usually not suggested for hyperthyroidism and thyrotoxicosis unless there is major eye or skin involvement or if the patient is in thyroid storm. Short-term use only for these conditions is suggested.

- **Iodine and iodine-containing compounds.** Pharmacologic doses of iodine as Lugol's solution or saturated solution of potassium iodide (SSKI) work by the following mechanisms:

  - Decreases iodine transport into the thyroid

  - Inhibits iodine organification and blocks the release of T4 and T3 from the thyroid gland

  - Decreases the vascularity of the thyroid in Graves' disease

  These affects are only transient, lasting only a few days to weeks.

  Thyrotoxicosis may return and even worsen. Consequently, iodine therapy is used only short term in preparation for surgery after a normal state has been achieved and maintained with the use of thionamides. Iodine is also used to treat thyroid storm since it can inhibit thyroid hormone immediately.

- **Oral cholecystographnic agents.** Oral cholecystographnic agents (iodine containing radiocontrast agents) such as iopanoic acid and sodium ipodate) produce a rapid fall in thyroid hormones. They act by inhibition of the peripheral conversion of T4 to T3 and by prevention of thyroid hormone secretion because of the inorganic iodine that is released from the drug. Both iopanoic acid and sodium ipodate, because of their rapid onset of action, are very effective treatments for thyrotoxicosis. They are not effective for long-term treatment because of the escape of thyroid hormone synthesis from the blocking action of iodine. Furthermore, iopanoic acid and sodium ipodate provide a load of iodine to the thyroid which makes the using of radioactive iodine not feasible for weeks. Therefore, these drugs are best used for emergency situations for a rapid decrease in thyroid hormone production, prior to surgery, or while waiting for the effect of radioactive iodine.

● **Perchlorate.** Perchlorate works by inhibiting the transport of iodine into the thyroid. Possible side effects include stomach irritation and aplastic anemia. These side effects are somewhat common; therefore, it stops the use of perchlorate as treatment for hyperthyroidism/thyrotoxicosis long-term. Used in conjunction with thionamides, perchlorate has been used successfully for depleting the thyroidal iodine overload in amiodarone-induced hyperthyroidism.

● **Thionamides.** There are three thionamide drugs, methimazole (MMI), carbimazole, and propylthiouracil (PTU), which are effective in their treatment of Graves'. Thionamides do not block the release of pre-formed thyroid hormone. Consequently, it takes one to six weeks for the thyroid hormones that are already stored and the iodine that is stored to be depleted, and the patient have total relief of symptoms and normalization of thyroid studies. Large goiters with large deposits of thyroid hormone may show a delayed response to thionamides.

The main problem with the use of thionamides is that there is a high relapse rate of thyrotoxicosis when the medications are stopped. Recurrence rate is 50 to 80 percent depending on the length of follow-up. Most relapses occur within 3 to 6 months, but it can occur much later. Remission rates have decreased over the last decade, perhaps due to an increased iodine supply in the diet of the average American. Relapse to hyperthyroidism after treatment suggests that another form of treatment may be necessary. Some patients become hypothyroid after therapy.

Mild side effects have been reported in 1 to 15 percent of patients that take thionamides.

● Hives (urticaria)

● Itching (pruritus)

● Joint pain (arthralgias)

● Slightly elevated liver enzymes

● Skin rash

Severe side effects of thionamides are rare and require prompt discontinuation of the medication.

- Cholestatic necrotic hepatitis
- Decrease of white blood cells (agranulocytosis)
- Inflammation of blood vessels (vasculitis)
- Lupus-like syndrome
- Toxic hepatitis

Thionamides can be used prior to thyroid surgery, with radioactive iodine, or as primary treatment. Treatment is usually for 1 to 2 years and then stopped.

- **Beta blockers (B-Adrenergic Antagonist Drugs).** Beta blockers were originally designed to reduce blood pressure by blocking the effects of epinephrine, also called adrenaline. It does this by slowing down the number of heart beats per minute as well as opening up blocked vessels. This, in turn, reduces tachycardia, palpitations, tremor, and anxiety. The effects of beta blockers are fast, so it is important for use early in the treatment of thyrotoxicosis. These drugs do not affect thyroid function, release, or synthesis. Beta blockers should not be used if you have asthma, emphysema, congestive heart failure, bradycardia (slow heartbeat), hypotension (low blood pressure), COPD (chronic obstructive pulmonary disease), or Raynaud's phenomenon.

- **Radioactive iodine therapy.** In order to function, the thyroid gland needs to absorb iodine on a daily basis. With this therapy, a radioactive form of iodine is orally taken by the patient. As the reactive iodine is absorbed, the low-level radiation is enough to destroy the overactive thyroid cells causing the thyroid to shrink and to produce less hormones.

Because this treatment involves destroying thyroid cells, it will likely have an effect on the amount of thyroid hormones produced in the future. For that reason, a patient's thyroid hormone levels must be checked regularly, and that individual may require thyroid medication to make up for a drop in thyroid hormone production.

This treatment may not be effective in people with large goiters; consequently, several treatments may be needed. If you have a large goiter then surgery may be the therapy of choice. In the elderly, radioactive iodine is usually the treatment of choice. In women that are of childbearing age, they should delay pregnancy for 6 to 12 months after receiving radioactive iodine.

- **Surgery.** Another possible treatment for hyperthyroidism is surgery. The goal of surgery is to decrease the excessive secretion of thyroid hormone and to prevent a relapse of thyrotoxicosis. For a long time, partial thyroidectomy was recommended. Recently, total thyroidectomy (the entire thyroid gland is removed) is more commonly performed. There is a higher rate of hypothyroidism associated with this procedure, but a lower rate of recurrence of hyperthyroidism.

Commonly your doctor will have you treated with thionamide, an anti-thyroid medication, to restore and maintain a normal thyroid state in preparation for surgery. Some surgeons may use inorganic iodine ten days before surgery to induce the involution of the thyroid gland and decrease the vascularity which makes the surgery easier.

Surgery is the best choice for individuals that have a larger goiter, if cancer cannot be ruled out, if cancer is present, and if multiple cold nodules are not expected to respond with shrinkage to radioactive iodine.

Some of the possible side effects of surgery include infection, bleeding, thyroid storm, injury to the recurrent laryngeal nerve, hypoparathyroidism, hypothyroidism, and hypocalcemia (low calcium level). With the partial or whole removal of your thyroid gland, a patient's levels of thyroid hormones must be carefully monitored.

■ Natural Therapies for Hyperthyroidism and Thyrotoxicosis

There are natural therapies for hyperthyroidism that have been shown to be clinically effective for mild disease. These may be used in conjunction with standard medical treatment. Before starting any, each natural option should be discussed with your healthcare provider.

- **Acupuncture.** Acupuncture, the use of small needles strategically placed in the skin, has been used as a treatment in China for thousands of years. Studies in China have shown it effective in treating hyperthyroidism.

- **Cold packs.** By placing ice packs over the thyroid gland, found at the base of your neck, three times a day you can reduce swelling. The cold will also help slow down the function of the thyroid gland.

- **Diet.** In treating your hyperthyroidism, it is important to learn how to get as much nutrition as possible from your food and to learn to make good food choices.

Eat Foods That Are Good for You

Whole fruits, vegetables, and nuts head the list. In addition, a high protein diet has been shown to be effective against mild Graves' disease. These foods contain goitrogens, a naturally occurring chemical, which has been shown to prevent or make it more difficult to utilize iodine. In so doing, they block thyroid synthesis. These goitrogenic foods include:

- Almonds
- Broccoli
- Brussels sprouts
- Cabbage
- Cassava root
- Cauliflower
- Kohlrabi (a vegetable)
- Millet
- Mustard
- Peaches
- Peanuts
- Pine nuts
- Rapeseeds
- Rutabagas
- Soybeans
- Sweet potatoes
- Turnips

However, it is important to understand these foods cannot be reliably used in place of medications in the treatment of Graves' disease since their goitrogen content is low. Furthermore, cooking inactivates the goitrogens. Likewise, no substantial documentation is available to show that dietary goitrogens interfere with thyroid function if the individual has adequate levels of iodine.

Studies have shown that individuals with hyperthyroidism should eat foods that contain flavonoids since they decrease serum T4 and inhibit both the conversion of T4 to T3 and 5'deiodinase activity. Fruits and vegetables of yellow, orange, red, and purple color—such as blueberries, purple grapes, and cherries—contain flavonoids.

Limit Some Food Choices

In addition to eating the right foods, you can minimize your hyperthyroid symptoms by avoiding certain foods and drink.

- **Avoid caffeine.** Caffeine can increase the severity of many Graves' disease symptoms, such as rapid heart rate, anxiety, and tremors. By eliminating products such as soda, coffee, tea, and chocolate from your diet, you can control some of these persistent issues.

- **Avoid foods that contain iodine.** Foods that are high in iodine content, such as seaweeds, iodized salt, fish from the sea, and shellfish, should be avoided.

- **Avoid foods that you are allergic to.** While it may be easy to identify foods and avoid the foods you are allergic to, some people have hidden food allergies that they may not be aware of. Many of these food allergies can aggravate Graves' symptoms. Make sure you are aware of all the foods you may have allergies to.

- **Avoid processed foods.** Cut down or stop consuming foods that are heavily processed, salted, and/or sugared. Also, make sure to consume foods low in iodine. Find a healthful diet that you can stick to.

■ Nutritional Supplements

Nutritional supplements may be helpful in the treatment of mild hyperthyroidism. Free radical injury occurs when the body is exposed to excess thyroid hormone. Low antioxidant status has been found in patients with excess thyroid production. In fact, the degree of cell damage in Graves' disease has been shown to be directly correlated with the amount of oxidative stress that is present. Taking antioxidants such as vitamins A, C, and E have been shown to be helpful alone or in conjunction with medications.

- **Calcium Citrate.** Calcium metabolism may be changed in hyperthyroidism where patients with Graves' disease have an increased risk of developing osteoporosis. Supplementing with calcium may be beneficial.

- **Coenzyme Q-10.** Similar to a vitamin, this substance is a cofactor in the electron-transport chain which is the energy producing cycle in the body. Q-10 levels have been shown to be low in adults and children with hyperthyroidism. Studies have also shown that coenzyme Q-10 levels may return to normal after treatment of hyperthyroidism with conventional therapies. It may be helpful to supplement with Q-10 in individuals with hyperthyroidism that have heart disease and also in people with long-standing uncorrected hyperthyroidism.

- **L-carnitine.** This amino acid is used for the transport of long-chain fatty acids into the mitochondria. L-carnitine is an antagonist of the thyroid hormone in peripheral tissues by inhibiting thyroid hormone entry into the nucleus of the cells. One study conducted over six months used carnitine in patients with hyperthyroidism. Patients taking L-carnitine improved their symptoms and liver profiles, but the patients that did not take L-carnitine were worse. The form of L-carnitine used should be L-carnitine alone or the acetic or propionic acid form and not the D-form. Individuals with elevated TMAO levels should not supplement with L-Carnitine because it can increase their risk of heart disease. Have your healthcare provider measure your TMAO levels and do not take L-carnitine if your TMAO level is high. In addition, if you have compromised kidney function, you may not be able to take L-carnitine or the dose may need to be decreased, therefore contact your physician before taking L-carnitine.

- **Selenium.** Subclinical hyperthyroidism may be due to low selenium intake. In fact, selenium deficiency alters the conversion of T4 to T3 in peripheral tissues, such as the kidney and liver. One study found men fed low selenium diets that their serum T3 levels were increased. A medical trial showed that subjects with autoimmune thyroiditis were given 200 micrograms of selenium for 3 months and their antibodies decreased or resolved. Selenium is one of the supplements that should be considered as a therapy for mild hyperthyroidism in people that are not high in selenium or selenium toxic. Consequently, have your healthcare provider measure your selenium level to make sure you are a candidate for selenium supplementation before beginning this important nutrient.

- **Vitamin A.** Given in large doses this antioxidant has an inhibitory effect on the thyroid gland. Vitamin A supplementation has been shown to decrease the symptoms of Graves' disease. The exact mechanism by which vitamin A works is unknown. If you smoke, then do not consider this therapy since large doses of vitamin A in smokers may be linked to an increased risk of developing lung cancer.

- **Vitamin C (Ascorbic acid).** Animal studies have shown that thyroid hormone in excess can reduce ascorbic acid levels in the blood, liver, adrenal glands, thymus, and kidney. Studies in human trials in patients with hyperthyroidism have also shown an increase in excretion of ascorbic acid. Furthermore, trials have shown that the medications thiourea and thiouracil also lower ascorbic acid levels. Consequently, supplementation with vitamin C is suggested in patients with hyperthyroidism.

Supplementation does not affect the course of the disease, but it may decrease the symptoms and metabolic effects.

- **Vitamin E.** The vitamin may be protective against the oxidative damage caused by hyperthyroidism. In an animal study, animals with hyperthyroidism were given vitamin E which helped to prevent the lipid peroxidation that is associated with hyperthyroidism. Human studies have shown that individuals with hyperthyroidism have low vitamin E levels. Therefore, supplementation with vitamin E is suggested.

- **Zinc.** Red blood cell zinc levels are lower in patients with hyperthyroidism since zinc needs are increased because of greater urinary zinc excretion in this disease process. Therapy with anti-thyroid medications has been shown to normalize RBC zinc levels two months after free T3 and free T4 were normalized.

Herbs

There are more than a few botanical supplements that may be helpful in some patients with mild hyperthyroidism. It is always advisable to work with a trained professional when using herbal supplementation.

- **Bugleweed.** In fact, the German Commission E, Germany's equivalent to the FDA, recognizes the use of bugleweed for mild hyperthyroid conditions associated with the dysfunction of the nervous system based on pharmacologic studies. However, they also stated that in rare situations high dosages have resulted in thyroid enlargement and sudden discontinuation has increased disease symptoms.

- **Club moss.** This herb has been studied for hyperthyroidism like bugleweed. Animal studies using club moss have shown its ability to block TSH activity at the receptor level, block the release of TSH from the thyroid, and suppress the iodine pump. It can also inhibit the peripheral T4-deiodination and conversion to T3.

- **Emblica officinalis.** Animal studies using this herb officinalis are promising. It was shown to reduce T3 and T4 concentrations by a significant amount. Human trials need to be done.

- **Flavonoids.** There are also botanical medicines that contain flavonoids, such as Hawthorne berry, astragalus, ginkgo biloba, licorice, and chamomile that may be helpful for mild hyperthyroidism.

- **Ginger.** It has been found that ginger has a positive effect on thyroid function. Ginger contains magnesium which has been proven to be a key factor in controlling thyroid disease. Since it aids in regulating inflammation, it is considered to also protect against thyroid conditions that are caused by inflammation. Ginger can be used in various ways. Fresh ginger root can be added when cooking or baking in the diced or powder form. In pill form, start with one capsule twice a day.

- **Lemon balm.** This herb has calming effects on the nervous system and has been used since ancient times for this issue. In vitro studies have confirmed that lemon balm's ability to block TSH receptors and inhibit both binding of bovine TSH to human thyroid tissue, and binding of autoantibodies in Graves' disease. Lemon balm has been used extensively in individuals with mild hyperthyroidism.

- **Motherwort.** This is used traditionally to treat anxiety, depression, heart palpitations, and tachycardia. Therefore, it may be good for relief of symptoms of mild hyperthyroidism. It can be used with bugleweed. The German Commission E supports the use of motherwort for the treatment of cardiac disorders associated with anxiety and for the symptomatic relief of mild hyperthyroidism.

- **Tumeric.** Tumeric is an herb that has been used for thousands of years. Like ginger, it can be beneficial in treating inflammation. It has anti-inflammatory properties which help to treat thyroid dysfunctions, such as Graves' disease. You can add turmeric when cooking or it can be taken in capsule form. Follow the dosage directions on the package.

Once the source of the hyperthyroidism has been identified and eliminated, the overproduction of thyroid hormones should stop. However, as a result of a number of treatments, there can now be a permanent underproduction of thyroid hormones which can lead to hypothyroidism. When this happens, patients are put on thyroid hormone for the remainder of their lives in order to normalize their thyroid hormone level. Once done, all the symptoms and signs of hypothyroidism should be reversed.

See also Graves' Disease

HYPOGLYCEMIA

See Premenstrual Syndrome (PMS).

HYPOPARATHYROIDISM

It is estimated that the prevalence of hypoparathyroidism in the United States is 77,000 cases diagnosed each year. The signs and symptoms of hypoparathyroidism are directly related to hypocalcemia (low calcium) or to hyperphosphatemia (high phosphate). They may also be due to treatment that is not effective. The diagnosis of hypoparathyroidism is confirmed by the presence of low concentration of serum or plasma calcium (total corrected for albumin or ionized) in the presence of a low or inappropriately normal level of PTH. A reduced PTH level leads to increased renal tubular phosphate reabsorption and a subsequent elevated level of serum phosphate, which also causes symptoms.

■ Signs and Symptoms of Hypoparathyroidism

❑ Cognitive changes

❑ Depression

❑ Dry hair and dry skin

❑ Hair loss

❑ Headaches

❑ Muscle spasms, cramps, and pain in the legs, feet, stomach, or face

❑ Pain with menstrual periods

❑ Tingling in your fingers, toes, and lips

❑ Weakness

■ Causes of Hypoparathyroidism

There are two forms of hypoparathyroidism, acquired and medical:

1. **Acquired hypoparathyroidism** usually occurs due to irreversible damage to the parathyroid gland or its removal. It may also be due to damage to the vascular supply of the gland. The incidence also depends on the expertise of the surgeon. In some centers, transient postsurgical hypoparathyroidism is common in patients after neck surgery.

2. **Medical hypoparathyroidism** is usually due to genetic, autoimmune, environmental, or other conditions that affect either parathyroid gland functioning or a mass.

Permanent hypoparathyroidism lasting for more than six months is rare post-operatively. Hypoparathyroidism is usually due to postsurgical complications in 75 percent of the cases of this disease. In 25 percent of cases, hypoparathyroidism is due to nonsurgical causes.

■ Etiologies of Medically Related Hypoparathyroidism

- **Autoimmune.** Autoimmune hypoparathyroidism is the most common cause of nonsurgical hyperparathyroidism and may occur as an isolated disease or part of the autoimmune polyglandular syndrome type I (APS-1).

- **Genetic.**

- **Idiopathic (arrives spontaneously without a known cause).**

- **Infiltrative.** Destruction of the parathyroid glands can occur secondary to granulomatous infiltration due to inflammatory disorders such as sarcoidosis, amyloidosis, and Riedel thyroiditis, which is a rare inflammatory disease of the thyroid that causes compression and fibrosis of adjacent tissues.

- **Magnesium imbalance.** Magnesium has a major impact on parathyroid function and on serum calcium level. Both low and high magnesium levels can result in hypocalcemia and altered parathyroid function. Hypocalcemia in association with hypomagnesemia (low magnesium) is resistant to treatment with calcium or vitamin D and requires magnesium supplementation. Deficiencies in intracellular magnesium may develop in the presence of normal serum magnesium. Intracellular magnesium is a key regulator of serum PTH. High levels of magnesium can cause hypocalcemia due to the inhibition of PTH release. Renal impairment decreases magnesium excretion and magnesium levels rise. Excessive intake can also cause hypermagnesemia (high magnesium) due to antacids, laxatives, cathartics, and total parental nutrition (TPN). Other severe illness can lead to transient hypoparathyroidism.

- **Metastatic cancer.** Rarely, metastases to the parathyroid glands can occur that results in hypoparathyroidism. A study revealed that the most common locations of cancers that metastasized to the parathyroid gland in order of occurrence are: breast, leukemia, malignant melanoma, lung, soft tissue (spindle cell sarcomas), and lymphomas.

- **Mineral deposition.** Hypoparathyroidism may be due to deposition of minerals in the parathyroid glands. For example, Wilson's disease can cause hypoparathyroidism secondary to the deposition of copper. Primary or secondary hemochromatosis with iron overload is associated with hypoparathyroidism. In recent years, there has been a decrease in cases due to the institution of chelation therapy.

- **Mitochondrial disorders.** Some mitochondrial disorders have been associated with hypoparathyroidism. They are due to mutations and deletions in mitochondrial DNA.

- **Radiation destruction.** In addition, exposure of the parathyroid glands to ionizing radiation (such as radioactive iodine) can rarely cause hypoparathyroidism.

- **Toxic agents.** The parathyroid gland is resistant to chemotherapeutic and cytotoxic mediations with rare exceptions. However, toxic agents can be an unusual cause of hypoparathyroidism.

- **Transient hypoparathyroidism.** Transient hypoparathyroidism can occur due to severe burn injury. Patients with severe burns can develop low magnesium levels (due to loss through the burn, abnormal intestinal secretion, and increased metabolic rate), hypocalcemia (low calcium), and hypoparathyroidism. Other severe illness can also lead to transient hypoparathyroidism.

As previously mentioned, morbidities of hypoparathyroidism are directly related to low calcium levels or hyperphosphatemia (high phosphorus) levels. This may lead to treatment that is not effective if these possible abnormalities are not taken into consideration. In addition, magnesium has a major impact on parathyroid function and on serum calcium levels. Both low and high magnesium levels can result in hypocalcemia and altered parathyroid function. Hypocalcemia in association with hypomagnesemia is resistant to treatment with calcium or vitamin D and requires magnesium supplementation.

Deficiencies in intracellular magnesium may develop in the presence of normal serum magnesium. Intracellular magnesium is a key regulator of serum PTH. Magnesium has many functions in the body. One of those is that it plays an important role in bone health. It increases the absorption of calcium, activates vitamin D, aids in parathyroid function (decreases bone breaking down), helps calcitonin function (increase the absorption of calcium), activates bone-building osteoblasts, and increases mineralization density. There are many symptoms of magnesium deficiency.

■ Signs and Symptoms of Magnesium Deficiency

- Aggressive behavior
- Anorexia nervosa/weight loss
- Anxiety/depression
- Neck or back pain or spasm
- Carbohydrate cravings
- Chest tightness
- Cold hands and feet
- Confusion/memory loss/ cognitive decline
- Constipation
- Decreased appetite
- Delirium
- Difficulty swallowing
- Fatigue
- Hyperexcitability
- Hyperventilation
- Insomnia
- Irritability
- Muscle cramps, soreness, or twitches
- Nausea/vomiting
- Numbness
- Palpitations
- Poor wound healing
- Salt cravings
- Sensitivity to light or noise
- Spontaneous carpopedal spasm (hand and feet spasm)
- Tingling
- TMJ
- Tremors
- Urinary spasm
- Vertigo
- Weakness

Furthermore, magnesium levels may become elevated. High levels of magnesium can cause hypocalcemia due to the inhibition of PTH release. Renal (kidney) impairment decreases magnesium excretion and magnesium levels rise. Symptoms of magnesium toxicity include drowsiness, lethargy, weakness, and loose stools.

Hyperphosphatemia (high phosphorus levels) are commonly also a cause of many of the problems associated with hypoparathyroidism. Symptoms of high phosphorus levels include extra-skeletal calcification with mineral deposition in the basal ganglia, cornea, renal parenchyma, and other tissues; decreased levels of iron, calcium, magnesium, or zinc; symptoms of diarrhea, fatigue, irritability, and numbness. If you have hypoparathyroidism, your healthcare provider will ask you to avoid foods that are high in phosphorus.

■ Foods High in Phosphorus

- Almonds
- Beef liver
- Brazil nuts
- Brewer's yeast
- Brown rice
- Cashews
- Cheddar cheese
- Chicken
- Dulse
- Eggs
- English walnuts
- Kelp
- Millet
- Peanuts
- Pearled barley
- Pecans
- Pinto beans
- Pumpkin and squash seeds
- Rye grain
- Scallops
- Sesame seeds
- Soybeans
- Wheat
- Wheat bran

Furthermore, low calcium levels are the cause of many of the symptoms of hypoparathyroidism. Common symptoms of hypocalcemia include abdominal pain, muscle spasm and twitching, paresthesias (burning and tingling) of the fingertips, toe tips, or lips, hypertension, depression, moodiness, and bone loss. There is a large variance of signs and symptoms that individuals will have due to hypocalcemia. Some individuals may not have any symptoms even though they are severely hypocalcemic (have low calcium level), while other people may have life-threatening manifestations, such as bronchospasm, laryngospasm, seizures, cardiac arrhythmias, or sudden death. The presence of symptomatic hypocalcemia is a function of not only how severe the hypocalcemia is but how quickly calcium levels declined.

A diagnosis of hypoparathyroidism is confirmed by the presence of low concentration of serum or plasma calcium (total corrected for albumin or ionized) in the presence of a low or inappropriately normal level of PTH. As mentioned, a reduced PTH level leads to increased renal tubular phosphate reabsorption and subsequent elevated level of serum phosphate which also causes symptoms. Your primary healthcare provider will order a serum calcium, serum magnesium, serum parathyroid level, and 24-hour urinary calcium to evaluate you to see if you have hypoparathyroidism. Secondary studies and scans are usually ordered by endocrinology.

Hypoparathyroidism can lead to other diseases, such as kidney stones, renal failure, heart problems, calcium deposits on the brain that can cause slowed movement, tremors, balance problems, and seizures. Cataracts, Addison's disease, and pernicious anemia can also occur. Moreover, many different organs in the body are affected by both acute and chronic manifestations of hypocalcemia and hypoparathyroidism.

■ Cardiovascular (Heart) Manifestations

- Bradycardia (low heart rate)
- Cardiomyopathy/congestive heart failure
- Hypotension (low blood pressure)
- Impaired cardiac contractility
- Increased risk of ischemic heart disease and all cardiovascular outcome in nonsurgical hypoparathyroidism
- Prolonged QT interval
- ST, QS, T-wave changes on ECG suggestive of having a heart attack
- Torsade de pointes or other arrhythmia

■ Dental Manifestations

- Defective root formation
- Dental aplasia or hypoplasia
- Enamel hypoplasia
- Failure of tooth eruption
- Severe dental caries (dental decay)

■ Dermatologic Manifestations

- Brittle hair and hair loss
- Brittle nails with transverse grooves
- Dry, rough, puffy, course skin

■ Immune Manifestations

- Increased risk of infection, particularly urinary tract infection

■ Neurologic and Neuromotor Manifestations

- Basal ganglia and other brain calcifications
- Extrapyramidal or cerebellar dysfunction

- Seizures, most commonly tonic-clonic or focal motor, less common are atypical absence of akinetic seizures

- Spikes and bursts of high-voltage, paroxysmal slow waves on EEG

■ Neuromuscular Manifestations

- Bronchospasm and laryngospasm

- Chvostek sign

- Fatigue

- Muscle cramping with carpal/pedal spasms or generalized muscle contractions

- Neuromuscular irritability

- Perioral/extremity numbness or tingling

- Trousseau sign

■ Neuropsychiatric Manifestations

- Bipolar disorder

- Cognitive changes

- Delirium

- Depression/anxiety

- Irritability

- Psychosis

- Reduced quality of life

■ Ophthalmologic (Eye) Manifestations

- Cataract

- Papilledema

■ Renal (Kidney) Manifestations

- Hypercalciuria

- Hypocalcemia

- Hypocalcemia and hyperphosphatemia due to the lack of PTH action on the kidney, which reflects the major role the kidneys play in setting normal circulating levels of both calcium and phosphate. In the absence of parathyroid hormone, the activity of the mechanisms transporting calcium and phosphate reabsorption become dysfunctional. This results in the chronically low calcium levels and elevated phosphate levels previously described.

- Nephrocalcinosis (too much calcium is deposited in the kidneys)

- Nephrolithiasis (kidney stones)

- Renal failure

- Renal insufficiency

- The product of calcium and phosphate concentration in extracellular fluid in conjunction with mineral crystal inhibitors and promoters is a major determinant of the propensity for calcium phosphate mineral to deposit in soft tissues.

- Vitamin D supplementation can be very complicated in hypoparathyroidism, since it can lead to adverse effects by inducing episodes of high calcium or hypercalciuria, which can lead to renal failure and ectopic mineralization.

■ Skeletal Manifestations

- Decreased bone remodeling   - Increases in bone mass

■ Treatment of Hypoparathyroidism

Treatment of hypoparathyroidism usually includes the following: calcium and judicious use of vitamin D. Your doctor may suggest a special form of vitamin D called calcitriol. The serum half-life of calcitriol is four to six hours, which is short compared with the biological half-life of other forms of vitamin D, which is about three weeks. High calcium levels can occur during your treatment with any form of vitamin D, but it only takes a few days to resolve with calcitriol rather than a few weeks after stopping vitamin D_2 or D_3. It is also recommended that you avoid foods that are high in phosphorus, and phosphate binders may further be recommended.

Moreover, you may be placed on a dietary restriction of sodium. Your healthcare provider will also monitor other functions in your body and look for complications of the disease. They may also prescribe parathyroid hormone and diuretics (water pills). Parathyroid hormone supplementation, like any hormone, can have possible side effects, which your doctor will closely monitor if you are prescribed parathyroid hormone.

■ Possible Side Effects of Parathyroid Hormone Therapy

- Headache
- Hypercalcemia (high calcium)
- Hypercalciuria (high calcium in the urine)
- Hypocalcemia (low calcium)

- Muscle spasm
- Nausea
- Paresthesia (tingling or pricking sensation)

These same side effects can, however, be seen in people that are not on parathyroid hormone but have hypoparathyroidism. In addition, initially therapy with parathyroid hormone was thought to increase an individual's risk of developing osteosarcoma (cancer of the bone), since it was a possible side effect seen in animal studies. The risk has been found to be dose related, and the dose of parathyroid hormone used in patients is much lower per body weight than that used in animal trials.

HYPOTHYROIDISM

Hypothyroidism—an underactive thyroid—is a more common disorder than you may think. As of 2014 the American Association of Clinical Endocrinologists (AACCE) has cited that about 27 million Americans suffer from either an overactive or underactive thyroid gland. Of these, around 80 percent of them are women. The AACCE has stated that a woman is five to eight times more inclined to have an underactive thyroid than a man, and women over the age of 50 are at a higher risk. While hypothyroidism can take several forms, the most common is Hashimoto's thyroiditis.

Hypothyroidism is defined as low thyroid function, or an underactive thyroid, where the thyroid gland does not make enough thyroid hormones to allow the body to function optimally. The main function of the thyroid hormone is to oversee your metabolism; therefore, people with this condition have symptoms associated with a low functioning metabolism. Hypothyroidism disturbs the normal equilibrium of the chemical reactions in the body. Unfortunately, the earliest signs and symptoms of low thyroid function can occur several years prior to laboratory results being abnormal. It is therefore important to be aware of this disorder's signs and symptoms.

Risk Factors for Hypothyroidism

There are a number of risk factors that can increase the possibility of developing hypothyroidism. The following factors may indicate if an individual is at increased risk:

- **Age.** Although, hypothyroidism can occur at any age, woman over the age of sixty are more likely to develop hypothyroidism.

- **Autoimmune Disorders.** Medical research has found that the majority of people with hypothyroidism produce antibodies that attack and destroy thyroid tissue. This process over time limits the amount of thyroid hormone being produced, which leads to hypothyroidism.

- **Genetics.** Statistics strongly indicate that genetics plays a role in a person's predisposition to develop hypothyroidism. While there is no evidence that only one gene is to blame, it is more likely that the presence of several specific genes increases the incidence of hypothyroidism. However, in order to turn these genes on, it may require one or more triggers, as listed below, to initiate this condition.

- **Gender.** Women are at a higher risk of developing hypothyroidism then men.

- **Ethnicity.** Statistically, Whites or Asians appear to be at greater risk for hypothyroidism than other people.

■ Causes of Hypothyroidism

The cause of hypothyroidism is commonly due to a problem with the thyroid gland. Less common etiologies may be related to problems in the brain or the pituitary gland. In addition, hypothyroidism may be due to a number of other factors, such as diet, Hashimoto's thyroiditis (see page 248), an unhealthy gut, thyroid surgery, radiation therapy, and medications. In addition, as deficiencies increase in certain minerals and vitamins that are factors that cause decreased production of T4, it can lead to symptoms of hypothyroidism.

■ Diet

Some studies have shown that a diet high in soy may decrease thyroid function. Natural-occurring chemicals in the soy may interfere with the absorption of thyroid hormones that you may be taking. This is controversial in the medical literature, but if you are on a high soy diet, and you are suffering from a thyroid problem, then you may want to decrease or stop your soy intake to see if it improves your thyroid function.

Naturally occurring chemicals are contained in many vegetables that disrupt normal function of the thyroid. Additionally, many foods may be deficient in several nutrients. (See related sections on nutritional deficiencies that follow.)

Iodine Deficiency. Iodine deficiency is a major cause of hypothyroidism. Iodine has therapeutic actions in the body. It is an antibacterial, anticancer, antiparasitic, antiviral, and mucolytic agent. The thyroid gland uses iodine on a daily basis. Iodine deficiency may affect other organs in the body as well, such as breasts, prostate, kidneys, spleen, liver, blood, salivary glands, and intestines.

There are many causes of iodine deficiency including the following:

- Soil your food is grown in is deplete in iodine

- Diets without ocean fish or sea vegetables, such as seaweed

- Inadequate use of iodized salt (low salt diet) in a region such as the Midwest which is low in iodine

- Diet that is high in pasta and breads which contain bromide (bromide binds to iodine receptors and prevents iodine from binding)

- Fluoride use (inhibits iodine binding)

- Vegan and vegetarian diets

- Sucralose (artificial sweetener that contains chlorinated table sugar)

- Medications (the following are some examples, but any medication that contains bromide or fluoride can lead to iodine deficiency):
  - Atrovent inhaler (contains bromide)
  - Ipratropium nasal spray (contains bromide)
  - Flonase (contains fluoride)
  - Flovent (contains fluoride)

The Importance of Iodine

Iodine is essential for everyone. It is a chemical element that is crucial for good health. Many conditions beside hypothyroidism may be improved with iodine supplementation including:

- Dupuytren's contracture
- Excess mucous production
- Fatigue
- Fibrocystic breast disease
- Headaches and migraine headaches

- Hemorrhoids
- Keloids
- Ovarian cysts
- Parotid duct stones
- Peyronie's disease
- Sebaceous cysts

Breast health is related to iodine levels. Studies have shown that areas of the world with high iodine intake like Japan have a lower rate of breast cancer. It is estimated that the breasts need approximately 150 micrograms of iodine per day in an average woman.

According to the World Health Organization, up to 72 percent of the world's population is affected by an iodine deficiency disorder. If you take thyroid hormone and you then start taking iodine you may need less thyroid medication. Therefore, it is best if you have your iodine levels measured before you start on thyroid hormone. In fact, sometimes your symptoms of hypothyroidism may resolve, and your labs may normalize with just taking iodine if you are low in this important nutrient. Most people do better when they take iodine supplements; take both iodine and iodide as one preparation. Lugol's solution would be one way of doing this. It is a liquid but has a metallic taste so you may opt to take the iodine/iodine supplement as a pill.

If you are on one of these medications do not discontinue their use. Instead see your healthcare provider and have your iodine levels measured to see if you are deficient in iodine. Then your physician can make appropriate recommendations.

It is very important that you have your iodine levels measured before you start taking iodine. Too much iodine in the diet, or by supplementation, has been associated with thyroiditis which is an inflammation of your thyroid gland. High levels of iodine can cause it to be trapped by thyroglobulin. Elevated levels of iodinated thyroglobulin then prompt the immune system to react and to cause inflammation. Furthermore, research has shown that in some areas of the world where there is high dietary iodine content or excessive supplementation that there is also an increase in not just thyroiditis but also thyroid cancer. Therefore, it is important that you have your iodine levels measured before you begin iodine replacement. If you are on an iodine supplement, taking vitamin B2 (Riboflavin) and vitamin B3 (Niacin) helps makes the iodine easier for the thyroid gland to absorb. Some studies suggest that if you have Hashimoto's thyroiditis (see page 177) that you should not supplement with iodine. More research needs to be done on this subject.

Iron Deficiency. One of the issues that may result from of an underactive thyroid is iron deficiency. In order for your thyroid to function optimally you have to have enough iron in your body. When the thyroid is underactive, the red blood cell production drops. It also plays a part in T4 to T3 conversion. In addition, iron is necessary for optimal immune system health, which is important if you are suffering from Graves' disease or Hashimoto's thyroiditis.

Iron deficiency can be caused by the following:

- Loss of blood
- Consuming too little iron
- Body's inability to absorb iron
- For women, pregnancy and blood loss during the menstrual cycle

Women are more likely to be deficient in iron, especially in their child-bearing years.

Magnesium Deficiency. Magnesium is an important supplement since most people are deficient in this mineral. Seven out of every ten Americans suffer from magnesium deficiency. Although there are several symptoms resulting from magnesium deficiency, one of the most common one is low thyroid function. Magnesium is necessary for the proper absorption of iodine. In addition, although magnesium is essential to every organ in your body, it is particularly important in the function of the heart, kidneys, and muscles.

Magnesium deficiency can result when you take large doses of vitamin C. The problem being that vitamin C competes with magnesium. In addition, healthy thyroid function relies on a balance of calcium and magnesium in the body.

Other causes of magnesium deficiency include:

- Alcohol abuse
- Certain medications
- Diarrhea
- Eating a diet high in trans fatty acids
- Excessive sugar intake
- Extreme athletic competition
- Gastrointestinal disorders
- High caffeine intake
- Increased consumption of foods and drinks high in oxalic acid (such as almonds, cocoa, spinach, and tea)
- Minimal intake of foods rich in magnesium
- Phosphates in soft drinks
- Poor absorption
- Stress
- Surgery
- Taking magnesium supplements while eating a high fiber meal
- Trauma

Selenium Deficiency. The mineral selenium is very important for your general health, as well as for your thyroid gland and thyroid hormones to function properly in your body. A deficiency in selenium can affect the conversion process of T4 to T3. Selenium deficiency can be rare, however, it can develop under certain conditions. The following are some of these circumstances:

- Foods that are grown on poor selenium soils
- Malabsorption, especially in the very elderly
- Severe gastrointestinal disorders

Vitamin B Deficiency. A deficiency in vitamin B_2 can contribute to a low functioning thyroid. A lack of Vitamin B_2 suppresses the production of T4 and the thyroid and adrenal glands from secreting their hormones. Vitamin B_3 is needed to keep the endocrine cells in efficient working order. It plays a role in the production of thyroid hormones. Vitamin B_3 is needed to produce tyrosine (an amino acid) in the body, and T3 and T4 are derived from tyrosine. Also, be aware that taking vitamin B2 (riboflavin) and vitamin B3 (niacin) is crucial if you are on iodine supplementation. It is also important in maintaining a healthy thyroid.

Vitamin D Deficiency. Like magnesium, many people are not aware that they have low levels of Vitamin D. Low levels of Vitamin D may interfere with the thyroid functioning properly. If you are suffering from an autoimmune thyroid condition, you can benefit from being tested for a deficiency in vitamin D. You can request your Vitamin D level to be checked when you have your next blood test. Besides taking daily vitamin D supplements, daily exposure to the sun is beneficial to your overall well-being.

Zinc Deficiency. Without the existence of zinc in the body the thyroid cannot convert the less active hormone T4 to the more active hormone T3. The hypothalamus also depends upon zinc to make the hormone it uses to cue the pituitary gland to switch on the thyroid. Too little zinc leads to a low functioning thyroid. In fact, zinc is a cofactor in over 100 reactions in the body. Chronic zinc deficiency can weaken your immune system.

■ Medications

Sometimes medications or nutrients are associated with a decrease in thyroid function. They may affect the thyroid function if your thyroid is intact, if you are dependent on levothyroxine, or it may suppress your TSH level. The following items lower absorption of thyroid hormone or elevate the excretion of thyroid hormone:

- Aluminum hydroxide
- Bile acid sequestrants
- Calcium
- Ferrous sulfate
- Lactose
- Sucralfate

The following are other medications that may also alter thyroid function:

- Amiodarone (inhibit conversion of T4 to T3)
- Cimetidine (can modify peripheral metabolism of thyroid hormones)
- Clomiphene
- Haloperidol
- Lithium (blocks iodine transport)

- Metoclopramide
- Oral contraceptives

There are also medications that increase the clearance of thyroid hormone so that it leaves the body sooner, such as:

- Carbamazepine
- Phenobarbital
- Phenytoin
- Rifampin
- Ritonavir
- Sertraline
- Tamoxifen, if used for more than one year

For those who rely on treatment with thyroid hormone medicine, taking certain supplements, for example calcium or iron, at the same time as the thyroid medication may decrease the amount of thyroid medicine that is being absorbed. It is recommended that calcium and iron supplements should not be taken at the same time as the thyroid hormone medication.

■ Signs and Symptoms of Hypothyroidism

Early diagnosis of hypothyroidism isn't always easy. Most people with an underactive thyroid aren't aware that they have this condition. They may suffer a number of symptoms without recognizing that the symptoms are thyroid-related or that there may be no symptoms early on in the disease process. Often times, the physician may minimize or misdiagnose the symptoms. The signs and symptoms of hypothyroidism normally progress slowly, over months or years, and quite often they may be confused with other disorders. The following are signs and symptoms of hypothyroidism:

- Acne
- Agitation/irritability
- Allergies
- Anxiety/panic attacks
- Arrhythmias (irregular heart rhythm)
- Bladder and kidney infections
- Blepharospasm (eye twitching) is more common
- Carpel tunnel syndrome
- Cholesterol levels that are high (hypercholesterolemia)
- Cognitive decline
- Cold hands and feet

- Cold intolerance
- Congestive heart failure
- Constipation
- Coronary heart disease/acute myocardial infarction (heart attack)
- Decreased cardiac output
- Decreased sexual interest
- Delayed deep tendon reflexes
- Deposition of mucin (glycoprotein) in connective tissues
- Depression
- Dizziness/vertigo
- Down turned mouth
- Drooping eyelids
- Dull facial expression
- Ear canal that is dry, scaly, and may itch
- Ear wax build-up in the ear canal (cerumen)
- Easy bruising
- Eating disorders
- Elbows that are rough and bumpy (keratosis)
- Endometriosis
- Erectile dysfunction
- "Fat pads" above the clavicles

- Fatigue
- Fibrocystic breast disease
- Fluid retention
- Gallstones
- Hair loss in the front and back of the head
- Hair loss in varying amounts from legs, axilla, and arms
- Hair that is sparse, coarse, and dry
- Headaches including migraine headaches
- High cortisol levels
- High C-reactive protein (CRP)
- Hoarse, husky voice
- High homocysteine levels (hyperhomocysteinemia)
- High insulin levels (hyperinsulinemia)
- Hypertension
- Hypoglycemia (low blood sugar)
- Impaired kidney function
- Inability to concentrate
- Increased appetite
- Increased risk of developing asthma
- Increased risk of developing bipolar disorder

- Increased risk of developing schizoid or affective psychoses

- Infertility

- Insomnia

- Iron deficiency anemia

- Joint stiffness (arthralgias)

- Loss of eyelashes or eyelashes that are not as thick

- Loss of one-third of the eyebrows

- Low amplitude theta and delta brain waves.

- Low blood pressure

- Low body temperature

- Menstrual cycle pain

- Menstrual irregularities including abnormally heavy bleeding

- Mild elevation of liver enzymes

- Miscarriage

- Morning stiffness

- Muscle and joint pain

- Muscle cramps

- Muscle weakness

- Muscular pain

- Nails that are brittle, easily broken, ridged, striated, thickened nails

- Need to get up and urinate in the middle of the night (nocturia)

- Nutritional imbalances

- Osteoporosis (bone loss)

- Abnormal sensation of feeling burning, tingling, and itching (paresthesia)

- Poor circulation

- Poor night vision

- Premenstrual syndrome (PMS)

- Puffy face

- Reduced heart rate

- Ringing in the ears (tinnitus)

- Rough, dry skin

- Shortness of breath

- Sleep apnea

- Slow movements

- Slow speech

- Swollen eyelids

- Swollen legs, feet, hands, and abdomen

- Tendency to develop allergies

- Vitamin B_{12} deficiency

- Weight gain

- Yellowish skin discoloration due to the inability to convert beta carotene into vitamin A

There are some conditions that may be or may not be signs and symptoms of hypothyroidism, such as growth hormone deficiency in children, retrograde uterus, vitiligo, skin cancer, dry eyes, TMJ, and teeth clenching. If you suffer from any one or a number of these health issues, and no root cause has not been found to alleviate the problem, perhaps it's time to consider looking at how well your thyroid is functioning.

■ Diagnosis

Early detection of hypothyroidism is not always easy. However, there are a number of steps you can take to discover if you are suffering from an underactive thyroid. This process can incorporate several factors, such as clinical evaluation and blood tests. In addition, since a thyroid condition or disease may encompass many factors, other tests may be administered as well, such as imaging tests and biopsies.

Self-Awareness. As you have seen on page 78, there are many signs and symptoms associated with the underproduction of thyroid hormones. A lack of these key chemicals can cause many health issues to occur. If you see that you suffer from a number of these problems, you can conduct a simple home test to see if there is a possibility of you having this condition.

Home Testing. If you are experiencing specific signs or symptoms that indicate you may have an underactive thyroid (see page 253), you can administer a safe and simple home test (see inset on page 257). You can determine the possibility of any potential thyroid dysfunction on your own, at your home, by measuring you basal temperature. Although this test is obviously not an official diagnosis of a thyroid dysfunction, it can give you some indication that you need to follow up with your physician for further testing to be administered.

■ Consult With Your Doctor or Other Healthcare Provider

If you feel a problem does exist, it is very important that you see your healthcare provider for an evaluation of your thyroid gland; and, that you have a complete workup done and not a partial workup.

Clinical Evaluation. Your physician will perform a complete physical exam of the gland, where he/she palpates your thyroid to determine if there are any lumps, nodules, growths (goiters), or masses. In addition, he/she will be checking the thyroid's size, and if it is solid and firmly fixed in place.

Simple Home Tests to Determine
If You Have a Potential Problem

The thyroid gland can be thought of as the body's thermostat. The hormones produced by the thyroid play a role in keeping you warm. Some patients will have normal or even optimal levels of thyroid hormone, but they still will have symptoms of hypothyroidism. For these individuals it is important to get a basal body temperature, since keeping the body at its optimal temperature setting cannot be achieved when the thyroid is struggling.

By measuring your basal temperature, yourself at home, you can determine if you have a thyroid issue. A basal body temperature is the temperature taken underneath your arm.

1. Place a mercury type thermometer within reach before bedtime.

2. Shake it down until you reach 96 degrees Fahrenheit.

3. In the morning as soon as you awake place the thermometer under your armpit for 10 minutes.

4. You take your temperature for three consecutive days and record the temperature.

A normal temperature is 97.8 to 98.2 degrees Fahrenheit. If you have an underactive thyroid, your average temperature will be lower than 97.8 degrees Fahrenheit. If you are a menstruating woman, then take your temperature during your menstrual cycle.

Blood Tests. The blood test is the most common test and plays an important role in diagnosing thyroid disease and treating thyroid conditions. A number of blood tests will be done in order to determine if you are suffering from hypothyroidism. Your physician will be evaluating your TSH, free T4, freeT3, rt3 (reverse T3), and thyroid antibodies (see page 165).

Thyroid binding globulin (TBG) can also be measured, see page 82. This is the amount of stored hormone. It is produced by the liver and is affected by illness, liver disease, and some medications. Sometimes estrogens can raise TBG, so this is another test that your doctor may order. Your healthcare provider may also order thyroid releasing hormone (TRH) also called thyrotropin-releasing factor (TRF), which is a hormone that stimulates the release of thyroid stimulating hormone (TSH) and prolactin from the pituitary. (See page 75.) Some individuals have an autoimmune process where their body is literally trying to attack its own thyroid gland and the body produces a normal amount of thyroid hormone or not enough. This is called Hashimoto's thyroiditis, where your test results reveal that your thyroid antibody levels are high.

Imaging Tests. Laboratory tests may not be enough to diagnosis thyroid dysfunction. Sometimes more tests are ordered. Imaging tests are administered for a diagnosis of various thyroid disorders. The following are other tests that may be performed:

- Iodine Uptake Scan: to measure the absorption of iodine in the thyroid.

- Thyroid Scan: a radioisotope is administered, usually given with the iodine uptake. Cells that do not absorb iodine will appear "cold (lighter on the scan)," a cell absorbing too much iodine will appear "hot (darker)."

- Thyroid Ultrasound: high frequency sound waves provide an image of the thyroid gland. It aids in performing fine need biopsies.

Fine Needle Aspiration (FNA). Fine needle aspiration is a type of biopsy that is commonly performed to detect or rule out cancer cells in the thyroid. It is commonly performed on swellings or lumps found in the thyroid. The fine needle aspiration can identify the type of cells contained in the abnormal tissue or fluid (see page 82).

Some patients have an autoimmune process where their body is literally trying to attack its own thyroid gland and the body produces a normal amount of thyroid hormone or not enough thyroid hormone. This is called Hashimoto's thyroiditis. Your test results reveal that your thyroid antibody levels are high.

■ Treatment of Hypothyroidism

There are several things to consider in looking at treatment for low thyroid function. You may benefit from detoxification of the liver or helping your gut stay healthy. You may have nutritional deficiencies and improving your nutritional status may improve your thyroid function. You may be taking a medication that causes your thyroid not to function as well as it could. This does not mean that you should stop your medication, but it does mean that certain medications may cause your thyroid not to function optimally. Therefore, you may have to replace a nutrient that is deplete due to the medication or you may have to take thyroid medication due to another drug that you are taking. Last, you may benefit from thyroid replacement as a medication.

■ Detoxification

Sometimes individuals with hypothyroidism do not need medication but would benefit from a quality detoxification program. There is evidence that elements in the environment and diet can lead to thyroid conditions. You can treat these thyroid problems by detoxing your thyroid. PCBs, dioxins, DDT, HCB (hexachlorobenzene), phthalates, and high levels of heavy metals, such as lead, arsenic, and mercury can cause dysfunction of your thyroid gland. It can affect both the production and conversion of thyroid hormones. It is possible to measure levels of most of these toxins and then have these removed. Cleaning out many of the toxins will not only address your thyroid symptoms, but it will give you an overall sense of well-being and good health. If you have never used detoxification supplements, it may be wise to consult with a doctor first.

The 5R program (Remove, Replace, Repopulate, Repair, and Rebalance) is an effective way to stabilize and treat gastrointestinal dysfunction and to further gastrointestinal health. Sometimes when the patient's GI tract health is improved by using the 5R program they no longer have symptoms of hypothyroidism, and their labs also normalize.

With any detoxification program you need to follow certain guidelines to make it most effective.

- Take a quality cleansing product

- Eat healthy and avoid refined foods, sugars, and junk food

- Drink purified water and avoid alcohol, sodas, and sugary drinks

- Be sure that you are eliminating the toxins

After your first detoxification program it is recommended that you go through detoxification once a year. (*See also* Diet on page 260.)

■ Diet

Besides nutritional supplements, your diet, and the kinds of foods you consume can provide you with some of the nutrients needed for a healthy thyroid gland. Whether or not you need a nutrient supplement in addition to your diet can be determined by a blood test that will indicate where you are deficient. (See reference section) Fortunately there are supplements, herbs, and nutrients that can boost the conversion of T4 to T3. The following should be considered:

- Ashwagandha (an herb)
- High protein diet
- Iodine
- Iron
- Melatonin
- Potassium

- Replacement of testosterone in men (decreases the concentration of thyroid binding globulin)
- Selenium
- Tyrosine (an amino acid)
- Vitamins A, B_2, E
- Zinc

Some studies have shown that a diet high in soy may decrease thyroid function. This is controversial in the medical literature, but if you are on a high soy diet then you may want to decrease your soy intake to see if it improves your thyroid function.

A diet consisting of processed foods and sodas leads to magnesium deficiency. Foods that are rich in magnesium consist of nuts and seeds, legumes, meats, and grains, such as rice and oats.

Iron can be found in foods such as meat, fish, and poultry. The iron found in these foods is absorbed easily. Plant-based, iron-containing foods, such as nuts, vegetables, grains, and fruits, are less absorbable. To keep your ferritin (a protein in the body that binds iron) levels at normal range it is crucial to either get enough iron from the foods you eat or from a supplement or from both.

To ensure you are consuming a rich source of vitamin B_2 you should include meat, mushrooms, almonds, whole grains, and leafy green vegetables in your diet. Foods high in vitamin B_3 are chicken, turkey, beef, and pine nuts. Some dietary sources of vitamin D include fish liver oils, beef liver, egg, alfalfa, and mushrooms. The mineral zinc can be found in protein-rich foods, such as meat, nuts, legumes, seafood, and whole grains.

If you have high or positive thyroid antibodies, then the best thing that you can do is to stop ingesting any gluten. The next best thing that you can do is to help your gastrointestinal tract (GI tract) be healthier.

■ Supplementation

There are several nutritional supplements you can take to stabilize your thyroid gland and restore its function, such as iodine, magnesium, selenium, vitamin B, vitamin D, and zinc. A deficiency in any of these nutrients can negatively affect your health. Not everyone with a hypothyroidism is deficient in the same nutrients, therefore it is necessary to be tested to determine what nutrients you may be deficient in. If you are lacking in basic nutrients, then starting a multivitamin may help your thyroid function improve.

- **Iodine.** Iodine has therapeutic actions in the body. It is an antibacterial, anticancer, antiparasitic, antiviral, and mucolytic agent. The thyroid gland uses iodine on a daily basis. Iodine is needed for the production of thyroid hormones.

- **Iron.** Iron and other minerals play an important role in hormone synthesis. Optimal levels of ferritin (storage iron) are 100 ng/ml. If you are a menstruating woman, then your ferritin levels should be at least 130 ng/ml since you lose iron every month when you menstruate. High levels of ferritin increase your risk of heart disease so ask your healthcare provider if you need to take iron.

- **Magnesium.** There is a direct link between magnesium and a healthy thyroid as well as heart related conditions, however, a magnesium deficiency is difficult to test for. You can boost your magnesium intake by eating a well-balanced diet, which includes dark, leafy vegetables, seeds and nuts, and eliminate caffeine from your diet. Magnesium supplements should be taken with caution since they may interact with certain medications. If you are taking any medications, check with your healthcare provider to see if there is a negative interaction.

- **Selenium.** One study looked at patients that were critically ill and showed that supplementation with selenium normalized thyroid lab results. Adding one or two Brazil nuts or garlic to your diet every day can help to provide you with the needed selenium supplementation.

You can get toxic with the use of selenium; therefore, see your doctor or other healthcare provider before starting high doses of selenium.

- **Vitamin B$_2$.** Make sure you are getting enough vitamin B$_2$. It is necessary in regulating thyroid enzymes and maintaining healthy thyroid function. Eating almonds, eggs in moderation, cashews, salmon, and broccoli help to boost your B$_2$ levels.

- **Vitamin B$_3$.** Vitamin B$_3$ is instrumental in building a strong immune system, and the cause of an underactive thyroid has often been associated with a weak immune system. For a mild vitamin B$_3$ deficiency, 50 to 100 mg per day in divided doses is recommended.

- **Vitamin D.** Vitamin D is key in keeping your bones strong; however, research suggests that low levels of vitamin D may have an effect on the thyroid working properly, as well as your immune system. See your healthcare provider to have your vitamin D levels measured to determine your exact dose.

- **Zinc.** Zinc supplementation has been shown to aid in a healthy thyroid hormone metabolism. Eating a healthy diet and zinc supplements can be taken to treat a zinc deficiency. Taking too much zinc can cause toxicity. Zinc deficiency in humans can result from a reduced dietary intake and an inadequate absorption of the mineral.

■ Disorders Caused By or Associated With Hypothyroidism

There are many diseases and conditions that have been associated with hypothyroidism. Depression has been strongly associated with hypothyroidism as have heart disease and memory loss.

- **Ankylosing Spondylitis (AS).** Ankylosing spondylitis is a kind of chronic rheumatic disease that affects the spine. The spine's vertebrae may fuse together causing pain and stiffness from the neck down to the lower back. Eventually it may result in a stooped-over posture. This condition affects men two to three times more than women. The inflammation in ankylosing spondylitis has been a subject of research. This inflammation has been linked to a low functioning thyroid and the activation of the body's immune system.

- **Arthritis.** Among the various hormonal influences that operate on the antioxidant balance, thyroid hormones play particularly important roles, since hypothyroidism has been shown to be associated with oxidative stress. Oxidative stress is defined as an imbalance between the production of prooxidant substances and antioxidant defenses which causes an inflammatory response. One of the manifestations of inflammation is arthritis and one of symptoms of hypothyroidism is arthritis. Interestingly, when the hypothyroidism is treated the pain tends to improve.

- **Attention Deficit Hyperactivity Disorder.** Attention deficit hyperactivity disorder is a condition characterized by impulsive symptoms, inattention, easily distracted, forgetfulness, and hyperactivity that affects everyday functioning. Some studies have shown that ADHD may be related to thyroid dysfunction. They found that increased levels of thyroid stimulating hormones correlated with an inability to sustain one's attention.

- **Cancer Mortality.** Thyroid hormone has been shown to be involved in carcinogenesis via its effects on cell proliferation pathways. However, the number of studies examining thyroid dysfunction and cancer risk and mortality is limited. One study revealed a significant increased risk of bone, skin, and breast cancer among patients with subclinical hypothyroidism.

- **Chronic Fatigue Syndrome (CFS).** Chronic fatigue syndrome has been associated with an underactive thyroid, however very often misdiagnosed. When diagnosed properly, the majority of cases are women in the age bracket of 25 to 45 years old. CFS is a medical condition where you suffer from long-term fatigue that is not due to exertion and this condition puts limitations on your ability to carry out normal daily activities. Research has indicated that a relationship exists between CFS and thyroid autoimmunity. These studies suggest that the immune system may be chronically active which would explain the fatigue and lack of energy you experience.

- **Diabetes.** Studies have found that diabetes and thyroid disorders tend to coexist in patients. Both conditions involve a dysfunction of the endocrine system. Thyroid disorders can have a major impact on blood sugar control, and untreated thyroid disorders affect the management of diabetes in patients. Several reports documented a higher-than-normal prevalence of thyroid dysfunction in the diabetic population. This is not surprising since thyroid hormones affect glucose metabolism via several mechanisms. Furthermore, both clinical and subclinical hypo-thyroidism have been recognized as insulin resistant states. Therefore, hypothyroidism is now considered a risk factor for developing diabetes mellitus.

Moreover, diabetes itself influences thyroid hormones and thyroid diseases. Altered thyroid hormones have been described in patients with diabetes, especially those with poor glycemic control. In diabetic patients, the nocturnal TSH peak is blunted or abolished, and the TSH response to TRH (*thyrotropin releasing hormone*) is impaired. Likewise, reduced T3 levels have been observed in uncontrolled diabetic patients. This "low T3 state" could be explained by impairment in peripheral conversion of T4 to T3 that normalizes with improvement in glycemic control. Also, higher levels of circulating insulin associated with insulin resistance have shown a proliferative effect on thyroid tissue resulting in larger thyroid size with increased formation of nodules. Furthermore, the evidence suggests a pivotal role of insulin resistance in underlining the relationship between type 2 diabetes and thyroid dysfunction.

- **Fibromyalgia (FMS).** Fibromyalgia is an arthritic related condition characterized by widespread musculoskeletal pain, soreness, and tenderness that rarely disappears. It is one of the most common chronic pain conditions also affecting women more than men. The most common symptoms of FMS mimics low thyroid symptoms and is therefore often misdiagnosed. Some experts suggest that FMS is also related to the immune dysregulation and others suggest that it is an indication of an underactive metabolism, a low thyroid disorder.

- **Kidney dysfunction.** Thyroid hormones influence renal (kidney) development, function, glomerular filtration rate, and sodium and water balance. A growing body of evidence suggests that hypothyroidism is a risk factor for chronic kidney disease, progression of chronic kidney disease, and higher death risk in individuals that have kidney disease. Conversely, patients with chronic kidney disease may be at higher risk for thyroid dysfunction via several pathways. In fact, primary and subclinical hypothyroidism and low T3 syndrome are common features in individuals with chronic kidney disease. In one study, elevated TSH, FT4, and reduced T3 concentrations were also associated with reduced kidney function. Most of the renal manifestations of thyroid dysfunction are reversible with treatment. This is important since low levels of thyroid hormones may predict a higher risk of cardiovascular and overall mortality in people with end-stage renal disease. In addition, even subclinical hypothyroidism is a risk factor for kidney disease and cardiovascular diseases in Type 2 diabetic patients.

• **Insulin Sensitivity or Insulin Resistance.** Insulin sensitivity indicates that the body has become resistant to the effects of insulin and can eventually lead to type II diabetes. One study showed that lower TSH and higher T4 levels are associated with improved insulin sensitivity, higher HDL, and better endothelial (pertaining to inner lining of blood vessels) function.

• **Nonalcoholic Fatty Liver Disease (NAFLD).** Thyroid hormones are very much involved in the regulation of body weight, lipid metabolism, and insulin resistance. Therefore, it is not surprising that thyroid hormones have a role in the pathogenesis of non-alcoholic fatty liver disease (NAFLD). In fact, subclinical hypothyroidism, even in the range of upper normal TSH levels, was found to be related to NAFLD in a dose-dependent manner in one study. This trial concluded that hypothyroidism is closely associated with NAFLD independently of known metabolic risk factors, confirming a relevant clinical relationship between these two diseases. Moreover, a meta-analysis provided strong evidence that hypothyroidism may play a vital role in the progression and the development of non-alcoholic fatty liver disease. Yet another meta-analysis also came to the same conclusion. In addition, a case report revealed that patients with subclinical hypothyroidism, compared to individuals with normal thyroid function, are at a higher risk of developing non-alcoholic fatty liver disease.

• **Weight Gain.** Thyroid hormones regulate your metabolism including your basal metabolic rate. Therefore, hypothyroidism may be the hidden cause of a weight problem. Thyroid hormones can have a major effect on your waistline. Low thyroid function can add pounds to your body while making it difficult to lose weight. This means that even if you watch what you eat, your body is less able to convert calories into energy. Those unused calories end up causing you to gain weight. Slowly, over time, you can gain 10 to 15 pounds without even realizing it. Furthermore, the combination of reduced metabolism and other symptoms of hypothyroidism makes losing weight seem like a losing battle. The depression and insomnia so often caused by hypothyroidism increase your likelihood of indulging in foods that are high in less desirous carbohydrates and "bad" fats. The fatigue associated with an underactive thyroid makes it harder for you to engage in the physical activity necessary to burn extra calories.

■ Thyroid Hormone Replacement

When you contemplate thyroid hormone replacement, it is important to look at how thyroid hormone is metabolized in the body. The body requires about 50 mg per year of iodine. About 70 percent of the T4 secreted daily is deiodinated to yield T3 and reverse T3 in equal parts. Eighty percent of circulating T3 comes from the peripheral monode-iodination of T4 at the thyrosol ring which occurs in the liver, kidney, and other tissues. Circulating reverse T3 is made the same way. Thyroid hormone is also metabolized in other pathways. It can be conjugated with glucuronate or sulfate and then excreted in the bile or it can be decarboxylated. Twenty percent to 40 percent of T4 is subsequently elim-inated in the stool.

Medical trials have shown that if you are diagnosed with hypothy-roidism, it is important that your doctor replace both T4 and T3 in 98 percent of individuals. If you only have your T4 pathway replaced, you may still experience low thyroid symptoms. Replacing T3 and T4 has been found to be more effective than replacing T4 alone in most people. One study revealed that 35 percent of people on T4 and T3 replacement scored better on mental agility tests than people who were just taking T4. Of these people, 67 percent stated they also had an improvement in mood and physical health. Likewise, benefits have been shown by adding T3 for patients already on T4, with the patients reporting better moods and brain function.

Let's take a closer look at prescribed thyroid medications that are available.

■ Prescriptions for Thyroid Replacement

There are different ways to take thyroid hormone replacement. They are all a prescription. You can take T4 alone, take T3 alone, or take both T4 and T3 which is commonly prescribed as desiccated thyroid, which is porcine (from a pig). If you have Hashimoto's thyroiditis, some studies in the medical literature suggest that porcine thyroid replacement may not be the best form to take. This problem can be solved by your doctor prescribing non-porcine thyroid hormone, which is compounded.

Common Desiccated Thyroid Hormones. The following are common desiccated thyroid hormones that are available in North America through a prescription. Most of them are close to four parts T4 to one-part T3.

- Armour thyroid (porcine) (ratio: T4 4 to T3 1)

- Euthyroid (ratio: T4 4 to T3 1)

- Liotrix (ratio: T4 4 to T3 1)

- S-P-T (pork thyroid suspended in soybean oil)

- Thyroid Strong (ratio: T4 3.1 to T3 1)

- Thyroid USP (ratio: T4 4.2 to T3 1) It may contain lactose sucrose, dextrose or starch— commonly more than 99 percent of the contents are not thyroid hormone

- Thyrolar (ratio: T4 to T3 1)

- Thyrar (bovine)

Synthroid and Levothyroxine are both comprised of only T4. *Armour Thyroid* is made up of T3, T4, T1, T2, and other substances that help the body convert T4 into T3, such as calcitonin, selenium, and diuretic effect. Some physicians feel that *Armour Thyroid* is not consistent from dose to-dose. However, there has never been a complaint to the FDA concerning the inconsistency of *Armour Thyroid* that was not generic. Therefore, it is important that your healthcare provider, when prescribing *Armour Thyroid*, see that it is written as DAW, meaning not generic.

Common Prescription T4. Listed below are the most common prescription T4 available in North America. All are immediate release and may contain lactose, which can interfere with thyroid hormone absorption. Absorption can vary from 48 to 80 percent.

- Eltroxin

- Levothyroid

- Levoxyl

- Synthroid

Common T3 Medications. The most common T3 medications available in North America, all of which are immediate release, include:

- Cytomel

- Liothyronine sodium (generic)

- Triostat (injectable)

Compound Thyroid Medication. Compounded thyroid medication is made by a compounding pharmacy that is specially trained to make compounded medications. The advantage to having your thyroid hormone compounded is that you then can have the ratio of your T4 and T3 to be any ratio that you want it to be. Four to one may not be the best ratio for you. In other words, with compounded prescription thyroid medication is customized to your own needs. It is personalized. One size does not fit all patients. Also, you are getting no fillers and the physician, when they write your prescription for compounded thyroid hormone, can also add selenium, chromium, zinc, iodine, or other nutrients if needed. Recent studies have shown that it is now time for personalized thyroid replacement to be prescribed for patients.

It is paramount that when you are started on thyroid medication that you have your thyroid levels re-measured in six weeks. Once you have an optimal dosage schedule, then your thyroid level should be re-measured every six months. There are things that can change your dose of thyroid medication, such as weight gain or weight loss. The amount of stress that you have also affects your thyroid dosage.

Thyroid medication should be taken on an empty stomach. Eat no food or vitamins for one hour prior to or after taking the medication, since calcium (which is in many foods) interferes with the absorption of thyroid replacement. It is not just dairy foods that are a problem—many other foods contain calcium. Additional things that alter thyroid absorption are ferrous sulfate (iron), aluminum hydroxide-containing antacids, and medications such as sucralfate and bile acid sequestrants.

You may have a hard time tolerating thyroid replacement if you have adrenal fatigue. Therefore, you should always have your adrenal health evaluated before you are prescribed thyroid medication. In other words, adrenal dysfunction treatment should begin before you start thyroid replacement. (For more on adrenal fatigue, see page 43.) For this reason, it is important you see a healthcare practitioner who is fellowship trained in Precision/Anti-Aging Medicine. (For information on how to locate a fellowship-trained/Master's Degree healthcare professional, see the Resources section on page 391.)

■ Outcome (Prognosis)

Once the source of the hypothyroidism has been identified and eliminated, any further damage to the thyroid gland should stop. Usually, most patients are put on a combination of T3 and T4 hormone for the rest of their lives to normalize their thyroid hormone level. Once done, all the symptoms and signs of hypothyroidism should be improved or resolved.

HYSTERECTOMY

See Menopause and Perimenopause.

INCONTINENCE

See Bladder Problems.

INSOMNIA

See Menopause and Perimenopause; Postpartum Depression; Premenstrual Dysphoric Disorder (PMDD); Premenstrual Syndrome (PMS).

INTERLEUKIN-6 (IL-6)

See Heart Disease.

IRREGULAR MENSTRUAL CYCLES

See Menopause and Perimenopause; Polycystic Ovarian Syndrome (PCOS); Premature Ovarian Decline (POD).

IRRITABILITY

See Menopause and Perimenopause; Postpartum Depression; Premature Ovarian Decline (POD); Premenstrual Dysphoric Disorder (PMDD).

LOW BLOOD SUGAR

See Cortisol (Part I), Premenstrual Syndrome (PMS).

MAGNESIUM DEFICIENCY

See Migraine Headaches: Hormonally Related; Osteoporosis.

MENOPAUSE AND PERIMENOPAUSE

Every day in the United States, 3,500 women enter menopause. Menopause is defined as the permanent end of menstruation and fertility for one year. It may just be the best time in a woman's life. You no longer have to worry about an unwanted pregnancy, your responsibilities of child rearing are gone, and you are still young and sexually interested. Menopause is a time you get to focus on yourself. Prior to this time, you have likely been busy taking care of other people. Now, "middle-age" begins at the age of sixty.

Menopause occurs naturally in women when the ovaries begin making less estrogen and progesterone. However, if your hormonal symphony is out of tune, you can begin to have symptoms of menopause as early as fifteen years prior to actual menopause.

The time just before menopause in your life is called perimenopause. This is the time when your body begins its transition into menopause, usually starting anywhere from two to eight years before menopause and lasting up until the first year after your final period. Your estrogen levels rise and fall unevenly during this time. You may still have menstrual cycles during perimenopause, but they might become more irregular. Also, the amount that you bleed during each cycle may be more or less than you previously experienced.

■ Diagnosing Menopause

The diagnosis of menopause is made by your physician when you have had no cycle for one year and your blood levels of FSH is elevated. When your FSH blood level is consistently elevated to 30 mIU/mL or higher, and you have not had a menstrual period for a year, it is generally accepted that you are in menopause. The average age to go through menopause ranges from thirty-five to fifty-five. Therefore, you may easily live one-half of your life without a menstrual cycle.

■ Symptoms of Menopause and Perimenopause

- ❑ Aching ankles, knees, wrists, shoulders, and heels
- ❑ Bloating
- ❑ Decreased sexual interest*
- ❑ Depression
- ❑ Dizzy spells
- ❑ Flatulence (gas)

- Frequent urination
- Hair growth on face
- Hair loss
- Hot flashes
- Indigestion
- Insomnia
- Irritability
- Lower back pain
- Memory lapses, lack of focus/ concentration

- Migraine headaches
- Mood swings
- Night sweats
- Osteoporosis or osteopenia
- Painful intercourse
- Palpitations
- Panic attacks
- Skin feeling crawly
- Snoring

- Sore breasts
- Urinary leakage
- Urinary tract infections
- Vaginal dryness
- Vaginal itching
- Vaginal odor
- Varicose veins
- Weight gain
- Weird dreams

* Loss of sexual interest can occur at menopause, but this is not really a "normal" finding if DHEA continues to make estrogen and testosterone after menopause. However, if DHEA is not making these hormones at sufficient levels, sexual interest can be decreased. Sexual interest may be lower due to lack of progesterone if you are not sleeping well. Furthermore, abnormal cortisol levels can cause sexual interest to decline as well as low testosterone levels.

Weight Gain and Menopause

Most women gain weight during menopause. The mechanism of the development of weight gain in menopausal women is commonly due to hormonal imbalance and an increase in the inflammatory process. The continuous depletion of the follicular ovarian pool during menopausal transition lowers estrogen production with a relative increase in androgen levels. This hormonal imbalance alters energy homeostasis by regulating hunger and satiety signals. The hormonal imbalance that occurs during menopause also promotes the higher accumulation of fat in the abdominal region. Moreover, low estrogen levels along with high androgen levels lead to redistribution of fat present in the gluteal and femoral regions to abdominal regions of the body, favoring abdominal obesity. Consequently, the hormonal changes during perimenopause and menopause substantially contribute to increased abdominal obesity, which leads to additional physical and psychological morbidity.

Estrogen inhibits the action of hunger signals, preventing events of excessive calorie consumption. It is postulated that during the menopausal transition because of fluctuating estrogen levels, its effectiveness to modulate hunger hormones is reduced. Menopausal women experience more intense hunger signals encouraging increased food intake which promotes weight gain. There is strong medical evidence that estrogen therapy may partly prevent this menopause-related change in body composition and the associated metabolic sequelae. In addition, transdermally applied estrogen also decreases inflammation which is another way that estrogen regulates adiposity.

It is the ratio of ovarian hormones that determines how much weight you will gain and where you will gain it. For example, if estradiol (E2) decreases and progesterone, testosterone, and DHEA are normal, then you may gain fat around the middle. Or, if the ratio of E2 to progesterone is high, you may gain weight around the hips.

Progesterone increases fat storage and decreases sensitivity to insulin. Therefore, if you only replace progesterone during menopause and you are also estrogen-deficient, you can predispose yourself to weight gain and diabetes. It is all about balance. If estrogen levels are low, then natural estrogen replacement should also be prescribed along with the progesterone provided you are a candidate for hormone replacement. Furthermore, a medical trial showed that women with PMS and perimenopause consumed more dietary fat, carbohydrates, and simple sugars and less protein. This is believed to be due to low progesterone levels.

Elevated testosterone levels that occur in some women perimenopausally, and after menopause, can cause you to gain weight, particularly around the waist as opposed to overall weight gain. Consequently, having your healthcare provider help you lower your testosterone levels, if they are elevated, is beneficial. Likewise, if your testosterone level is low at menopause, testosterone replacement helps the body burn fat.

A double-blind, placebo-controlled human study provided evidence that DHEA reduced body fat and age-related skin atrophy stimulating procollagen/sebum production. It also had numerous other positive effects. Therefore, DHEA replacement at perimenopause and menopause is also important for weight loss.

Cortisol, one of your sex hormones, facilitates the storage of body fat. If cortisol levels increase, you will store more fat, increase muscle breakdown, and increase insulin resistance. If your cortisol levels remain high, your body goes into the "flight or fight" response, and you gain weight. (For more on this subject, see the section on cortisol on page 40.)

■ Additional Facts About Hormones and Weight Gain

- Women who use HRT and are hormonally balanced gain less weight than those who don't.

- Prolonged stress can decrease the function of the ovaries and hormone production, which can also cause weight gain.

- Obesity leads to higher levels of estrone (E1), the estrogen associated with an increase in breast cancer risk.

■ Treating Menopause

The treatment you need at menopause is as individualized as is your own fingerprint. The goal is to not only alleviate symptoms but to also prevent disease. Some healthcare providers do not understand the intricacies of hormone replacement. They believe that one size fits all. Therefore, it is paramount that you see a practitioner that is fellowship trained in Metabolic, Anti-Aging, and Regenerative Medicine for hormone replacement. Also, compounding pharmacists that are fellowship trained can make recommendations to your healthcare provider as to dosing of hormones.

For women who are still cycling, progesterone is usually given days fourteen to twenty-five of the cycle. For postmenopausal women, low dose hormones are recommended. Doses that are low help you maintain vision, memory, and mobility, aid in preventing heart disease, and also help alleviate symptoms associated with menopause. There is not a reason postmenopausally to use higher dose hormones. If you choose to, then you must cycle. If you use low dose hormonal therapy, then the choice to cycle or not is up to you.

Most commonly, physicians and other healthcare practitioners recommend that for the first year of menopause—while you are trying to balance all of your hormonal levels—you take the medications daily. After the first year, your symptoms will likely have improved. In this case, most healthcare practitioners recommend a hormonal holiday. This can be done by taking all of your hormones days one to twenty-five and no hormones on days twenty-five to twenty-eight. If your hormones are balanced when you do this, you will not have a cycle.

However, many women describe that their memory is not as sharp when they do not take their hormones for a couple of days. Consequently, most postmenopausal women take their prescription hormone replacement Monday through Saturday, taking no hormones on Sunday. This still gives you a weekly hormonal holiday during the month. See part III of this book for a detailed description of hormone replacement therapy.

Risk Factors for Early Menopause and Perimenopause

Generally, menopause occurs naturally. However, certain treatments can speed up the process. For example, a partial or total hysterectomy (sometimes called surgical menopause) can cause menopause to occur earlier than anticipated. Chemotherapy and radiation therapy can have similar effects. Additionally, women who suffer from premature ovarian failure (POF) sometimes experience menopause at earlier ages. (For more on POF, see the section on premature ovarian failure, starting on page 312.)

■ Surgical Menopause

Surgical menopause is the removal of the ovaries in women who haven't yet experienced natural menopause. It almost always occurs with a hysterectomy, which is the removal of the uterus.

One-third of women in the United States have had a hysterectomy. The average age for this operation is thirty-five. Women who have had a partial hysterectomy, which is when the ovaries are left in, can still have a change in hormonal function. Research has shown that about 60 to 70 percent of women experience a decrease in hormones (to menopausal levels) within three to four years of the operation. For some women, progesterone levels may fall within several months of the surgery and estrogen levels may decline within one to two years. The changes in hormone levels occur because your uterine artery is cut and tied off during the hysterectomy, which decreases blood flow to your ovaries. Surgical menopause reduces testosterone levels to a greater degree than natural menopause does in most patients.

MIGRAINE HEADACHES— HORMONALLY RELATED

Many women that get migraine headaches suffer from ones that are hormonally related. Some women get headaches just before they ovulate, and some women get hormonally related migraines just before they cycle. Migraines that are hormonally related are linked to 60 percent of migraines that occur in women.

Causes of Hormonally Related Migraines

Some women get headaches when their estrogen and/or progesterone levels drop just before the start of their cycle. At ovulation, estrogen levels decrease, and progesterone levels elevate. This causes some women to get migraine headaches. Additionally, the fluctuating levels of estrogen at perimenopause may cause migraine headaches in women who have never had them or increase the intensity and frequency of headaches in women who already suffer from hormonally related headaches. Estrogen levels affect headaches in several ways:

- Declining estrogen can cause vasoconstriction, which increases migraine pain.

- Declining estrogen levels lower a woman's pain threshold, which makes nerve endings more sensitive to pain-causing stimuli.

- Decreasing estrogen levels cause an increase in norepinephrine in the brain, which is a neurotransmitter that enhances vasoconstriction and decreased blood flow to the parts of the brain that can produce an aura experienced by many migraine sufferers. This also intensifies the pain from the migraine headache.

- Declining estrogen levels can lower beta-endorphins, which help relieve pain.

- Lower estrogen levels decrease serotonin levels at serotonin receptor sites, which are paramount in decreasing migraine pain. When serotonin levels fall, blood vessels in the brain can spasm. If this occurs, the result may be a migraine headache. Even worse, a blood vessel spasm can be a causative factor for a stroke.

- Stress can also play a role in hormonally related migraines.

■ Conventional Therapies

In some studies, oral contraceptives have been used. This is not a suggested therapy. There may be an increased incidence of stroke with oral contraceptive use in patients with migraines, particularly if the patient has an aura before they get a migraine headache. In addition, menstrual migraines tend to be less responsive to traditional migraine therapies.

■ Precision Medicine Therapies

Herbal and hormonal therapies along with magnesium have proven to be the mainstay of therapies for hormonally related migraine headaches.

Herbal Therapies

Chasteberry has an effect on neurotransmitters and on hormones. It is most effective when used if you have estrogen dominance (high estrogen/ low progesterone). Dose: 20 to 40 mg a day for 4 to 12 weeks. Possible side effects include GI upset, nausea, acne, and an increase in menstrual bleeding.

Hormonal Therapies

Estrogen dominance occurs when estrogen levels are not balanced with the amount of progesterone in the body. In other words, there is too much estrogen in relationship to progesterone. See the section on Estrogen/Progesterone ratio. See your healthcare provider or pharmacist to have saliva testing done.

If you have migraines just before you ovulate, then your healthcare provider will start you on progesterone on day 12 of your cycle and continue it until day 25 instead of starting the progesterone on day 14 of your cycle. If your migraine headache occurs just before your menstrual cycle, then your healthcare provider will prescribe you progesterone so that you take the dose that is right for you days 14 to 22 of your cycle and then ½ that dose days 23 to 25 of your menstrual cycle. This way you will not have a sudden drop in your progesterone level, which can precipitate a migraine headache.

Migraine headaches that occur once a month may become more frequent and/or more intense during perimenopause due to estrogen levels constantly changing. Your healthcare provider will order a saliva test and can prescribe a very small amount of biest cream daily and progesterone days 14 to 25 of your cycle to help control the increase in frequency and severity of your headaches.

Stress can make hormonally related migraines worse. Studies have shown that women are more susceptible to stress in the premenstrual time of their cycle. Cortisol levels can be measured by saliva testing and treated according to lab results if they are abnormal.

Neurotransmitter imbalances related to hormonal dysfunction may also contribute to migraine headaches that are hormonally related and non-hormonally related. Balancing your hormones will improve neurotransmitter function as will improving the health of your GI tract.

Magnesium

Topical magnesium that is a compounded prescription can be very helpful when applied to the site of migraine. It aids in decreasing spasming.

OSTEOPOROSIS (WOMEN)

Osteoporosis is a systemic skeletal disorder characterized by low bone mass and microarchitectural deterioration of bone tissue, resulting in an increase in bone fragility and susceptibility of fracture. Osteoporosis is a disease in which bones become more fragile and more likely to break. If untreated, the disease can progress painlessly until a bone breaks. The most common places patients with osteoporosis experience fractures are the hip, the spine, and the wrists. Mild bone loss is called osteopenia. Major bone loss is called osteoporosis.

In North America, Europe, Australia, and Asia, it is estimated that one in every three women fifty-five years old and older will have a fracture from osteoporosis in their lifetime. Globally, about 1.7 billion hip fractures occur each year. Of the women who break a hip, half will never walk again. This number is expected to increase four-fold by 2050 with the greatest increases expected in Africa and Asia. In the United States, almost half of women over sixty have osteoporosis. In addition, the rate of hip fracture is projected to increase by 240 percent in women by 2050.

Bone mineral density is not enough. Bone strength is also important. Almost 50 percent of bone fractures occur in people who have normal bone density. Bone strength is equally as important as bone density. Bone strength involves geometry, microarchitecture, and material properties.

■ Symptoms of Osteoporosis

❏ Back pain   ❏ Loss of height

❏ Bone fractures

Risk Factors for Osteoporosis

Osteoporosis does not have a single cause. The many risk factors for developing osteoporosis include:

- Abnormal cortisol levels

- Alcohol abuse

- Acid-base imbalance is important. A diet higher in fruits and vegetables produces a more alkaline environment which reduces urinary calcium excretion. Furthermore, whether a food is acid or alkaline before it is eaten does not necessarily determine how it contributes to acid-base balance after it is eaten. Moreover, foods that are higher in sulfur amino acids, phosphorus, or chloride (for example meat, grains, nuts, and dairy products) contribute to the acidic load. Likewise, foods that are potassium and magnesium salts of organic acids like fruits and vegetables contribute to the alkali load.

- Caffeine increases calcium loss. If an individual drinks three cups of coffee daily, they lose 45 mg of calcium. Coffee also contains twenty-nine different acids which also draw calcium out of bones. In fact, more than 1,000 over-the-counter medications contain caffeine, including weight loss products, cold preparation, pain relievers, and allergy products.

- Calcium deficiency

- Decrease in level of estrogen

- Electrolyte balance is also important, particularly potassium.

- Excessive alcohol intake

- Excessive intake of vitamin A

- Excessive protein intake

- Excessive zinc supplementation

- Fluoride in drinking water

- Genetic predisposition. It is also estimated that 50 percent to 80 percent of the individual variability in bone mass is determined by genetics, such as fair complexion and thin bone structure.

- High fat diets

- Hyperparathyroidism

- Hyperthyroidism

- Lack of exercise

- Menopause

- No menstrual cycle for more than 6 months prior to menopause

- Oxidative stress has a negative influence on bone structure.

- Poor diet. The DASH trial revealed that people who ate a diet higher in fruits and vegetables had lower bone turnover markers.

- Smoking

- Soft drink use

- Surgeries. Some surgeries increase the risk of bone loss including total thyroidectomy (complete removal of the thyroid gland) and removal of part, or all, of the intestines including intestinal bypass surgery for weight control.

- Vitamin D deficiency

Medications can also increase the risk of bone loss. The following are some of these medications.

- Androgen suppressive medications for prostate cancer

- Aromatase inhibitors

- Corticosteroids

- Cyclosporine

- Dilantin and other anticonvulsants

- Excessive thyroid medication

- Gonadotrophin-releasing hormone agonists

- Heparin

- Isoniazid

- Lasix

- Lithium

- Medroxyprogesterone

- Methotrexate

- PPIs. A case-controlled study of over 13,000 people with hip fractures showed that taking high doses of PPIs (antacids) long-term, for more than a year, were 2.6 times more likely to break a hip. Taking modest doses of PPIs regularly for 1 to 4 years increased the risk of hip fracture 1.2 to 1.6 times.

- SSRIs. The 5-year CAMOS study was conducted on 5,000 adults over the age of 50. The use of SRRIs for at least five years was associated with twice the risk of fractures and a reduction of bone density of 4 percent in the hip and 2.4 percent in the spine.

- Tetracycline

■ Medical Conditions That Are Commonly Associated With Osteoporosis

- Anorexia nervosa

- Celiac

- COPD

- Crohn's disease

- Cushing's disease

- Diabetes mellitus

- Fat malabsorption

- Gallbladder disease

- History of chronic low back pain for more than ten years

- History of stress fractures

- Hypercalciuria

- Hypochlorhydria

- Kidney disease

- Lactose intolerance

- Multiple myeloma

- Nulliparous

- Primary biliary cirrhosis

- Rheumatoid arthritis

- Scoliosis

Causes and Treatment for Osteoporosis in Women

Bones are constantly breaking down and reforming, reabsorbing and depositing calcium as this occurs. As people age the ratio of breakdown and reformation changes, with bone breakdown eventually exceeding bone formation. This change in ratio is higher in postmenopausal women.

To maintain your bone health, your body needs calcium, magnesium, boron, zinc, copper, silicon, phosphorus, manganese, vitamins B_6, B_{12}, D, K, and folate. Additionally, your body has to have an optimal amount of bioflavones and amino acids to maintain and build bone.

Therapies for Osteoporosis

Conventional Therapies

The following are conventional therapies for osteoporosis.

- Bisphosphonates are by far the most common conventional therapy for bone loss. The following are possible side effects of this class of drugs:
  - Acute phase reaction (transient flu-like symptoms)
  - Atrial fibrillation (irregular heartbeat)
  - GI symptoms
  - Hypocalcemia (low calcium level)
  - Increase in hip fracture after five years of use
  - Musculoskeletal pain
  - Ocular (eye) side effects
  - Osteonecrosis of the jawbone
- Calcium
- Exercise
- Parathyroid hormone (PTH) is FDA approved to build bone. It is a prescription and is to be used for severe osteoporosis in postmenopausal women.

It is not to be used for mild osteoporosis. In addition, it is not to be used for more than 24 months in the patient's lifetime. It is a subcutaneous (SQ) daily injection. Possible side effects include the following.

- Active Paget's disease
- Back spasms
- Depression
- Heart burn
- Increased risk of developing osteosarcoma (cancer of the bone).
- Itching, swelling, redness at site of injection
- Leg cramps
- Skeletal malignant conditions
- Unexplained elevations of alkaline phosphatase (blood study)
- Reduce alcohol intake
- Vitamin D

Precision Medicine Therapies

The following are Precision Medicine therapies for osteoporosis:

- Decrease the amount of sugar in your diet. Sugar decreases the rate the body absorbs and increases the elimination of calcium and magnesium which can lead to bone loss.

- Exercise 3 to 4 times a week.

- Reduce alcohol intake.

- Nutrients: Boron, Calcium, Copper, Magnesium, Phosphorus, Silicon, Strontium, Vitamin B_6, B_{12}, and folate, Vitamin D, Vitamin K, Zinc

    Boron. Boron along with vitamin D increases the mineral content in bone and also increases cartilage formation.

▪ Food Sources of Boron

- Almonds
- Apples
- Broccoli
- Cauliflower
- Dates
- Grapes

- Green leafy vegetables, such as kale
- Hazelnuts
- Honey
- Legumes

- Peaches
- Peanuts
- Pears
- Prunes
- Raisins
- Tomatoes

    Calcium. Calcium has many beneficial effects on bone structure.

▪ Factors That Decrease Calcium Absorption

- Aging process
- Caffeine
- Celiac disease
- Chronic alcoholism
- Cigarette smoking (nicotine)

- Glucocorticoid excess
- Hyperthyroidism
- Hypoparathyroidism
- Malabsorptive bariatric surgery
- Menopause

- Oxalate
- Phytates
- Sugar
- Vitamin D deficiency
- Weight gain

Calcium

Calcium is the most abundant mineral in the body. More than 99 percent of the body's calcium is in its bones and teeth. Calcium has many functions in the body, including the important role it plays in supporting bone and tooth structure. Calcium reduces bone loss and decreases bone turnover. Numerous studies have shown that calcium supplementation can help decrease bone loss by 30 to 50 percent.

Important Facts About Calcium

- Calcium carbonate is not the best form of calcium to use. Calcium citrate or hydroxyapatite are now the preferred forms.

- Calcium intake helps lower cholesterol.

- Calcium is also needed for the absorption of vitamin B_{12}.

- Calcium should be taken throughout the day for maximum absorption because your body can only absorb 500 mg at a time. It is best taken with meals and at bedtime.

- Consuming Tums is not a good way to intake calcium, due to poor absorption.

- Hydrochloric acid, citric acid, glycine, and lysine all help increase calcium absorption.

- Milk is not the best source of calcium since pasteurization destroys up to 32 percent of the available calcium.

- Use only pharmaceutical grade calcium supplements. Lower grade products may be contaminated with lead, mercury, arsenic, aluminum, or cadmium. (For suggestions on companies that use pharmaceutical grade supplements see the Resources section on page 391.)

- Vitamin C increases calcium absorption by 100 percent.

- You can take too much calcium.

■ Factors That Increase Calcium Absorption

- B-cell lymphoma and other active cancers
- Carbohydrates
- Crohn's disease
- Estrogen
- Fat
- Food
- Growth
- Lactation
- Lactose
- Lysine
- Obesity
- Prebiotics
- Pregnancy
- Primary hyperparathyroidism
- Probiotics
- Protein
- Sarcoidosis
- Tuberculosis (TB)
- Vitamin D

Excessive calcium consumption or elevated calcium levels due to a disease process may have negative effects.

- Blocks the uptake of manganese in the body
- Causes kidney stones
- Clogs arteries (predisposes to heart disease)
- Decreases iron absorption
- Decreases thyroid function
- Interferes with the absorption of magnesium
- Interferes with the absorption of zinc
- Interferes with the making of vitamin K

Additionally, calcium supplementation can interact with medications. It increases the toxicity of digoxin (a heart medication) and decreases the absorption of ciprofloxacin and most fluroquinolone antibiotics. Calcium can also inhibit the absorption of tetracycline, another antibiotic.

■ Food Sources of Calcium

Besides supplementation, there are many foods you can eat to get calcium.

- Almonds
- Barley
- Beet greens

- Black beans
- Bluefish
- Brazil nuts
- Brick cheese
- Broccoli
- Chicken
- Chinese cabbage
- Dandelion greens
- Dates
- Eggs
- English walnuts
- Garbanzo beans
- Ground beef
- Halibut
- Hazelnuts
- Kale
- Kelp
- Mackerel
- Mustard greens
- Olives, ripe
- Parsley
- Pecans
- Pinto beans
- Prunes, dried
- Rice, brown
- Salmon
- Sesame seeds
- Shrimp
- Soybeans
- Sunflower seeds
- Tofu
- Turnip greens
- Watercress
- White beans
- Yogurt

When you're looking to increase your calcium, there are a few things you should avoid. The items on the following list all decrease calcium absorption.

Foods that decrease calcium absorption

- Cocoa, chocolate
- Diet high in breads
- Excessive zinc supplementation
- Heavy exercise
- High fat diet
- High fiber cereals, fiber supplements (wait two hours after eating before taking calcium)
- Rhubarb
- Soft drinks
- Spinach
- Swiss chard
- White flour
- Whole wheat

Copper. Copper should be supplemented if zinc is supplemented. Copper and zinc have to sit in appropriate ratios in the body. Usually, 10 to 15 mgs of zinc to 1 mg of copper are needed. Copper plays an important role in bone metabolism and turnover.

■ Food Sources of Copper

- Almonds
- Barley
- Beef liver
- Brazil nuts
- Buckwheat
- Butter
- Carrots
- Clams

- Coconut
- Cod liver oil
- Garlic
- Hazelnuts
- Lamb chops
- Olive oil
- Oysters
- Peanuts

- Pecans
- Pork loin
- Rye grain
- Shrimp
- Split peas, dry
- Sunflower oil
- Walnuts

Magnesium. Magnesium has 300 functions in the body. It is very much needed for bone health. The following are roles magnesium plays in bone health.

- Activates bone-building osteoblasts
- Activates vitamin D
- Aids in parathyroid function (decreases bone break down)

- Helps calcitonin function (increases the absorption of calcium)
- Increases mineralization density
- Increases the absorption of calcium

■ Causes of Magnesium Deficiency

- Alcoholism
- Antibiotics (gentamicin, carbenicillin, or amphotericin B)
- Asthma medications (beta-agonists or epinephrine)
- Caffeine intake
- Cyclosporine, which prevents organ transplant rejection

- Diarrhea
- Digoxin use (heart medication)
- Diuretics (water pills)
- Drugs used for chemotherapy (cisplatin, vinblastine, or bleomycin)
- Excessive fiber intake
- Excessive sugar intake

- Extreme athletic competition
- Foods high in oxalic acid (almonds, cocoa, spinach, tea)
- Laxatives
- Phosphates in soft drinks
- Steroids
- Stress
- Surgery
- Trans fatty acids
- Trauma

Like calcium, you can also get magnesium through some magnesium-rich foods.

Acid-Creating Foods

The average American diet includes many foods that, once eaten, create acid in your body. If you eat mostly acidic foods and not enough alkaline foods, your body must find alkalizing materials elsewhere to neutralize its pH levels. It often must resort to using the calcium and protein in your bones. As a result, your bones can become weakened, possibly irrevocably, and your body systems can age at an accelerated pace, resulting in a slew of related problems. The following foods create particularly high acidity levels in your body.

- Chocolate
- Dairy products, such as butter, cheese, ice cream, milk, and yogurt
- Drinks, such as beer, black tea, coffee, and soft drinks
- Fish, such as haddock
- Fruit, such as blueberries, cranberries, and dried fruit
- Grains, such as barley, oats, rice, wheat, and white bread
- Honey
- Meat products, such as beef, chicken, ham, turkey, and veal
- Nuts, such as peanuts and walnuts
- Processed soybeans
- Sugar
- Vegetables, such as corn
- White vinegar

■ Food Sources of Magnesium

- Almonds
- Apricots, dried
- Avocados
- Brazil nuts
- Buckwheat
- Cashews
- Cheddar cheese
- Coconut
- Collard leaves
- Corn
- Dandelion greens

- Dark green vegetables
- Dates
- Figs, dried
- Kelp
- Parsley
- Peanuts
- Prunes, dried
- Pumpkin seeds
- Rice, brown
- Rye

- Sesame seeds
- Shrimp
- Soybeans
- Spinach, raw
- Sunflower seeds
- Swiss chard
- Tofu
- Wheat bran
- Wheat germ
- Wheat grain
- Yeast, brewer's

Manganese. Manganese is needed for the repair of soft bone and connective tissue and is used for bone growth and maintenance. Excessive calcium supplementation can decrease the absorption of manganese.

■ Food Sources of Manganese

- Avocados
- Bay leaves
- Brazil nuts
- Buckwheat
- Cloves

- Ginger
- Hazelnuts
- Oatmeal
- Pecans

- Seaweed
- Tea
- Thyme
- Whole wheat

Phosphorus. Phosphorus regulates bone formation, inhibits bone re-absorption, and affects the regulation of calcium. Most Americans eat enough phosphorus-containing foods that low phosphorus levels are rarely seen.

■ Food Sources of Phosphorus

- Almonds
- Beef liver

- Brazil nuts
- Brewer's yeast

- Brown rice
- Cashews

- Cheddar cheese
- Chicken
- Dried pinto beans
- Dried soybeans
- Eggs
- English walnuts
- Garlic

- Hulked sesame seeds
- Kelp
- Millet
- Peanuts
- Pearled barley
- Pecans
- Pumpkin seeds

- Rye grain
- Scallops
- Squash seeds
- Sunflower seeds
- Wheat
- Wheat bran
- Wheat germ

Silicon. Silicon is a trace mineral that has been shown to increase bone mineral density. It is found in many forms, but the only form that is useful to humans is orthosilicic acid. Foods that are high in fiber usually contain silicon. The recommended dose is 1 to 5 mg a day. High dosages can cause kidney stone production.

■ Food Sources of Silicon

- Apples
- Celery
- Cherries
- Endive

- Legumes
- Oats
- Onions
- Oranges

- Rice bran
- Root vegetables
- Unrefined grains

Strontium. Strontium is a wonderful trace mineral that promotes bone formation and decreases bone resorption. Studies found a reduction in vertebral fractures of 37 percent and 40 percent and a reduction in non-vertebral fractures of 14 percent and 16 percent. The dose is 2 grams for two years and then discontinue taking it.

Vitamin B_6, B_{12}, and Folate. Levels of vitamins B_6, B_{12}, and folate are commonly low in individuals with osteoporosis. Low levels of these nutrients are associated with elevated homocysteine levels. High homocysteine levels interfere with collagen cross-linking, which leads to a defective bone matrix. This may be since high amounts of homocysteine are associated with vitamin B_{12} deficiency. Therefore, people with elevated homocysteine levels have an increased risk of developing osteoporosis. For information on homocysteine, see the inset (page 195) on secondary risk factors for heart disease.

Vitamin D. Vitamin D is a prohormone that has many functions in the body.

- 1,25(OH)2D3 has been shown to directly accelerate osteoblast-mediated mineralization by stimulating the production of ALP-positive mature matrix vesicles.

- 1,25(OH)2D3 also has a direct effect on bone resorption since it acts as a calcium-regulating hormone and induces receptor activator of nuclear factor kappa-beta ligand (RANKL) expression in osteoblasts.

- A study concluded that vitamin D supplementation decreased the risk of vertebral fractures by 37 percent and non-vertebral fractures by 23 percent.

- Vitamin D supplementation reduced the relative risk of hip fracture by 26 percent and any non-vertebral fracture by 23 percent compared to taking calcium alone or placebo in another medical trial.

- A study showed a link between deficient levels of vitamin D and premature aging of bone.

- Optimal vitamin D status: 55 to 80 ng/mL (120 to 160 nmol/L). Also get calcium level. If calcium levels are elevated, find the cause of the high level. Vitamin D excess alone is rarely the case.

- 25-OH vitamin D levels may be normal in patients who are vitamin D toxic and have high calcium levels due to vitamin D hypersensitivity syndrome. Hypersensitivity syndrome is commonly seen in the following cases:
  - Cancer
  - Crohn's disease
  - Granulomatous diseases
  - Hyperparathyroidism
  - Sarcoidosis
  - TB

- Optimal supplementation should be with vitamin D3 not vitamin D2.

■ Diseases Associated With Suboptimal Vitamin D Levels

- Ankylosing spondylitis
- Back pain
- Breast cancer
- Colon cancer
- Depression
- Diabetes

- Epilepsy

- Grave's disease

- Heart disease

- Hypertension (high blood pressure)

- Lupus

- Migraine headaches

- Multiple sclerosis (MS)

- Osteoarthritis

- Parkinson's disease

- PCOS

- Rheumatoid arthritis

Vitamin D is mainly available through sunlight. You make it in your skin from exposure to the sun. Topical sunscreens block vitamin D production by 97 to 100 percent. Dairy products, fish and fish liver oils, liver, sweet potatoes, and dandelion greens also contain some vitamin D. Supplementation with vitamin D is best done with vitamin D3. New studies have shown that you may need more vitamin D than healthcare providers previously thought. Therefore, it is very important to have your vitamin D levels measured regularly.

Vitamin K. Vitamin K has six major purposes in the body and there are three forms of vitamin K that the body can take in from diet. Twenty-five percent of your vitamin K comes from what you eat. Seventy-five percent of vitamin K used by the body is produced in our intestinal tract by friendly bacteria.

- K_1: found in leafy green vegetables.

- K_2: (MK-4): found in meats, eggs, and dairy products.

- K_2: (MK-7): found in fermented soybeans and other fermented foods.

- Vitamin K is important for bone mineralization. Osteocalcin, the chief bone matrix protein, is a Gla-protein that is dependent on vitamin K to be produced. Low levels of vitamin K impair activation of osteocalcin and decrease the activity of bone-forming cells. Therefore, low intake of vitamin K has been associated with bone loss. The good news is that vitamin K supplementation has been effective in preventing and treating osteoporosis.

- A recent study has shown that daily vitamin K intake must be at least 100 micrograms to maintain optimal bone health.

- The following are causes of vitamin K deficiency:
  - Consumption of medications that cause malabsorption of fat
  - Hydrogenated fat intake
  - Lack of adequate beneficial bacteria in the intestine
  - Lack of dietary intake
  - Use of broad-spectrum antibiotics

- Low bone density has been found in people treated with warfarin. There is an association between fracture risk and warfarin use. Studies have shown a benefit and the safety of patients taking warfarin and low-dose vitamin K (100 micrograms a day).

- Dosages of vitamin K for healthy people: 2.5 to 45 mg a day. Consider supplementing with K_1 and K_2. Up to 10 mg per day of vitamin K_1 or 45 mg of vitamin K_2 have been used in clinical trials for osteoporosis. MK-4 is chemically synthesized. MK-7 is better absorbed and stays in the body longer. The half-life is 3 days compared to a few hours for other forms of vitamin K.

■ Food Sources of Vitamin K

- Asparagus
- Beef
- Broccoli
- Cheese
- Egg yolks
- Green beans
- Green cabbage
- Ham
- Lettuce
- Liver (beef, pork, chicken)
- Oats
- Peaches
- Potatoes
- Raisins
- Spinach
- Tomatoes
- Turnip greens
- Watercress
- Whole wheat

If you are on an anticoagulant such as *Coumadin*, consult your doctor as to how much vitamin K-rich foods or supplementation you may need. Studies have revealed that bone density is reduced in some patients who take *Coumadin*. Likewise, an increased risk of bone fracture has been associated with long-term use of *Coumadin*. Research has shown that taking *Coumadin* with a low dose of vitamin K (100 micrograms a day) can be beneficial and safe. Still, you should consult your healthcare practitioner before beginning vitamin K supplementation if you are taking *Coumadin*.

A recent study also revealed that supplementation of vitamin K_2 improves the effectiveness of bisphosphonates, which are medications used to treat osteoporosis.

Zinc. Zinc is used in many enzymatic reactions in the body. In fact, 100 enzymes use zinc as a cofactor. It is needed for the formation of bone and skin.

■ Symptoms of Zinc Deficiency

- ❏ Acne
- ❏ Anemia
- ❏ Anorexia
- ❏ Arthritis
- ❏ Behavioral disturbances
- ❏ Brittle nails
- ❏ Craving for sugary foods
- ❏ Dandruff
- ❏ Decreased ability to taste
- ❏ Decreased desire for protein-rich foods
- ❏ Decreased sense of smell
- ❏ Decreased sexual function
- ❏ Delayed sexual maturation
- ❏ Diarrhea
- ❏ Eczema
- ❏ Enlargement of the spleen and liver
- ❏ Fatigue
- ❏ Frontal headaches
- ❏ Growth retardation
- ❏ Hair loss
- ❏ Immune deficiencies
- ❏ Impaired nerve conduction
- ❏ Impaired wound healing
- ❏ Impotence
- ❏ Infertility
- ❏ Low sperm count
- ❏ Memory impairment
- ❏ Negative nitrogen balance
- ❏ Nerve damage
- ❏ Night blindness
- ❏ Poor appetite
- ❏ Psoriasis
- ❏ Reduced salivation
- ❏ Sleep disturbances
- ❏ Stretch marks
- ❏ White spots on nails

■ Factors that Can Predispose You to a Zinc Deficiency

- Aging (zinc absorption decreases with age)
- AIDS
- Alcoholism
- Anorexia nervosa
- Caffeinated beverages
- Calcium supplementation
- Celiac disease
- Certain medications, such as: Cortisone, some diuretics (water pills), Tetracycline
- Chronic renal (kidney) failure
- Cirrhosis
- Cystic fibrosis
- Excess copper
- Food rich in phytic acid, such as unleavened bread, raw beans, seeds, nuts, and grains
- Hemolytic anemia
- Infection
- Inflammatory bowel disease
- Iron supplementation
- Nephritic syndrome
- Pancreatic insufficiency
- Pancreatitis
- Rheumatoid arthritis
- Short bowel syndrome
- Smoking
- Surgery
- Teas containing tannin

■ Food Sources of Zinc

- Almonds
- Beef
- Black pepper
- Brazil nuts
- Buckwheat
- Chicken
- Chili powder
- Cinnamon
- Egg yolk
- Ginger root
- Ground round steak
- Hazelnuts
- Lamb chops
- Lima beans
- Milk, dry; nonfat
- Mustard
- Oats
- Oysters, fresh
- Paprika
- Peanuts
- Pecans
- Rye
- Sardines
- Soy lecithin
- Split peas
- Thyme
- Walnuts
- Whole wheat

- Decrease stress. See the section on cortisol. You can do all the things suggested in this chapter, but if you stay stressed you may still break down bone!

- See a Precision Medicine/Anti-Aging specialist to have your hormones replaced if they are low and you are a candidate for hormone replacement. Estrogen replacement therapy has been shown to help build bone structure and to help maintain bone. Progesterone also helps build bone. A new study suggested that progesterone is effective to prevent and treat bone loss. Furthermore, testosterone not only builds bone but also improves the strength of bone. Yet another study revealed that transcutaneous (on the skin) hormone therapy with micronized estradiol and progesterone is the treatment of choice in postmenopausal osteoporosis, as evidenced by bone mineral density and biochemical markers.

- 5R program for GI health. If your gut is not healthy, it is hard to absorb the minerals and other nutrients you need to build bone. Likewise, low stomach acid in the gut decreases absorption of minerals. Have your healthcare provider order a gut health test to determine the health of your GI tract.

OVARIAN CANCER

Ovarian cancer is the most lethal gynecologic cancer. Less than one-half of patients survive for more than five years after diagnosis. Ovarian cancer affects women of all ages but is mostly diagnosed after menopause. More than 75 percent of affected women are diagnosed at an advanced stage because early-stage disease is usually asymptomatic, and symptoms of late-stage disease are nonspecific. Unfortunately, only about 20 percent of all cases of ovarian cancer are detected before the tumor growth has spread beyond the ovaries. High-grade serous carcinoma (HGSC) is the most commonly diagnosed form of ovarian cancer. A woman's chance of surviving ovarian cancer is better if the cancer is found early on.

The cause of ovarian cancer is unknown. However, substantial progress has been made in identifying genes that are associated with a high risk of ovarian cancer (such as BRCA1 and BRCA2), as well as a precursor lesion of HGSC called serous tubal intraepithelial carcinoma. This holds promise for identifying individuals at high risk of developing the disease and for developing prevention strategies. In addition, women with Lynch syndrome (hereditary nonpolyposis colorectal cancer) have the highest risk of developing ovarian cancer, but account for only approximately 10 percent of those with the disease. Other less common genetic syndromes may increase the risk of ovarian cancer, but their contribution to genetic risk is small.

Risk Factors for Ovarian Cancer

- **Age.** Ovarian cancer is not common in women under the age of forty. Therefore, age is considered a risk factor for this type of cancer.

- **Diet.** Nutrition and diet also play a role in whether you have an increased risk of developing ovarian cancer. Studies have shown that women who consume dairy (quantities vary depending on the study) have a 44 percent greater risk of developing ovarian cancer.

- **Inflammation.** Studies have shown that elevated levels of COX-2 (an inflammatory marker) are present in people with ovarian cancer. Additionally, if one of your close family members had ovarian cancer, you are at a higher risk of developing it yourself.

- **Family history.** A family history of ovarian and/or breast cancer is a risk factor for ovarian cancer.

- **Toxins.** Avoiding substances such as talcum powder, which has been found in everyday products such as baby powder, vaginal deodorants, and makeup, may decrease your risk of ovarian cancer.

- **Tobacco.** Avoiding the use and exposure of tobacco products can not only lower your risk for ovarian cancer but also lower the risk of any other long-term health consequence.

- **Weight.** Being overweight or obese may increase your risk of developing ovarian cancer.

If you have an increased-risk family history, you should see your healthcare provider to refer you for genetic counseling. If genetic mutations (for example, BRCA mutations) are identified, bilateral salpingo-oophorectomy (removal of both ovaries and fallopian tubes) can be considered for risk reduction. In both average- and high-risk women, long-term hormonal contraceptive use reduces risk by about 50 percent according to some studies. However, the overall strength of evidence for ovarian cancer prevention was moderate to low, primarily because of the lack of randomized trials and inconsistent reporting of duration of use and other factors.

A study concluded that the combined increase in risk of breast and cervical cancers and vascular events was likely to be equivalent to or greater than the decreased risk in ovarian cancer with oral contraceptive use. Consequently, the use of oral contraceptives is not recommended as a strategy to prevent ovarian cancer.

Preventing Ovarian Cancer

Women who have had a least one child, especially before the age of 30, have a lower risk of developing ovarian cancer. In fact, the risk lowers for each child you have. Also, breastfeeding decreases your risk of developing this disease process.

■ Foods and Drinks That May Decrease Your Risk of Developing Ovarian Cancer

- **Tomato Juice.** Drinking eight ounces of tomato juice every day has been shown to cut your risk of developing ovarian cancer by 50 percent.

- **Ginger.** The active compounds in ginger (gingerols) have been shown to destroy cancerous ovarian cells according to a University of Michigan study. Use one teaspoon fresh ginger or one-half a teaspoon of ground ginger every day.

- **Green tea.** Swedish scientists revealed that women who sipped 16 ounces of green tea daily were 46 percent less likely to develop ovarian cancer. Also, each additional cup they drank decreased their risk another 18 percent.

- **Nuts.** A study revealed that eating 1/3 cup of any type of nuts daily could reduce your risk of developing ovarian cancer by 18 percent. This study was published in the Journal of the National Cancer Institute. Nuts have nutrients that decrease inflammation.

- **Peppers.** One-half a cup of red, orange, yellow, or green peppers increases the ability of the liver to break down carcinogens before they can harm the ovaries due to their quercetin content.

Other foods such as red onions, apples with the skin on them, purple grapes, blueberries, and tea also contain quercetin. Asparagus, broccoli, and cherries are also quercetin-containing foods.

- **Endive.** Eating three cups a week of endive may decrease your risk of getting ovarian cancer by as much as 75 percent according to the Journal of the National Cancer Institute.

- **Flaxseed.** Sprinkling two tablespoons of ground flaxseed over your food or putting it in a smoothie can cut your ovarian cancer risk by 38 percent. Flaxseeds are rich in lignans, which are compounds that protect the ovaries from surges in estrogen.

- **Cruciferous vegetables.** Cauliflower, cabbage, broccoli, Brussels sprouts, and kale are cruciferous vegetables that are thought to lower women's risk of ovarian cancer.

Some foods and drinks may increase your risk of developing ovarian cancer, such as sugar, alcohol, and foods with saturated and trans fats. Limit your intake. Supplementation with certain nutrients may play a preventive role against ovarian cancer.

Vitamins C and E may reduce your risk of developing ovarian cancer by 68 percent according to one medical trial. The dose of vitamin C is 500 mg and dose of vitamin E is 400 IU. Both nutrients decrease the enzymes that fuel the growth of abnormal cells according to scientists at Stanford.

Large numbers of epidemiological studies have shown that vitamin D plays an important role in cancer prevention by regulating cellular proliferation and metabolism. Studies suggest that it exhibits protective and anti-tumorigenic activities through genomic and nongenomic signal transduction pathways. These results indicate that vitamin D deficiency results in an increase in the risk of developing ovarian cancer and that vitamin supplements may potentially be an efficient way of preventing cancer.

Last, getting enough sleep boosts your immune system. A study conducted at the Fred Hutchinson Cancer Research Center showed that going to bed by 11 pm every night reduced your risk of developing ovarian cancer by 32 percent. Melatonin, your hormone of sleep, is also a powerful immune builder and anticancer hormone. See the chapter on melatonin.

PAINFUL INTERCOURSE

See Endometriosis.

PAINFUL MENSTRUAL CYCLES

See Dysmenorrhea and Menstrual Cramps; Endometriosis.

PELVIC PAIN

See Endometriosis.

POLYCYSTIC OVARIAN SYNDROME (PCOS)

PCOS, which is otherwise known as polycystic ovarian syndrome, is the most common endocrine disorder in women of reproductive age worldwide. It affects nearly 10 percent of women in the United States and accounts for 75 percent of the women with amenorrhea (no menstrual cycle). PCOS also accounts for 85 percent of women with androgen excess and hirsutism.

The definition of PCOS has changed over time. Three criteria were set up by the National Institutes of Health.

- Irregular or absence of menstruation

- Excess androgen production

- Lack of other reasons for irregular or absence of cycles and excess androgen

Initially, having ovarian cysts was not one of the three criteria for the diagnosis of PCOS. Therefore, ovaries with many cysts do not necessarily mean that the patient has PCOS. Then the Consensus workshop sponsored by the European Society of Human Reproduction and Embryology (ESHRE) and the American Society of Reproductive Medicine (ASRM) in 2003 agreed upon a new definition of PCOS. Two out of three criteria must be present: oligoovulation (ovulation that is irregular or infrequent) and/or anovulation (ovulation does not occur, so an egg is released from the ovary), clinical or biochemical signs of excess androgen activity, and polycystic ovaries on ultrasound (greater than or equal to 12 follicles 2 to 9 mm or volume greater than 10 mL).

■ Signs and Symptoms of PCOS

The following are common signs and symptoms of PCOS.

- ❑ Acanthosis nigricans
- ❑ Acrochordons (skin tags)
- ❑ Alopecia
- ❑ BMI (greater than 30)
- ❑ Depression/irritability/tension
- ❑ Epilepsy connection
- ❑ Gray-white breast discharge
- ❑ High hip to waist ratio (greater than 0.85)
- ❑ Hirsutism
- ❑ Infertility/recurrent miscarriage
- ❑ Irregular or absent menstrual cycles
- ❑ Obesity/inability to lose weight
- ❑ Oily skin/acne
- ❑ Pelvic pain
- ❑ Sleep apnea
- ❑ Thinning scalp hair

The following are laboratory testing abnormalities that may be present in PCOS.

- ❑ Abnormal lipid profile
- ❑ Decreased SHBG (sex hormone binding globulin)
- ❑ Elevated DHEA levels
- ❑ Elevated insulin level/insulin resistance
- ❑ Elevated LH to FSH ratio (elevated LH and decreased FSH)
- ❑ High estrone
- ❑ High testosterone level and other androgens such as androstenedione

■ Disease or Disorders Associated with PCOS

PCOS patients are at risk of developing other disease processes including the following.

- **Cancer.** Women with polycystic ovarian syndrome have an increased risk of developing hormonally related cancers. In fact, women who had a history of PCOS and irregular periods have a five-fold increase in endometrial cancer. In addition, women who have a history of PCOS may have an increased risk of developing ovarian cancer. Likewise, women with a history of PCOS may be at risk for breast cancer since they tend to be overweight and have hormonal changes that can lead to unopposed estrogen in the body.

- **Diabetes.** If you have PCOS you are seven times more likely to get diabetes. About half of all women with PCOS have insulin resistance. Some studies suggest that women with PCOS who have irregular cycles, or no cycles, may have double the risk for diabetes. The risk factor for diabetes in patients with an irregular cycle increases even more if an individual is obese. The risk of getting diabetes is also increased in people with PCOS that are not overweight or insulin resistant.

- **Heart Disease.** Women with PCOS have an increased risk of heart disease compared to women without PCOS. Up to 70 percent of women in the U.S. with PCOS have dyslipidemia. Women with PCOS frequently have elevated total cholesterol, LDL (bad cholesterol), and triglycerides. They also tend to have low HDL (good cholesterol) and apoprotein A-1. In addition, women with PCOS have a sevenfold risk of having a heart attack. Likewise, homocysteine levels may be increased in people with PCOS, which increases their risk of heart disease as does a higher than usual rate of elevated c-reactive protein (CRP). Moreover, women with PCOS frequently have decreased total antioxidant status and increased oxidative stress. This pattern may be one of the contributing causes of heart disease in women with PCOS.

- **Hypertension.** Women with PCOS have four times the rate of hypertension than women who do not have PCOS.

- **Infertility.** Higher than normal levels of testosterone are also found in PCOS patients. High levels of testosterone inhibit ovulation.

- **Obesity.** Studies have shown that women with PCOS store fat better and burn calories at a slower rate than women who do not have PCOS.

Therapies for PCOS

Conventional Therapies

There are many medical and surgical treatments that are used conventionally to treat PCOS.

Causes of PCOS

The exact cause of PCOS in unclear. Etiologies of PCOS are varied.

- Many scientists believe that PCOS has a hereditary component. Forty percent of women with PCOS have a sister with PCOS and 35 percent of women with PCOS have a mother with PCOS. There is some suggestion in the medical literature that women with PCOS are born with a gene that triggers higher than normal levels of androgen or insulin.

- Women that are overweight and women that are not that have PCOS, both have a higher rate of insulin resistance and hyperinsulinemia than controls. Insulin decreases SHBG levels, which increase the level of circulating testosterone. Furthermore, insulin works with LH to increase androgen production in the ovarian theca cells.

- In addition, it is suggested that women with PCOS have a hyperactive production of CYP17 enzyme, which is responsible for forming androgens (testosterone and androstenedione) from DHEA-S at those sites. High DHEA is due to stimulation with ACTH produced by the pituitary mainly due to stress. The excessive DHEA is then converted into androgens via adrenal metabolism. This contributes to high androgen levels in PCOS.

- High testosterone levels correlate to the high LH (luteinizing hormone) levels. High androgen levels in the ovary inhibit FSH, which then inhibits the development and maturation of the follicle. The metabolism of estrogens then changes by way of the 2-hydroxylation and 17-alpha-oxidation pathways which are decreased. Estrogen levels increase due to peripheral aromatization of androstenedione. This results in estrogen dominance due to the over production of estrogen.

- Skin and adipose tissue are also postulated to contribute to the etiology of PCOS. Women who have hirsutism have an elevated sensitivity to androgen activity in the skin so they may develop abnormal patterns of hair growth. Aromatase and 17-beta-hydroxysteroid activities are increased in the fat cells and peripheral aromatization increases with the increase in weight.

- Phthalates, bisphenol-A, cadmium, and mercury toxicities have all be related to PCOS.

- The imbalance in the HPO axis that occurs in POCS is part of the cause of this disease. Twenty-five percent of women with PCOS have hyperprolactinemia (high prolactin level). The hyperprolactinemia is due to the abnormal estrogen negative feedback from the pituitary. Elevated prolactin can contribute to high estrogen levels.

- In addition, stress may be a contributing factor to PCOS. A study showed that many women with PCOS cannot process cortisol effectively, leading to elevated cortisol levels in the body. When women are under stress, too much prolactin may be released. This may affect the ability of the ovaries to produce the right balance of hormones.

- Likewise, hypothyroidism (low thyroid function) may be a cause of PCOS.

- Anti-androgen medications
  - Aldactone (spironolactone)
  - Tagamet (cimetidine)
  - Ketoconazole
- Testosterone metabolism blockers
  - Propecia (finasteride)
- Medications to lower blood sugar
  - Glucophage (metformin) is the most successful
- Gonadotropin-releasing hormone antagonists
- Lupron (leuprolide)
- 5-alpha reductase inhibitors

- Finasteride
- Hair metabolism inhibitors
  - Vaniqa cream (eflornithine)
- Menstrual regulators
  - Oral contraceptives. Oral contraceptives work by suppressing pituitary LH, increasing SHBG, and decreasing androgen section. Choose ones that are least androgenic. Combination pills may worsen insulin resistance and should not be used.
  - Progesterone
  - Ovulation Inducers
- Surgery

Precision Medicine Therapies

There are many Precision Medicine therapies for polycystic ovarian disease.

Diet. Increase fiber intake in your diet, which lowers blood sugar, blood pressure and cholesterol. Also start a low glycemic index eating program. Weight loss in patients with PCOS can improve the following: signs of hyperandrogenism, menstrual irregularity, hyperinsulinemia (high insulin level), restore ovulation and fertility, improve gonadotrophin pulsatile secretion, may prevent diabetes and coronary heart disease, and deceases ovarian P450c17 alpha activity.

Essential fatty acids. They slow down the absorption of carbohydrates into the blood stream. They also decrease inflammation. PCOS has an inflammatory component. Dose: EPA/DHA 1,000 mg a day.

Exercise. Exercise is very important in women with PCOS. Several studies showed that women with PCOS who exercised improved ovulation, reduced insulin resistance, and promoted weight loss.

NAC. Studies revealed that using n-acetyl cysteine (NAC) in conjunction with clomiphene citrate increased ovulation and pregnancy rates in women with infertility that had PCOS and that could not conceive with the use of clomiphene citrate alone. NAC depletes the body of zinc and copper. Therefore, make sure you are taking prenatal vitamins.

Nutrients. There are many nutrients that are beneficial for patients with polycystic ovarian syndrome.

Vitamin D deficiency is common in women with PCOS. Vitamin D plays a physiologic role in reproduction, including ovarian follicular development and luteinization with altering anti-mullerian hormone (AMH) signaling, follicle-stimulating hormone sensitivity, and progesterone production in human granulosa cells. It also affects glucose homeostasis.

A study supports the beneficial effects of vitamin D supplementation on liver markers and modest improvements in insulin sensitivity in vitamin D deficient women with PCOS. A current meta-analysis demonstrated that vitamin D supplementation in women with PCOS resulted in an improvement in hs-CRP. In addition, a randomized, double-blinded, placebo-controlled clinical trial was carried out on 60 subjects. It revealed that the administration of vitamin D and a probiotic for 12 weeks to women with PCOS had beneficial effects on mental health parameters, serum total testosterone, hirsutism, hs-CRP, plasma total antioxidant capacity, glutathione, and malondialdehyde (MDA) levels. Also, a study revealed that the co-administration of vitamin D and omega-3 fatty acids for 12 weeks had beneficial effects on mental health parameters, serum total testosterone, hs-CRP, plasma total antioxidant capacity and malondialdehyde (MDA) levels, and gene expression of IL-1 and VEGF among women with PCOS.

Another study revealed that magnesium and vitamin E co-supplementation for 12 weeks in PCOS women had beneficial effects on parameters of insulin metabolism and some markers of cardio-metabolic risk.

Probiotics/Synbiotics. Probiotics and synbiotics have been shown to be helpful in individuals with PCOS. A study suggested that probiotic/synbiotic supplementation may improve glucose homeostasis parameters, hormonal, and inflammatory indices in women with PCOS. In addition, synbiotic pomegranate juice in the form of a beverage has been shown to improve insulin resistance, insulin, testosterone level, BMI, weight, and waist circumference in PCOS.

Selenium supplementation may be beneficial in people with low selenium levels. A study revealed that 200 micrograms a day of selenium supplementation for 8 weeks among PCOS women had beneficial effects on insulin metabolism parameters, triglycerides, and VLDL-C levels; however, it did not affect fasting glucose and other lipid profiles. You can become toxic on selenium. Have your healthcare provider measure your selenium level.

Herbal Therapies. There are many herbal therapies that have also been shown to be beneficial for patients with PCOS.

- Adaptogens for stress to improve the stress response and HPA function have been shown to be effective.
  - American ginseng
  - Ashwagandha

- Eleuthera
- Ginseng
- Rhaponticum
- Rhodiola
- Schizandra

These herbal therapies have been shown to lower testosterone in women with PCOS.

- Camellia sinensis (green tea) increases SHBG which decreases testosterone and promotes weight loss. A placebo-controlled trial of women with PCOS showed that the body weight of the group that used green-tea decreased by 2.4 percent. Dose: 270 mg a daily

- Cimcifuga racemosa (black cohosh) binds to estrogen receptors and lowers LH.

- Glycyrrhiza glabra (licorice root) can decrease testosterone synthesis. A study using 3.5 grams of licorice containing 7.6 percent glycyrrhizic acid (0.25 grams total glycyrrhizic acid a day) for 2 months showed a reduction in testosterone levels. Do not take if you have high blood pressure. If you develop hypertension while taking it then discontinue.

- Maitake mushroom extract (Grifola frondosa) in a study was very effective in inducing ovulation. The proposed mechanism of action is that maitake mushroom enhanced insulin sensitivity.

- Serenoa repens (saw palmetto) inhibits 5-alpha reductase, which inhibits the conversion of testosterone to DHT and reduces androgen effects at the hair follicle and pilosebaceous unit, which decreases hirsutism and acne. Dose: 200 to 250 mg twice a day.

- Spearmint tea lowers testosterone levels and may raise FSH and LH. It may also improve hirsutism.

- Urtica dioica (nettle) is nettle root. It binds to and increases SHBG decreasing the amount of testosterone available for the body to use. Dose: 300 mg twice a day. Nettle leaf does not work.

- Vitex agnus castus (chaste berry) reduces prolactin secretion since it has dopamine agonist activity at the hypothalamic-pituitary level. It also lowers the estrogen-progesterone ratio and indirectly increases progesterone. Dose: 30 to 40 mg of dried herb. Vitex should be standardized to 0.5 percent agnuside and 0.6 percent aucubin per dose.

- White peony (Paeonia laterflora) has several actions that are beneficial for patients with PCOS.
  - Increases progesterone
  - Reduces elevated testosterone
  - Modulates estrogen
  - Modulates prolactin
  - Affects the ovarian follicle by its action on aromatase. A study using white peony revealed that it lowered testosterone, regulated LH and FSH ratios, and increased ovulation and rate of conception.

Hormones. PCOS, as you have seen, may cause hormonal imbalances.

- Cortisol. When you are stressed your cortisol levels elevate as does your insulin level. Moreover, if cortisol is increased. it decreases the making of progesterone and its activity. Cortisol competes with progesterone for common receptors. Consequently, if cortisol levels are elevated, the symptoms of PCOS can be exacerbated. The adaptogenic herbs discussed previously are beneficial to balance cortisol levels.

- Elevated testosterone. Women with PCOS have high androgen levels. The herbal therapies described on page 35 have been shown to lower testosterone.

- Many women with PCOS have low progesterone levels. Have your practitioner order a 28-day saliva test. If your progesterone level is low, then your doctor may start you on progesterone transdermally (on the skin) days 14 to 25 of your cycle. This does increase fertility. If you are not wanting to initiate a pregnancy, then discuss with your doctor birth control options.

- Estrone levels may be elevated. Weight loss commonly lowers estrone levels as does liver detoxification.

- Acupuncture can have a positive effect on PCOS patients since it influences the sympathetic nervous system, endocrine system, and neuro-endocrine system.

- A cognitive behavioral therapy (CBT) lifestyle program for pre-conceptional weight-loss in women with polycystic ovary syndrome was found to be effective.

- A study examined women with PCOS having bariatric surgery. Resolution of menstrual irregularity occurred in 100 percent of the women. Bariatric surgery causes nutritional depletions that are permanent. Make sure the nutrients that are deficient are replaced.

The good news is that there are many conventional and Precision Medicine approaches to the treatment of PCOS that have been found to be beneficial.

POSTPARTUM DEPRESSION

After a pregnancy, your body resets its hormonal levels, which sometimes results in an imbalance in hormonal function. Because of this, some women experience postpartum depression. Postpartum blues/depression has been reported to occur in 15 to 85 percent of women within the first 10 days after childbirth, with a peak incidence on day five.

■ Symptoms of Postpartum Depression

The following are symptoms of postpartum depression:

- ❑ Decreased appetite
- ❑ Difficulty bonding with the baby
- ❑ Fatigue, overwhelming at times
- ❑ Feeling shameful or guilty without cause
- ❑ Increased irritability and anger

- ❑ Insomnia
- ❑ Loss of sexual interest
- ❑ Mood swings which may be severe at times
- ❑ Social withdrawal
- ❑ Thoughts of harming themselves or their babies

■ Causes of Postpartum Depression

After a pregnancy, the body resets its hormonal levels. Postpartum depression is commonly due to an imbalance in hormonal function.

- When a woman delivers, the decrease in estrogen is two thousand times greater than the decline in estrogen that she experiences just before her cycle begins.

Risk Factors for Postpartum Depression

Postpartum depression is not exclusive to first-time moms. It can occur after the birth of any child. A new mother's risk of developing postpartum depression increases if the mom:

- Did not want or expect the pregnancy
- Experienced a great deal of stress during the year before the pregnancy
- Experienced a marital conflict
- Had postpartum depression after a previous pregnancy
- Has a history of depression
- Has a weak support system from family and friends

- Progesterone levels fall abruptly at delivery which can trigger depression as well.

- After delivery, thyroid hormone can also be dysfunctional. In fact, postpartum thyroid disorders occur in 5 percent to 10 percent of women. It is important to measure hormonal levels since some of the symptoms of hypothyroidism are very similar to the symptoms of estrogen and/ or progesterone loss. Furthermore, postpartum thyroid dysfunction can occur up to three years after delivery.

Therapies for Postpartum Depression

Conventional Therapies

Conventionally an antidepressant is prescribed for postpartum depression. Psychological counseling is also helpful. In addition, oral contraceptives are commonly given.

Precision Medicine Therapies

Precision Medicine therapies for postpartum depression are centered on the cause of the disease process. Complete thyroid studies are measured, and thyroid hormone replacement is prescribed if needed.

A 28-day salivary test to measure your female hormones may be ordered to determine if your estrogen, progesterone, and testosterone levels are optimal. If your progesterone and/or testosterone levels are low, your healthcare provider can prescribe natural hormone replacement. Your levels should be remeasured again in three months using a one-day saliva test which is done on day 21 of your cycle. This same test also measures your DHEA and cortisol levels. If your DHEA level is low, you may also be prescribed a small dose of DHEA, or your doctor may decide to see if your body is able to start making your own DHEA by helping your cortisol levels balance with the other hormones. A low DHEA level is commonly secondary to cortisol levels being too high or too low. See the section on DHEA and cortisol.

In addition, studies have also shown that omega-3-fatty acids (fish oil) have been an effective treatment for postpartum depression. Dose: 1,000 to 2,000 mg a day.

If the depression continues to be severe, oxytocin therapy has been shown to be helpful with or without an antidepressant. Psychological counseling and eating a healthy diet that is low in sugar also is beneficial.

With appropriate treatment, symptoms usually improve and alleviate after a few months, but have been known to last up to a year in some cases.

PREMATURE OVARIAN DECLINE (POD)

Premature ovarian insufficiency (POI) is a condition associated with female infertility that affects about 1 percent of women under the age of 40. Premature ovarian decline (POD) and premature ovarian failure (POF) are similar ailments. A less perceptible decline in ovarian activity, known as premature ovarian aging (POA) occurs in about 10 percent of women. With POD, hormone production begins to decrease at an early age. However, women with POD still have follicles in their ovaries and still experience menstrual cycles. Women with premature ovarian failure have loss of normal hormonal function at an early age and do not cycle.

Premature ovarian decline is commonly due to hormonal dysregulation. Some studies have shown that women can have low estrogen or testosterone levels even though their progesterone and FSH levels are normal, and the women are still menstruating. Another reason for POD is estrogen dominance where women have low progesterone with normal or elevated levels of estrogen.

■ Causes of POD

The term premature ovarian decline was coined by Dr. Elizbeth Vliet in her ground-breaking book: It's My Ovaries, Stupid. The following are causes of POD as described by Dr. Vliet in her book:

- Chronic dieting

- Cigarette smoking which damages ovarian follicles

- Compulsive exercise

- Discontinuing birth control pills after long-term usage (especially high-progestin pills)

- Eating disorders, such as anorexia or bulimia that suppress the hypothalamus and its regulation of the ovaries

- Hypothalamic dysfunction due to high intake of soy or other excitotoxins, such as glutamate, MSG, or aspartame

- Hysterectomy without ovarian removal

Risk Factors for POD

The following are risk factors for premature ovarian dysfunction:

- Body weight—thinner women have earlier onset
- Living at high altitudes
- Malnutrition
- Mother had an early onset of menopause
- Nulliparous—a women who has not birthed a child
- Vegetarian diet

- Polycystic ovarian disease
- Postpartum (after delivery)
- Thyroid disorders

- Toxic exposures, such as black widow spider bites, Lyme disease, or pesticides
- Viral oophoritis (inflammation of an ovary)

Newly, your mitochondria which are the engines in your body, can age prematurely which may cause mitochondrial DNA mutations in the egg leading to early deterioration in function.

Therapies for POD

Conventional Therapies

Conventional therapies are usually centered around treating the cause of the problem and starting synthetic hormone replacement.

Precision Medicine Therapies

Precision Medicine therapies center on treating the cause of the problem and also achieving hormonal balance through natural hormone replacement. A 28-day saliva test to determine the hormone levels throughout the entire month along with adrenal function is the best place to begin to determine what treatment course you should follow if you have POD. In addition, stress has been shown to impact ovarian function. The following blood levels are also important to determine the best course of therapy.

- Complete thyroid studies:
  - TSH
  - T3
  - Free T4
  - Reverse T3
  - Thyroid antibodies

- FSH and LH
- Gonadotropin releasing hormone (GnRH) to determine hypothalamic function
- Prolactin
- Ultrasound of the pelvis.

From these labs, your doctor can then develop a personalized approach to the treatment of premature ovarian decline.

Consider refueling the mitochondria under your healthcare provider's direction to see if your hormonal function improves with daily use of the following.

- Alpha lipoic acid: 300 mg
- Coenzyme Q-10: 300 mg
- D-ribose: 15 grams

- L-carnitine: 2 grams a day if you have a normal TMAO level (See section on Heart Disease).
- Magnesium glycinate: 400 mg
- NADH: 10 mg twice a day

See also Premature Ovarian Failure (POF).

PREMATURE OVARIAN FAILURE (POF)

Premature ovarian failure is defined as a primary ovarian defect characterized by absent menarche (the first occurrence of a menstrual cycle) before the age of 40. It is also characterized by low estrogen levels as well as other decreased levels of sex hormones. It affects approximately: one in 10,000 women by age 20; one in 1,000 women by age 30; one in 100 women by age 40. The symptoms of premature ovarian failure are the same as you would see in a menopausal woman. Up to 50 percent of individuals with POF will have intermittent and unpredictable ovarian function which may persist for some years.

Premature ovarian failure (POF) is not entirely the same as POD. POF is defined as the end of menstrual cycles before the age of thirty-five while follicle-stimulating hormone (FSH) levels are elevated (above 20 mIU/

mL). FSH is the hormone that regulates the development, growth, pubertal maturation, and reproductive process in the human body.

■ Symptoms of POF

Many of the symptoms of POF are similar to symptoms of menopause.

❏ Decreased sexual desire   ❏ Irritability

❏ Difficulty concentrating   ❏ Night sweats

❏ Hot flashes   ❏ Shorter life span

❏ Irregular menstrual cycles   ❏ Vaginal dryness

■ Causes of POF

POF can develop when there are few or no responsive follicles left in the ovaries. ("Responsive" follicles are the follicles that release estrogen while maturing and eventually release an egg. When there are few or none left, it is called follicle depletion.) It can also result from follicles that don't respond properly (follicle dysfunction). However, more often than not, there is no definitive cause of POF that is found.

● Follicle depletion. Follicle depletion can be caused by chromosomal defects or by exposure to toxins.

● Follicle dysfunction. Follicle dysfunction usually arises from autoimmune disease. A woman's body sometimes produces antibodies against her own ovarian tissue, which can harm the follicles that contain eggs.

To be more descriptive, premature ovarian failure may be due to a primary or secondary failure.

● Primary premature ovarian failure is an ovarian defect defined by absent menarche (the first occurrence of menstruation) which is in 50 percent of the cases and is due to ovarian dysgenesis—disorder of the reproductive system. X chromosome abnormalities, such as Turner syndrome, are most of the cases of primary amenorrhea (absence of menstruation).

● Secondary premature ovarian failure is an ovarian defect due to premature depletion of ovarian follicles or arrested follicular development.

Risk Factors for POF

There are many reasons why women may experience POF, such as early loss of follicles in the ovaries, viruses, endocrine disruptors, autoimmune diseases, or any other disorder that prevents the ovaries from functioning normally. However, there are only two main risk factors for POF:

- Age. The older you get, the higher your risk of developing POF will be. At age thirty-five, the average woman's risk of developing POF is one in 250.

- Family history. If POF runs in your family, your risk of developing the disease is greater. However, in her book *It's My Ovaries, Stupid,* Dr. Elizabeth Vliet looks at many other possible reasons why the ovaries stop functioning at an early age.

Additional Causes of POF

- Autoimmune process. The risk of premature ovarian failure increases in association with alteration in immunological parameters and oxidative stress.

- Cessation of birth control pills after long-term use

- Chemotherapy

- Chronic dieting and eating disorders (anorexia, bulimia)

- Cigarette smoking

- Compulsive exercise

- Damage before you were born (in utero) from smoking, alcohol, pesticides, and other chemical exposures

- Genetic abnormalities

- High intake of excitatory items (glutamate, MSG, aspartame)

- High intake of soy

- Hysterectomy without removal of ovaries

- Living at high altitudes

- Malnutrition

- Medications that disrupt the hypothalamic-pituitary-ovarian pathways (antidepressants, antipsychotics, and anticonvulsants)

- Never having been pregnant (more pregnancies lead to later menopause)

- PCOS

- Postpartum (may happen to women who are older when they deliver)

- Radiation exposure

- Recreational drug use (marijuana, cocaine, ecstasy)

- Thin body structure (thinner women have earlier onset)

- Thyroid disorders

- Toxic exposures (black widow spider bites, Lyme disease, pesticides)

- Tubal ligation

- Vegetarian diet

- Viral oophoritis (viral infiltration of the ovary). Herpes zoster and cytomegalovirus are two of the most common infectious causes.

Therapies for POF

Conventional Therapies

- Addressing infertility. Infertility is a common complication of POF, and unfortunately, there is no treatment to restore fertility to women who have POF. However, one thing that can be viewed as a type of treatment for infertility is to investigate alternate forms of childbirth, such as in vitro fertilization with donor eggs.

- Estrogen therapy. Replacing estrogen can help relieve vaginal dryness and hot flashes. However, if your doctor prescribes estrogen for you, he or she will likely also recommend you take progesterone in order to protect the lining of your uterus. Using these two hormones together can restart menstruation in women who may have stopped.

Precision Medicine Therapies

After all appropriate tests are performed, your healthcare provider will better be able to discuss possible treatment options for you. If you have premature ovarian failure, a wonderful option is to be started on prescription natural hormones. Natural hormones, as you have seen in this book, help not only with symptoms, but clinical trials have shown that they also help prevent and treat heart disease and cognitive decline. In addition, hormones are needed to help maintain bone structure and help prevent osteopenia/osteoporosis.

See also Premature Ovarian Decline (POD).

Diagnosing POD and POF

There are several studies that your healthcare provider will order to help with the diagnosing of POD and POF.

- The gold standard to evaluate POD or POF is to have a twenty-eight-day salivary test done. This measures your levels of estrogen, progesterone, and testosterone throughout an entire month. Your DHEA, cortisol, and melatonin levels are also measured with this test since they are also part of your hormonal symphony. This way, your healthcare practitioner will be able to develop a treatment program that is individualized to your own needs. No two women are alike, so the hormones you need at whichever stage in life you are at are unique to you.

- Karyotype. This test examines all forty-six chromosomes for abnormalities. Sometimes women with POF have only one X chromosome instead of two. There are other chromosomal disorders that are related to POF, which is why the karyotype is useful.

- Complete thyroid studies
  - TSH
  - Free T3
  - Free T4
  - Reverse T3
  - Thyroid antibodies

- FSH and LH

- Gonadotropin releasing hormone (GnRH) to determine hypothalamic function)

- Prolactin

- Ultrasound of the pelvis.

- Nutritional testing to determine levels of nutrients that may be deficient. Adequate intake of trace elements is required to prevent oxidative stress and immune dysfunction.

PREMENSTRUAL DYSPHORIC DISORDER (PMDD)

Premenstrual dysphoric disorder (PMDD) is a condition that is associated with severe emotional and physical symptoms that are linked to the menstrual cycle. PMDD is considered to be a severe form of PMS that affects about 5 to 10 percent of menstruating women.

PMDD is distinguished from PMS by the intensity and severity of its symptoms. The symptoms of PMDD are often so severe that they are considered disabling, meaning they get in the way of daily activities and relationships. By definition, the symptoms of PMDD start during the last week of your menstrual cycle and usually cease during the week following your cycle.

There are different types of PMDD. Some examples of PMDD are listed below.

- Symptoms start at mid-cycle (ovulation) and become worse as the cycle approaches and end shortly after the cycle begins.

- Symptoms start during the week before the menstrual cycle starts and end shortly after the cycle begins.

- Symptoms occur at ovulation and resolve after a few days but reoccur as the cycle approaches.

- Symptoms start at ovulation, become progressively worse, and continue until the menstrual cycle concludes.

Furthermore, these symptoms occur every month or almost every month.

■ Diagnosing PMDD

In order to be diagnosed with PMDD, your symptoms must be severe enough to really disrupt your life. In other words, the symptoms interfere with work, school, relationships, and/or social activities.

■ Symptoms of PMDD

The following are the symptoms that meet the criteria for the diagnosis of PMDD. The symptoms PMDD sufferers experience may change from month to month, but at least five of the following symptoms need to be present to make the diagnosis of PMDD.

❑ Difficulty concentrating and staying focused

❑ Fatigue, tiredness, or loss of energy

❑ Feeling out of control or overwhelmed

❑ Insomnia or sleeping too much

❑ Loss of interest in usual activities (work, school, or social activities)

❑ Marked anxiety, tension, or edginess

❑ Marked appetite change, overeating, or food cravings

❑ Persistent, marked irritability; anger; increased conflicts

❑ Physical symptoms such as weight gain, bloating, breast tenderness or swelling, headache, and muscle or joint pain

❑ Sudden mood swings (crying easily or extreme sensitivity)

❑ Very depressed mood, feeling hopeless

■ Causes of PMDD

The cause of PMDD isn't clear. The current theories related to the cause of PMDD focus on the fact that it may not be due to a hormonal imbalance but rather to an imbalance of the neurotransmitters in your body. One neurotransmitter that is being looked at is serotonin, your "happy" neurotransmitter. Additionally, a number of women with severe PMS may have an underlying psychiatric disorder, and major depression is very common in women who have PMDD. However, PMDD can and does also occur in women who do not have depression.

■ Treating PMDD

PMDD treatment is designed to minimize or eliminate symptoms. Since symptoms vary, treatment will depend on the individual and the symptoms she is experiencing.

● Certain medications, such as:

• Anti-anxiety medications

• Diuretics (water pills)

● *Paxil CR* (parozetine controlled release)

- YAZ (drospirenone ethinyl estradiol, an oral contraceptive)
- *Zoloft* (sertraline)
- Eating five to six small meals per day
- Exercise
- Increasing your complex carbohydrate and protein intake
- Limiting your intake of alcohol, caffeine, salt, and refined sugar
- Psychotherapy
- Hormonal therapy (usually progesterone, but testosterone and estrogen levels can be suboptimal)
- Chaste tree (Vitex agnus castus given as part of an herbal combination.)

PREMENSTRUAL SYNDROME (PMS)

Premenstrual syndrome (PMS) is a hormonal disorder that is characterized by the monthly recurrence of physical or psychological symptoms. It can be difficult to diagnose, because there are so many signs and symptoms associated with PMS. The only thing all the symptoms have in common is they all affect you two weeks before your monthly period. They usually subside when your menstrual cycle begins.

PMS affects between 60 and 75 percent of women in the United States, which means that as many as three of every four women who menstruate experience some form of PMS. The problems are more common in women who are between their late twenties and early forties. Generally, the problems and symptoms reoccur in predictable patterns, but some months may be more severe than others.

Diagnosing PMS

There is no test to positively diagnose PMS from a conventional medicine viewpoint. Doctors sometimes attribute symptoms to PMS based on your premenstrual pattern, which is established by keeping a record of your symptoms for at least two months (or however long your doctor requests). Show your record to your doctor, who will then determine the proper method of treatment. From a Precision Medicine perspective, a 28-day salivary test is imperative to help diagnose PMS.

■ Symptoms of PMS

PMS has many symptoms associated with it. Some of these symptoms affect weight gain, such as abdominal bloating, appetite changes, and salt and sugar cravings. However, there are many other symptoms of PMS.

❑ Abdominal bloating

❑ Aches and pains

❑ Acne flare-ups

❑ Alcohol sensitivity

❑ Angry outbursts

❑ Anxiety

❑ Asthmatic attacks

❑ Avoidance of social activities

❑ Backache

❑ Bladder irritation

❑ Bleeding gums

❑ Blood pressure increases during the luteal phase

❑ Breast tenderness

❑ Bruising

❑ Changes in appetite

❑ Clumsiness

❑ Confusion

❑ Conjunctivitis

❑ Constipation

❑ Cramps

❑ Craving salty foods or sweets

❑ Crying spells

❑ Decreased hearing

❑ Decreased productivity

❑ Decreased sex drive

❑ Depression

❑ Diarrhea or constipation

❑ Difficulty concentrating

❑ Dizziness

❑ Drowsiness

❑ Eye pain

❑ Facial swelling

❑ Fatigue

❑ Fear of going out alone

❑ Fear of losing control

❑ Food sensitivity

❑ Forgetfulness

❑ Headaches

❑ Herpes (cold sores)

❑ Hives or rashes

❑ Hot flashes

❑ Indecision

❑ Inefficiency

❑ Insomnia

❑ Irritability

❑ Joint pain

❑ Leg cramps

❑ Leg swelling

❑ Mood swings

❑ Muscle aches

❑ Nausea

❑ Palpitations

❑ Panic attacks

❑ Poor coordination

❑ Poor judgment

❑ Poor memory

❑ Poor vision

❑ Restlessness

❑ Ringing in ears

❑ Runny nose

❑ Seizures

❑ Sensitivity to light and noise

❑ Sinusitis

❑ Social withdrawal

❑ Sore throat

❑ Spots in front of eyes

❑ Suspiciousness

❑ Swollen fingers

❑ Tearfulness

❑ Tension

❑ Tingling in hands and feet

❑ Tremors

❑ Visual changes

❑ Vomiting

❑ Weight gain

Additionally, women with PMS tend to have low zinc levels. Zinc is involved in over 300 reactions in the body, including the production of the sex hormones. Thus, low zinc levels can lead to a host of problems including infertility, hypothyroidism, and elevated blood sugar levels.

The number of symptoms may seem overwhelming, but in actuality, most women who have PMS experience only a few.

■ Causes of PMS

As of yet, the cause of PMS is not known. Changes in hormones during the menstrual cycle are definitely an important consideration. There are, however, several theories and factors that contribute to PMS.

● Caffeine consumption

● Low blood-sugar levels

● Low estrogen levels. Estrogen levels change during your twenty-eight-day cycle, but not as dramatically as progesterone levels do. Your estrogen levels decrease at ovulation. They also decrease just before and during your cycle. When estrogen levels decline, your neurotransmitters change. Serotonin and dopamine levels decline, which can lead

Twenty-Eight-Day Menstrual Cycle

Every month, women who are of a reproductive age and who are not pregnant experience a menstrual cycle, which results in either pregnancy or menstruation. The average menstrual cycle is twenty-eight days long.

Days one to five of the cycle are considered the menstrual phase. The first day of a woman's period is considered the first day of the monthly menstrual cycle. If the egg has not been fertilized, it disintegrates. Low levels of estrogen and progesterone at this time cause the endometrium (the lining of the uterus) to break down and leave the body in the form of blood. This is known as a period, or a menstrual cycle. On average, the bleeding lasts about five days.

Expanding past the menstrual phase, days one to thirteen are considered the follicular phase. During this time, the brain releases follicle-stimulating hormone (FSH), which promotes the development of several follicles in the ovaries. Only one of these follicles, which each contain an egg, will reach maturity. As day thirteen approaches, the ovaries release more and more estrogen, thickening the uterine lining in case an egg gets fertilized.

Days ten to eighteen are the ovulatory phase. During this phase, the brain releases an abundance of luteinizing hormone (LH), which causes the mature follicle to bulge out from the surface of the ovary and burst, releasing the egg. This usually occurs around day fourteen. After this, the egg begins to travel down the fallopian tube and into the uterus. Fertilization, and therefore pregnancy, is most likely to occur during this phase.

Days fifteen to twenty-eight are the luteal phase. Having released the egg, the follicle develops into a corpus luteum, which secretes more and more progesterone, causing the endometrium to thicken further in case embryonic development takes place. If the egg is fertilized, the corpus luteum will begin to make human chorionic gonadotropin (HCG), which helps maintain the corpus luteum and its release of progesterone. Human chorionic gonadotropin is also the hormone that pregnancy tests detect.

The fertilized egg continues down the fallopian tube until it reaches the uterus, where it implants itself to the endometrium. This is where it develops into a fetus.

to depression. Also, when estrogen levels decrease, your norepinephrine levels may increase, which can make you feel more anxious and
irritable.

- Low progesterone levels. Low progesterone levels on days twelve to
fourteen of the menstrual cycle, which can be confirmed by saliva testing, are very commonly associated with PMS. There is no clear course
of development when it comes to PMS. However, something in the
person's life interferes with the pituitary-ovarian feedback loop, and it
decreases the supply of progesterone.

- Neurotransmitter changes are a common cause of PMS. Decreased
serotonin activity has been seen in the late luteal phase of the cycle and
therefore may be related to the increase in appetite, psychomotor activity, and depression that may occur in PMS. In addition, the serotonergic
system in women who have PMS has been shown to have abnormal
functioning. This is related to altered serotonin levels and altered serotonin transmission. Additionally, some women who experience severe
PMS symptoms have undiagnosed depression, but depression by itself
does not cause all the PMS symptoms.

- Oral contraceptives. Taking oral contraceptives may contribute to PMS,
due to the progestin (synthetic progesterone) they contain.

- Partial hysterectomies. A partial hysterectomy may be a precipitating
factor for PMS due to the decreased supply of blood to the ovaries post
hysterectomy.

- Pregnancies, miscarriages, abortions, and tubal ligations (a procedure
where the fallopian tubes are cut, burned, or blocked to prevent pregnancy) are also considered contributing factors to PMS. Studies have
shown that after a tubal ligation, women have higher estrogen levels
and lower progesterone levels in the second half of their cycle each
month.

- Women with PMS may also have a decreased effectiveness in their
stress response compared to women without PMS. They may experience a blunted cortisol response. Consequently, stress can aggravate
some symptoms.

Additionally, some women who experience severe PMS symptoms
have undiagnosed depression, but depression itself does not cause all

PMS symptoms. Likewise, while stress can aggravate some symptoms, it does not cause them on their own.

Nutrition can also play a role. Deficiencies in certain vitamins and minerals, such as vitamin B_6, calcium, and magnesium, can make the symptoms of PMS worse. Eating a lot of salty foods can cause fluid retention, which can worsen symptoms. Drinking alcohol can cause mood and energy disturbances, which can also aggravate symptoms.

■ Precision Medicine Therapies for PMS

Precision Medicine approaches to PMS include the following: dietary factors, nutritional supplements, exercise, thyroid medication if indicated, botanicals, progesterone replacement, and mind-body therapy.

Dietary factors. A study showed that women with PMS eat a diet that is worse than the standard American diet compared to women without PMS.

- 62 percent more refined carbohydrates

- 275 percent more refined sugar

- 79 percent more dairy products

- 78 percent more sodium

- 53 percent less iron

- 77 percent less manganese

- 52 percent less zinc

Another study comparing women with and without PMS showed that women with PMS consumed fivefold more dairy products and threefold more refined sugar than those that did not have PMS. Some women with PMS find that their symptoms improve if they avoid dairy products.

Yet another trial showed that women with PMS consumed more dietary fat, carbohydrates including simple sugars, and less protein. Improving the patient's eating habits will help their symptoms of PMS. Women should decrease caffeine and alcohol intake, which are antagonists to B vitamins, and eat six small meals a day avoiding refined sugars even though many women crave them just prior to their cycle.

The sugar cravings that some women have may be a physiological response to serotonin deficiency, because eating carbohydrates increases the brain uptake of tryptophan, which then increases serotonin synthesis in the brain.

Eating refined carbohydrates relieves the symptoms short-term but in the long run makes the symptoms of PMS worse. Sugar decreases magnesium from the body and causes fluid retention. To decrease the edema that may occur with PMS, also avoid foods with a high sodium content and incorporate foods into your diet that are natural diuretics like strawberries and parsley.

Evening primrose oil (500 to 3,000 mg a day) and increasing your intake of water has been also shown to be beneficial to decrease the occurrence of edema during PMS, along with exercising and eating a good fat diet. Progesterone can also be an effective diuretic. Likewise, if you eat a poor diet, it sets up an inflammatory response in the body. Elevated c-reactive protein (CRP) has been correlated with the physical and psychological symptoms of PMS. Eating a Mediterranean diet, which is anti-inflammatory, is the best choice.

■ Nutritional Support

- **Magnesium.** Women with PMS may have low magnesium levels. Some of the symptoms of PMS are the same as magnesium deficiency: anxiety, depression, irritability, and headaches. Individuals should eat foods that are high in magnesium. Supplementing with magnesium glycinate (400 to 600 mg with normal renal function) has been shown to help with the symptoms of PMS. One trial, where patients with PMS were given magnesium, the patients had the following results: reduction of nervousness in 89 percent, decreased breast tenderness in 96 percent, and weight loss in 95 percent. In a double-blind study, using magnesium 360 mg three times a day, the patients had a dramatic relief in PMS-related mood changes. Another study showed that the combination of magnesium and vitamin B_6 improved PMS symptoms better than either nutrient by itself.

- **Pyridoxine (vitamin B_6) is a cofactor for more than 100 enzymatic reactions in the body.** Many of the reactions are related to neurotransmitter function: dopamine, serotonin, epinephrine, norepinephrine, taurine, and histamine all need vitamin B_6 for production. Vitamin B_6 also reduces some of the negative effects of estrogen dominance and increases progesterone. Furthermore, B_6 enhances the accumulation of magnesium in the cells. Vitamin B_6 helps resolve symptoms of PMS, such as bloating, headache, breast pain, depression, irritability, and possibly acne. Many studies have shown a positive effect with B_6 supplementation for all PMS symptoms. The most common dose prescribed is 100 mg a day. Some patients may need to take the active form of pyridoxine, which is pyridoxal-5-phosphate. However, some trials showed that vitamin B$_6$ supplementation was not effective.

- **Vitamin E.** In a medical trial, women with fibrocystic breast disease took vitamin E at 150, 300, or 600 IU daily versus placebo. Symptoms of PMS also improved, such as anxiety, depression, and sugar cravings.

- **Tryptophan** is a precursor to serotonin. In a double-blind study, cyclic administration of L-tryptophan (2 grams three times a day) improved mood disturbances in women with PMDD. Studies have shown that L-tryptophan used in patients with PMS had reductions in the following symptoms: mood swings, insomnia, carbohydrate cravings, tension, irritability, and dysphoria. Lower doses may be effective (500 to 1,000 mg a day) if taken on an empty stomach or with carbohydrates. Start the tryptophan at ovulation and use until day three of menses. Tryptophan should be avoided if you are taking an MAOI. It should be used with caution if you are taking on SSRIs or amitriptyline. Therefore, contact your healthcare provider before starting tryptophan.

- **Calcium.** Studies have shown that calcium supplementation improves PMS symptoms.

- **Manganese.** Another study using manganese and calcium supplementation improved mood, concentration, and behavior in patients with PMS.

- **Zinc** levels have been shown in clinical trials to be low in patients with PMS. Zinc is needed for the control of the synthesis and secretion of sex hormones. When zinc levels are low prolactin levels increase, which lowers progesterone levels. Taking a multivitamin with adequate zinc and eating foods high in zinc can be beneficial if you have PMS.

- **Evening primrose oil.** Some women with PMS have been shown to have abnormalities of prostaglandin metabolism. A study found that women with PMS may have a defect in the conversion of linoleic acid to gamma-linolenic acid (GLA). Evening primrose oil (EPO) contains preformed GLA so it can bypass this metabolic block in prostaglandin synthesis. Double-blind studies have shown that EPO improved symptoms of PMS in doses of 3 to 6 grams a day. Other studies did not show a benefit with the use of EPO.

- **Omega-3-fatty acids.** Dietary or supplemental omega-3-fatty acids have been found to be beneficial for depression. Furthermore, omega-3-fatty acids have also been shown to help with menstrual pain. The most common dose is 2,000 mg day 14 until the menstrual cycle concludes.

Exercise

Exercise helps with PMS symptoms: painful muscles and joints, tension headaches, low back pain, lower body bloating, tiredness, and irritability. Studies have shown that women who exercise regularly do not have PMS as often as women who do not exercise. Women with PMS should do a regular exercise program. Exercise has the following effects that help with PMS: elevates endorphin levels, improves glucose tolerance, decreases catecholamines, and modulates estrogen levels. A medical trial showed that the frequency of exercise, rather than intensity, aids more in the prevention and alleviation of the physical and emotional symptoms of PMS.

Botanicals

- **Black cohosh** (Cimcifuga raccmosa) has the following effects which may improve PMS symptoms: may have a balancing effect on estrogen, is a relaxant, sedative, anti-spasmotic, and has serotonergic and dopaminergic effects. A study in women with PMS showed that black cohosh was effective in reducing anxiety, tension, and depression. The most common dosage is 20 to 40 mg of standardized extract twice a day. Researchers found that compounds in black cohosh bind 5-HT7 receptors, which may be why it is effective for mood. The German Commision E endorses the use of black cohosh for PMS. Use this botanical with caution if you have liver disease. It is always a great idea to discuss with your healthcare provider any vitamins and herbal therapies you are considering.

- **Chasteberry** (Vitex agnus castus) is the most popular and efficacious herb for PMS. It acts like a diuretic, binds opiate receptors, affects gonadotropin-releasing hormone, affects follicle-stimulating hormone-releasing hormone, decreases LH and prolactin (a dopamine agonist), and raises progesterone and facilitates its function. Studies of 1,500 women in Germany treated with Chasteberry revealed that 33 percent had complete resolution of symptoms and 57 percent reported significant improvement. In a randomized clinical study comparing chaste tree standardized extract (20 mg tablet standardized for casticin) versus placebo in women with PMS, it revealed a 52 percent decrease in PMS symptoms in women who used Chasteberry and a 24 percent decrease in PMS symptoms in women that were the control. A common suggested dosage of Chasteberry is: 250-500 mg a day of dried fruit or 20 to 40 mg a day of extract.

- **St. John's Wort** (*Hypericum perforatum*) was used in a randomized double-blind placebo-controlled crossover trial looking at women with PMS. They were given Hypericum perforatum capsules (900 mg a day and standardized to 0.18 percent hypericin and 3.38 percent hyperiforin) or placebo. St. John's wort was of more benefit than placebo in relieving the following: anxiety, irritability, pain, depression, nervous tension, mood swings, and feeling out of control. An uncontrolled study using Hypericum perforatum in women with PMS found that two-thirds of the women in the study had at least a 50 percent decrease in the severity of their symptoms. The recommended dose is 300 to 600 mg three times a day of standardized extract (0.3 percent hypericin content). Precautions: If you are taking drugs that increase photosensitivity, protease inhibitors, cyclosporine, or other medications that are metabolized by the cytochrome P-450 CYP3A4 system or affect P-glycoprotein, you should not take St. John's wort.

- **Ginkgo biloba** has shown to help with PMS symptoms. The suggested dose is 80 to 160 mg a day of extract (24 percent ginkgoflavonglycosides). Ginkgo is a blood thinner, so it should not be used with other blood thinners.

- **Saffron (Crocus sativus L.)** has a serotonergic mechanism. A study using 15 mg of Saffron twice a day versus placebo showed that women using the Saffron had a much higher rate of resolution and improvement of PMS symptoms than placebo.

- **Lavender** has been shown to be very good for the following symptoms of PMS: anxiety, irritability, depression, and insomnia. The German Commission E suggests lavender for mood, sleep disturbances, and restlessness.

- **Motherwort** is used for symptoms of PMS, such as nervous exhaustion, irritability, hysteria, dysmenorrhea, and nervous excitability.

- **Dandelion leaf** can be helpful for fluid retention that occurs with PMS. The dose is 200 mg capsule twice a day.

SUPPLEMENTATION FOR PMS		
Supplements	Dosage	Considerations
Angelica sinensis	Given as part of an herbal combination	Helps treat painful cycles (dysmenorrheal), absence of cycles (amenorrhea), and abnormal menstruation (metrorrhagia). Start supplementation on day fourteen of your cycle and continue until end of cycle. If you are taking it for abnormal cycles, stop before your cycle starts.
Borage oil	500 to 1,000 mg	Can help reduce breast tenderness, fluid retention, cramps, and psychological PMS symptoms.
Calcium	600 to 1,000 mg	Can help reduce breast tenderness, fluid retention, cramps, and psychological PMS symptoms.
Evening primrose	1,000 to 2,000 mg	Can help reduce breast tenderness, fluid retention, cramps, and psychological PMS symptoms.
Ginkgo biloba	120 to 180 mg	Helps relieve breast pain and tenderness.
Licorice (glycyrrhlza glabra)*	Varies (see doctor for dosage)	Lowers estrogen levels and raises progesterone levels. Decreases water retention. Do not use if you have high blood pressure.
Magnesium	300 to 600 mg	Can help reduce breast tenderness, fluid retention, cramps, and psychological PMS symptoms.
Omega-3	1,000 to 2,000 mg	Can help reduce breast tenderness, fluid fatty acids retention, cramps, and psychological PMS symptoms.
St. John's wort (Hypericum perforatum)	500 mg twice a day	Do not take if you are on an antidepressant.
Taurine	1,000 mg	Can help reduce breast tenderness, fluid retention, cramps, and psychological PMS symptoms.
Vitamin A	5,000 to 8,000 IU (can use up to 25,000 under the direction of a physician)	Can help reduce breast tenderness, fluid retention, cramps, and psychological PMS IU symptoms.
Vitamin B_6	100 mg in a B complex	Can help reduce breast tenderness, fluid retention, cramps, and psychological PMS symptoms.
Vitamin B_{12}	1000 micrograms in a B complex	Can help reduce breast tenderness, fluid retention, cramps, and psychological PMS symptoms.
Vitamin E	400 to 800 IU	Can help reduce breast tenderness, fluid retention, cramps, and psychological PMS symptoms. Do not use if you take Coumadin.

■ Medications

- **Progesterone.** Since PMS is a state that is affected by low progesterone levels, progesterone supplementation has been found to be helpful. Supplementation should be with bio-identical progesterone, which is compounded to be the same chemical structure as the progesterone your body makes. This is also called natural progesterone. It is a prescription made by a compounding pharmacy to be used on days fourteen to twenty-five (starting twelve days after your first day of bleeding) of the menstrual cycle.

  This progesterone is applied as a cream, which is derived from wild yams and soybeans. However, if you have insomnia, progesterone is best taken as a pill so that it affects the GABA receptors in the brain, which will produce a calming effect and allow you to sleep better. Otherwise, transdermally (on the skin) applied progesterone is usually prescribed. Progesterone has been found to be effective for many women with PMS. It is important to do salivary testing to determine the dosage. Progesterone can be given transdermally (on the skin) or orally for PMS and is given days 14 to 25 of the menstrual cycle.

- **Thyroid Medication.** Some of the symptoms of PMS are similar to symptoms of hypothyroidism. Studies have shown that subclinical hypothyroidism was common in women with PMS and that they did better when placed on a small amount of thyroid medication if they have hypothyroidism. Therefore, it is important to have your doctor check your thyroid levels. If they are low or suboptimal, then consider taking a small dose of prescription thyroid medication. As you have seen, it is also important to have iodine levels measured prior to starting thyroid medication.

- **Other Hormones and Neurotransmitters.** There is also a subset of women who have low estradiol (E_2, a form of estrogen) levels and normal progesterone levels associated with PMS. For these women, progesterone will not work. Low levels of E_2 are associated with neurotransmitter changes, including dopamine, norepinephrine, and epinephrine depletion. Furthermore, a rapid rise and fall in estrogen levels can affect serotonin production. This may trigger depression and changes in eating patterns. If you are one of these women, the herbal therapies discussed previously may be more effective.

■ Mind-Body Therapy

Many mind-body therapies have been shown to be effective for PMS: cognitive-behavioral therapy, group therapy, hand reflexology, massage, hypnotherapy, biofeedback, guided imagery, and yoga.

STRESS

See Heart Disease; Osteoporosis; Polycystic Ovarian Syndrome (PCOS); Postpartum Depression.

STROKE

See Heart Disease.

SURGICAL MENOPAUSE

See Menopause and Perimenopause.

THYROTOXICOSIS

See Hyperthyroidism.

URINARY LEAKAGE

See Bladder Problems.

UTERINE CANCER

Uterine cancer is cancer of the uterus. It is the most common form of cancer of the female tract with over 60,000 new cases being diagnosed each year. Endometrial cancer is a form of uterine cancer. It occurs in the lining of the uterus and is the most common form of cancer of the uterus. It usually occurs after menopause.

Endometrial Cancer

Endometrial cancers can be divided into two subtypes: type 1, which are estrogen dependent and comprise about 80 percent of all endometrial cancers, and type 2, which are non-estrogen dependent. Abnormal vaginal bleeding is the most common symptom, but a woman may also experience discharge, weight loss, abdominal or pelvic pain, dysuria (painful urination), or dyspareunia (painful intercourse). Vaginal bleeding in any postmenopausal woman should be considered uterine cancer until proven otherwise. Most endometrial cancers are slow-growing and are discovered at an early stage. These cases can be successfully treated, usually by hysterectomy, with better than 90 percent cure rates. Advanced cases that spread beyond the uterus more commonly have a bad outcome.

■ Preventing Uterine Cancer

You can decrease your risk of uterine cancer by normalizing your weight and following a good diet that is anti-inflammatory and low in sugar. Also, regular physical activity is associated with a 20 percent to 30 percent reduction in risk. Having normal melatonin levels or supplementing with melatonin when your levels are low also lowers your risk. Melatonin levels can be measured by a salivary test (see page 377 for details).

Eating a healthy diet helps to prevent all forms of cancer. Studies have shown that avoiding or reducing meat, dairy products, and saturated fats decrease your risk of developing uterine cancer. In fact, one study revealed that saturated fat increased your risk of developing this disease more than three times that of other types of fat. In addition, previous research found that a higher fat intake, particularly saturated fat, was associated with elevations of endometrial cancer risk by approximately 60 to 80 percent.

Avoid sugar and high glycemic-index carbohydrates. The Iowa Women's Health Study found a 78 percent greater risk for endometrial cancer in women who consumed the most sugar-sweetened beverages, compared to those who consumed the lowest amount. Likewise, a meta-analysis comparing women whose diets had the highest compared with the lowest glycemic load found a roughly 20 percent higher risk for those in the former category.

Risk Factors for Uterine Cancer

Women between the ages of 50 and 70 are at an increased risk for cancer of the uterus. Some of the other major risk factors are:

- Antidepressant use

- Diabetes/chronic hyperinsulinemia (high insulin level)

- Early age of menarche (when your cycles started)

- Estrogen secreting tumors are rare, but they increase the risk of developing endometrial cancer.

- Genetic variants in hormone metabolism

- Genetics/Family history. Uterine cancer may run in families where colon cancer is hereditary. Women who have a first-degree relative with endometrial cancer are at increased risk of developing endometrial cancer. A family history of (HNPCC) hereditary nonpolyposis colorectal cancer (Lynch syndrome) greatly increases the risk as well. Women in families with Lynch syndrome, also called hereditary non-polyposis colorectal cancer (HNPCC), have a higher risk for uterine cancer. It is therefore recommended that all women under the age of 70 with endometrial cancer should have their tumor tested for Lynch syndrome, even if they have no family history of colon cancer or other cancers. The presence of Lynch syndrome has important implications for women and their family members. About 2 percent to 5 percent of women with endometrial cancer have Lynch syndrome. In the United States, about 1,000 to 2,500 women diagnosed with endometrial cancer each year may have this genetic condition.

- High androgen levels (testosterone, DHEA, androstenedione) increase your risk by inducing chronic anovulation (ovaries do not release an egg during the menstrual cycle) and progesterone deficiency in premenopausal women. In menopausal women, low progesterone levels and excess weight may increase the risk through elevated plasma levels of androgen precursors and increasing estrogen levels through the aromatization of the androgens in adipose tissue (body fat). The ovarian androgen excess may be because of an interaction between obesity-related, chronic hyperinsulinemia with genetic factors predisposing to the development of ovarian hyperandrogenism.

- Hormone replacement with estrogen alone and no progesterone to balance (unopposed estrogen)

- Lack of physical exercise

- Low sex hormone binding globulin level (SHBG)

- Menopausal women who have increased levels of estrone and estradiol (estrogen dominance)

- Menopause after the age of fifty-five

- Moderate-to-high alcohol intake

- Obesity. Obesity accounts for more than 50 percent of all cases of endometrial cancer. It is presumably due to the peripheral conversion of androgens to estrogen in adipose tissue, which leads to greater endogenous estrogen concentrations in obese persons. Obese women have a much greater risk of being diagnosed with endometrial cancer, which rises progressively with higher body weight. An obese woman with BMI equal to or greater than 40 is 7 times more likely to develop endometrial cancer compared with a normal-weight woman. The rising incidence of obesity in recent decades has increased endometrial cancer diagnoses in women less than 50 years of age.

- Other cancers. Women who have had breast cancer, colon cancer, or ovarian cancer may have an increased risk of uterine cancer.

- PCOS (polycystic ovary syndrome). Individuals with PCOS have high estrogen levels but low levels of progesterone, which creates an imbalance, along with high levels of androgens, which increases the risk.

- Race. White women are more likely to develop uterine cancer than women of other races. However, Black women have a high rate of being diagnosed with advanced disease. Black and Hispanic women also have a higher risk of developing tumors that are aggressive.

- Radiation therapy. Women who have had previous radiation therapy for another cancer in the pelvic area, which is the lower part of the abdomen between the hip bones, have an increased risk of uterine cancer.

- Tamoxifen. Previous treatment with tamoxifen to prevent or treat breast cancer presents an increased risk of developing uterine cancer. The benefits of tamoxifen use usually outweigh the risk.

- Unhealthy eating program

- Use of biphasic estrogen high-dosed oral contraceptives

■ Foods and Drinks That Decrease Your Risk of Developing Uterine Cancer

- Eat more fruits, vegetables, and legumes.

- Soy. A study showed that a high soy intake is associated with a 20 percent lower endometrial cancer risk. This may be due to soy helping to stop the conversion of other steroids like testosterone into estrogen.

- Coffee and green tea drinking. Women who consume the most coffee were found to have a 20 percent lower risk for endometrial cancer when compared to those who consumed the lowest amount. High coffee consumers who had never been treated with HRT were found to have a 40 percent lower risk. Similarly, green tea drinkers had a nearly 20 percent lower risk for endometrial cancer in the highest compared with lowest intake group. These effects may be due to the ability of caffeine and other methylxanthines in coffee to increase sex hormone-binding globulin (SHBG) and increase insulin sensitivity. For green tea, actions may include promotion of apoptosis (programed cell death), cell cycle arrest, up-regulation of glutathione-S-transferases that inactivate carcinogens, and anti-estrogen effects.

See also Cervical Dysplasia (Abnormal Pap Smear)

UTERINE FIBROIDS

Uterine fibroids, which are known as *leiomyomata*, are benign (non-cancerous) growths on or within the walls of the uterus. They are the most common gynecologic tumors occurring in about 20 to 25 percent of women over 30 years of age. These tumors can be a variety of different sizes and quantities. The resulting symptoms depend upon these factors. If the fibroids are small and do not cause any symptoms (80 percent of women are asymptomatic), a doctor may recommend that no course of action be taken. However, larger—or multiple—fibroids can cause pain, excessive bleeding, and problems urinating, as well as infertility and premature labor. When uterine fibroids cause serious problems such as these, treatment options include surgery (hysterectomy or myomectomy).

Medical management is mainly based on the use of progestogens, antifibrinolytics agents, non-steroidal anti-inflammatory drugs, Gonadotropin-releasing hormone analogs, and selective progesterone receptor modulators. However, current treatments are primarily surgical and interventional; approximately three-quarters of all fibroid treatments are hysterectomies. Clinically, fibroids account for one-third to half of

Causes of Uterine Fibroids

The exact etiology of uterine fibroids is unknown.

- Leiomyomas (benign tumors) are sex hormone dependent. Fibroid tissue has an increased number of estrogen and progesterone receptors, and fibroid tissue is hyperestrogenic (high estrogen level) and hypersensitive to estrogen. In addition, fibroid tissue does not have the normal regulatory mechanism that limits the estrogen response. Your healthcare provider can measure hormone levels by serum or saliva to determine hormonal balance.

- Thyroid dysfunction may also play a role in the development of fibroids. Low progesterone-to-estradiol ratios are associated with decreased conversion of T4 to T3. Furthermore, hypothyroidism with normal levels of T4 and low levels of T3 may be an indicator of sex hormone imbalance and estrogen dominance.

- Adrenal gland function also affects sex hormone production and regulation. Have your healthcare provider or compounding pharmacist order salivary testing of DHEA and cortisol and treat according to lab results.

- There may be a genetic component to the development of fibroids. Chromosomal abnormalities may play a role as well as chromosomal translocations, deletions, inversions, and breakpoints are associated with familial patterns of fibroid growth.

all hysterectomies and are associated with substantial morbidity and healthcare costs for women of reproductive age. Alternative techniques to surgery are mainly based on the uterine artery embolization. This is a procedure where an interventional radiologist uses a catheter to deliver small particles which block the blood supply to the uterine body. This is considered a minimally invasive procedure.

A risk for fibroids is associated with race; black women have a higher risk of developing fibroids earlier in life than their white counterparts and develop more-severe forms of the disease. New information is rapidly accumulating concerning the genetic subgroups that lead to fibroid formation, which might aid further understanding of this disease and lead to individualized treatments.

Fibroids have estrogen receptors and are thus responsive to the body's

- Obesity and inflammation may also play a role in the development of uterine fibroids. Fibroids are more common in obese women. Adipocytes are endocrine organs that can produce estrone. Inflammatory markers are also produced in the adipocytes (cell specialized for the storage of fat) and contribute to fibroid formation, such as: IL-2, IL-6, TNF-alpha, leukotriene B4 (LTB4). Studies have shown a connection between systemic inflammation and fibroid growth. Growth factors, such as fibroblast growth factor, vascular endothelial growth factor, and transforming growth factor, are concentrated in fibroid cells. They respond to inflammatory mediators. These stimulated growth factors increase blood vessel growth or angiogenesis (development of new blood vessels) in the fibroid which increases growth of the fibroid.

- It is important to control the vascularity with anti-angiogenesis factors, which can then reduce the growth of the tumor or fibroid by decreasing its blood supply.

- There may be a gut connection to the development of fibroids. If the intestinal tract is dysbiotic (has more bad bacteria than good bacteria), it creates gut-associated inflammatory markers, which when added to estradiol stimulate the growth of atypical cells that develop into fibroids. Also, intestinal dysbiosis with bacterial and yeast overgrowth may contribute to estrogen dominance through the effects of bacterial toxins and yeast mycotoxins, which may have estrogenic effects.

level of estrogen. During periods of pregnancy, when estrogen levels increase, fibroids tend to grow in size. After menopause, on the other hand when estrogen levels drop significantly, fibroids usually become smaller. For this reason, doctors will often recommend a medication with an estrogen-lowering effect, which will artificially create this situation. Similarly, you may find it effective to take natural progesterone to balance the estrogen in your body. Uterine fibroids are commonly an estrogen dominant state. Your doctor will be able to prescribe a specific dosage. Furthermore, you should avoid drinking coffee. Although no substitute for necessary surgery or other medical action, the nutrients on page 346 may allow these procedures to be avoided by shrinking the uterine fibroids naturally.

Fibroids are classified according to their location, which includes the following:

- Cervical fibroids (in the cervix)
- Interligamentous fibroids (between the uterine broad ligaments)
- Intramural
- Pedunculated fibroids (attached to a stalk)
- Submucosal
- Subserous

Therapies for Uterine Fibroids

Conventional Therapies

The following are conventional therapies for uterine fibroids:

- High-intensity focused ultrasound
- Leuprolide acetate (Lupron) pre-operatively
- Oral contraceptives
- Selective progesterone receptor modulators
- Surgery

Precision Medicine Therapies

Precision Medicine therapies commonly revolve around managing symptoms. The therapy usually will not shrink fibroids but may keep a fibroid from growing larger. Furthermore, as estrogen levels decline in peri- and post-menopause, the fibroids may get smaller. It is important to control factors that promote estrogen dominance and subsequent fibroid growth. The following are Precision Medicine therapies for uterine fibroids:

Diet

A healthy diet will not shrink fibroids, but different eating plans have been associated with higher or lower levels of estrogen and better or worse estrogen metabolism. If you are eating red meat more than two or three times a week, decrease your intake. Also add more fiber to your diet. Low fiber diets are associated with higher estrogen levels. In addition, saturated fats, sugar, caffeine, alcohol, and "junk foods" have been shown to interfere with the body's ability to metabolize estrogen. It can also deplete the body of B vitamins, which likewise affect the body's ability to breakdown estrogen. Furthermore, whole grain fiber also helps to excrete estrogens through the bowel and hence helps to lower estrogen levels.

Nutritional therapies

Lipotropic factors

- Inositol and choline have a lipotropic effect which means that they help with the removal of fat from the liver. Do not supplement with choline without having your healthcare provider measure TMAO levels in your blood. If you have a high TMAO level, then do not take choline. Also do not eat egg yolks or red meat.

- Pancreatic enzymes aid in the digestion of fibrous/smooth muscle tissue and may help to dissolve fibroids. More studies need to be done to determine if this is an effective therapy for fibroids. Pancreatic enzymes for this purpose should be taken between meals.

- Vitamin C and citrus bioflavonoids are helpful for uterine fibroids. Vitamin C strengthens capillary desmosomes (maintains cell-cell adhesion) and also helps reduce menorrhagia (abnormally heavy or prolonged menstrual cycle). Citrus bioflavonoids rutin and hesperidin increase vitamin C's effects and are very mildly estrogenic. This has a tonic effect which can reduce the effects of estrogen dominance. Some vitamin C supplements contain citrus bioflavonoids. Dose: 1,000 to 2,000 mg a day.

- B vitamins as B complex, helps to support methylation, aids in liver detoxification, and adrenal gland function. B complex should be taken twice a day. In addition, niacin (vitamin B_3) can be used for menstrual cramping that can be associated with fibroids.

- Calcium D-glucarate reduces the activity of beta-glucuronidase which is produced by an imbalance in intestinal bacteria. Beta-glucuronidase cleaves the glucuronic acid-estrogen bond on estrogens that are meant to be extracted and instead puts the estrogen back into the circulation. Dose: 500 mg twice a day.

- Vitamin D. Studies have shown that low levels of vitamin D are associated with increased inflammatory cytokines which can further aggravate fibroids. Have your healthcare provider measure your vitamin D level so that you know how much vitamin D_3 to take.

- EPA/DHA (fish oil) decreases inflammation. Fibroids are associated with an increase in inflammatory markers. Dose: 1,000 to 3,000 mg a day.

Botanicals

Traditional herbal therapies have been used for many years in the hopes of reducing fibroids or slowing their growth. Medical trials need to be done since there are few studies available to document that they work, but traditionally they have been used.

- Black alder bark (Alnus serrulata)

- Corydalis tubers (Dicentra canadensis)

- Figwort flowering herb (Scrophularia nodosa)

- Mayapple root (Podophyllum peltatum)

- Scudder's Alterative: Should be used at 30 to 40 drops TID in a small amount of warm water. It may help with pelvic lymphatic drainage.

- Yellow dock root (Rumex crispus)

- Compounded Echinacea Red Root

  - Baptisia root (Baptisia tinctoria)

  - Blue flag root (Iris versicolor)

  - Echinacea (Echinacea spp.)

  - Prickly ask bark (Xanthoxylum clava-herculus)

  - Red root (Ceanothus americanus)

  - Stillingia root (Stillingia sylvatica)

  - Thuja leaf (Thuja occidentalis)

- Compounded Fraxinus/ Ceonothus

  - Ginger root (Zingiber officinalis)

  - Goldenseal root (Hydrastis canadensis)

  - Helonias root (Chamaelirium luteum)

  - Life root (Senecio aureus)

  - Lobelia (Lobelia inflata)

  - Mayapple root (Podophyllum peltatum)

- Mountain ash bark (Fraxinus americanus)

- Red root (Caenothus americanus)

- Compounded Gelsemium/ Phytolacca (Turska formula)

  - Aconite (Aconitum napellus)

  - Bryonia root (Bryonia dioica)

  - Gelsemium root (Gelsemium sempervirens)

  - Poke root (Phytolacca americana)

Other possible extracts that can be used:

- Burdock root (Arctium lappa)

- Chaste tree (Vitex agnus castus)

- Crila (Crinum latifolium)

- Dandelion root (Taraxacum officinalis)

- Nettles (Urtica dioica)

- Oregon grape (Berberis aquifolium)

In a Vietnamese Crila study conducted over 3 months, Crila decreased the size or stopped the growth of the fibroid tumors in almost 80 percent of the women that took it. It also helped decrease heavy menstrual flow in some of the women. Possible side effects which commonly decrease over time include nausea, headache, vaginal dryness, and hot flashes.

Topical Applications

- Castor oil packs as hot packs work through the lymphatic system and decrease inflammation. Apply over the pelvis three to five times a week for 20 to 60 minutes.

- Poke root oil can be rubbed onto the stomach over the uterus nightly before bed for one month then two or three times a week thereafter.

Herbal phytoestrogens. There are two kinds of phytoestrogens that are found in medicinal plants, as seen on the following page.

- **Steroids and sterols.** Estradiol and estrone are found in small amounts in apple seeds, date palms, and pomegranate seeds. Diosgenin is a steroid derivative found in at least 20 varieties of plants including wild yams. Beta-sitosterol is the most common phytosterol. It is found in plant oils, in wheat germ oil, cottonseed oil, and soybean oil, and is also the dominant phytosterol in garlic and onions. Additionally found in herbal sources such as licorice root, saw palmetto, and red clover. Stigmasterol also falls in this category and is closely related to beta-sitosterol and is sourced from soybean oil. Other sources include burdock, fennel, licorice, alfalfa, anise, and sage.

- **Phenolic phytoestrogens** are flavonoids. Questions are always being asked about phytoestrogens possibly increasing the risk of breast or uterine cancer. No definite conclusion has been reached in the medical literature. **Therefore, use with caution.** They include the following: isoflavones which are present in higher concentrations in legumes, and coumestrol, which is a member of the coumestans class and is 6 times more estrogenic than isoflavones. Red clover also contains coumestrans. Last, ligans found in grains and cereals, and are highest in flaxseed, act as a phytoestrogen.

Homeopathy

The following homeopathy therapies may be beneficial to relieve symptoms.

- Aurum muriaticum: to reduce size of fibroids

- Belladonna: for heavy, red bleeding

- Hydrastinum muriaticum: for large anterior wall fibroids with bladder symptoms

- Ignatia: for grief associated with fibroids

- Medorrhinum 200 C: for fibroids

- Phosphorus 6C, 200C: for bright red bleeding with no clots

- Sabina: for bright red bleeding with clots and for severe cramps

- Secale: for almost black blood and for profuse bleeding

- Sepia: for pressure and anger

- Silicea 6C: for heavy bleeding, for cold, thin, and fatigued patients

- Thlaspi bursa pastoris 6C: (Shepherd's purse): for frequent heavy dark bleeding.

Progesterone

- Several studies suggest that progesterone replacement will help to decrease the growth of fibroids. Have your healthcare provider order a salivary test to determine if your progesterone level is suboptimal.

Acupuncture

- Acupuncture along with deep pelvis massage may be helpful.

VAGINAL DRYNESS AND VAGINAL ATROPHY

Vaginal dryness is the reduction in lubrication of the luminal surface of the vagina. It occurs in 14 to 31 percent of women and can occur at any age. More, specifically, 50 percent of postmenopausal woman have vaginal dryness and 63 percent of women with breast cancer experience this symptom. There are two types of vaginal dryness: simple and complex. Simple vaginal dryness occurs in healthy patients and resolution of symptoms occurs with treatment. Complex vaginal dryness occurs in people that have pelvic floor dysfunction and resolution of the symptom may not occur. This is seen in individuals with diseases such as diabetes and hypertension.

Vaginal atrophy is also called atrophic vaginitis. It is an inflammatory condition of the vagina and outer urinary tract and is associated with thinning and shrinkage of the tissue and/or decreased lubrication. Vulvovaginal atrophy is a common condition associated with decreased estrogen levels of the vaginal tissue. Symptoms of vaginal atrophy include the following: vaginal dryness, irritation, itching, soreness, burning, dyspareunia (painful sexual intercourse), vaginal discharge, urinary frequency, and urgency. It can occur at any time in a woman's life cycle, although more commonly in menopause where the incidence is about 50 percent.

Vaginal lubrication is very dependent on the availability of nitric oxide. The enzymatic activity of nitric oxide synthase is increased by estrogen and other sex hormones.

Causes of Vaginal Dryness and Atrophy

The following are risk factors for vaginal dryness:

- Low estrogen levels can occur after delivery and during breast feeding. Low estrogen is common in women that are menopausal, have premature ovarian failure, have had their ovaries removed and also in women that have had radiation to the pelvis.

- Other medical conditions are associated with vaginal dryness. They include the following:

  - Dermatoses
  - Diabetes
  - Lichen sclerosis
  - Metabolic syndrome
  - Neuropathies (particularly autonomic neuropathy)
  - Pituitary disorders
  - Psoriasis
  - Sjogren's syndrome
  - Type I
  - Type II
  - Untreated hypertension

- Prescription medications can also cause vaginal dryness.

  - Antidepressants
  - Anti-estrogen therapy for chemotherapy
  - Anti-estrogen therapy for endometriosis or fibroids
  - Antihistamines and decongestants
  - Atypical
  - Chemotherapy
  - Diuretics
  - Progestin predominant oral contraceptives
  - SSRIs
  - TCAs

- Environmental factors furthermore are an etiology of vaginal dryness.

  - Dehydration including the use of alcohol
  - Lack of sufficient arousal before intercourse
  - Smoking
  - Use of douches, very hot baths, or strong detergents and dehydrating soaps
  - Use of highly absorptive tampons
  - Use of male condoms with not enough external lubricant

Therapies for Vaginal Dryness and Atrophy

Conventional Therapies

- Estradiol vaginal cream

- Topical vaginal lubricants

  - Water-based lubricants increase moisture, but if they have a high pH then they can also dehydrate. So, choose a vaginal lubricant that hydrates and glides but does not have a high pH.

  - Polymer-based lubricants, which seal in moisture, may be hard to remove from the skin. There are two types: silicone-based and oil-based. Petroleum-based oils are strong solvents and may dissolve latex in condoms. Oils that contain fatty acids (olive, avocado, coconut) are weaker solvents and do not tend to degrade latex. A few things to remember if you choose to use polymer-based lubricants: Olive oil can become rancid, avocado may stain the sheets green, and coconut is hard to clear the vaginal area with long-term use.

  - Liquid silk lubricants are both water-based (moisturizing) and moisture sealing (dimethicone) and are made from propylene glycol and parabens, which can cause skin irritation. It has been shown to be very useful for lichen sclerosis and psoriasis. Dose: massage into vulva and vagina as needed up to three times a day.

  - Pink silicone lubricants are more useful as a moisture sealer than moisturizer and are more useful than water-based lubricants to decrease friction during intercourse. It contains aloe which may cause dermatitis in some people. The pH is more acidic, and some individuals may get an irritation using this kind of lubricant.

  - Liquid organic silk lubricant is water-based with silicone. It is preserved with phenoxyethanol. The pH is a little high, which works well for some women and for others it may be irritating. Massage it into the vulva and vagina as needed up to three times a day. In addition, it contains aloe, which may be irritating for some people.

- Vaginal renewal program

  - It helps you recondition the health and flexibility of the skin of the vulva and vagina by increasing blood flow through dilation and reduces friction tearing of the skin. It also increases blood flow to the vulva and vaginal canal. It is suggested for women just starting hormone replacement, women who have had pelvic radiation therapy, and women who have vaginal atrophy who have skin tearing and pain with intercourse. It can be used with topical estrogen, which may be more effective than estrogen or the vaginal renewal program alone. If the pelvic floor muscles are not flexible, then have your healthcare provider send you to a physical therapist that specializes in pelvic floor conditioning. Vaginal renewal program is contraindicated for patients with vaginismus, which is involuntary tensing of the vagina.

Precision Medicine Therapies

Precision Medicine therapies for vaginal dryness and atrophy have been proven to be beneficial and range from: lifestyle changes, to nutrients and botanicals, to medications. There is no single therapy that has been shown to be helpful for all individuals.

Lifestyle

- Stop smoking if you are a smoker. Smoking increases the risk of vaginal dryness.

- A consistent exercise program is very beneficial. It is a good method to help decrease the rate of vascular aging. It also increases the function of small vessel blood flow and increases the perfusion of the vagina. Furthermore, it affects nitric oxide positively, improves endothelial health including heart health and improves lubrication if you exercise just before intercourse.

- Diet is important. Eating a Mediterranean diet is ideal for vaginal dryness since it decreases inflammation.

Nutrients

Nutrients have also been shown to be beneficial for vaginal dryness and atrophy.

- **L-arginine** is an amino acid that acts as the protein substrate for nitric oxide production. The dose is 500 to 1,000 mg a day if you have normal kidney function. Possible side effects of this nutrient include low blood pressure, nausea, and high blood sugar. Try and eat foods that are high in arginine first before supplementing. Too high of levels can inhibit nitric oxide production. Do not take if you have kidney disease. Use only under a doctor's direction if you have heart valve disease.

- **Vitamin D** has many functions in the body. In relationship to vaginal dryness, it helps the formation of the calmodulin cofactor needed for nitric oxide production and elevates the bioavailability of nitric oxide after production. Have your healthcare provider measure your vitamin D levels before starting this supplement. You can become vitamin D toxic since it is stored in the body. See the section on Osteoporosis for further discussion.

Botanicals

- **Alfalfa** is a phytoestrogen that contains genistein, biochanin A, and daidzein. It may have a beneficial effect on estrogen, but do not use if you have or have had a hormonally related cancer.

- **Calendula** is a cream that you apply to the affected area twice a day. It soothes vaginal tissue and heals abrasions and helps to prevent viral and bacterial infections. It is suggested by ESCOP and the German Commission E for skin and mucosal injuries and abrasions.

- **Comfrey** moistens, heals, and soothes irritated and inflamed tissues. Some of its components have anti-inflammatory activity and promote tissue healing, such as allantoin and rosmarinic acid. When used as a vaginal salve, comfrey oil has been shown to increase epithelial cell growth and tissue integrity. The German Commission E approves topical use of comfrey only on unbroken tissue. It is to be used for only 4 to 6 weeks.

- **Ginkgo** promotes vasodilation and inhibits platelet activation. It is a blood thinner, therefore, do not take if you are on a prescription blood thinner. Also use with caution if you are on a natural blood thinner, aspirin or non-steroidal anti-inflammatory medication or over-the-counter product. The dose is 60 to 120 mg a day of standardized extract.

- **Ginseng** (Panax ginseng) facilitates endothelial nitric oxide release and is an antioxidant. Taken orally or used on the skin it may be effective for vaginal dryness. Dose: 1 to 2 grams root tea infusion three times a day or taken orally as a capsule or tablet or used on the skin as a compounded prescription cream. Possible side effects of ginseng are agitation and insomnia. Therefore, do not take just before bedtime. It is also a phytoestrogen, therefore, do not use if you have or have had a hormonally related cancer.

- **Hops** has estrogenic effects since it contains 8-prenylnaringenin. It also has strong estrogen receptor-binding bioactivity. Do not use if you have or have had a hormonally related cancer. It may help with vaginal dryness, and hops may also help with hot flashes and night sweats. It may also decrease insomnia since it has a sedating effect. In some individuals it may exacerbate depression. It may also interfere with barbiturates.

- **Red clover** contains phytoestrogens. It may help with vaginal dryness and also other menopausal symptoms. Do not use red clover if you have or have had a hormonally related cancer.

- The following botanicals have NOT been found to be effective for vaginal dryness, including Black cohosh, topical genistein, and Damiana (Turnera diffuse).

Medications

- DHEA cream vaginally applied is yet another treatment modality for vaginal dryness and atrophy. This is a compounded prescription. See your doctor to discuss this potentially beneficial therapy. It can be mixed with estriol vaginal cream.

- Hyaluronic acid vaginally is an excellent choice for individuals that have vaginal dryness, and they cannot use estriol vaginal cream. See your healthcare provider since this is a compounded prescription.

- Phosphodiesterase-5 inhibitors prolong vasodilation, which has a good effect on genital perfusion. The oral form is not recommended for vaginal dryness. Do not use if you are taking prescription nitrates or alpha1 blockers. Possible side effects include nausea, headache, nasal congestion, kidney impairment, liver impairment, low blood pressure, change in vision, and hearing toxicity.

- Vaginal applied estriol (E3) helps maintain muscle tone of the vagina and urethra. It reduces vaginal irritation and prevents drying and thinning of the vaginal tissues and improves symptoms that are already present. It may be used with the vaginal renewal program. See your healthcare provider since this is a compounded prescription.

VAGINITIS

See Diethylstilbestrol (DES) Babies.

VULVODYNIA

Vulvodynia is chronic vulvar (outer part of the female genitals) pain that impacts quality of life issues, such as physical disabilities, psychological distress, and sexual function. The pain can be localized and occur in just one area of the vulva or vestibule (entrance to the vagina) or can be generalized and occur in different areas of the vulva at different times. The prevalence rate is 9 to 12 percent of women.

Causes of Vulvodynia

For some women, food triggers an attack of vulvodynia. Foods that contain chemicals, such as citric acid, salicylic acid, and oxalates, may increase pain related to vulvodynia. The following is a list of foods that have been implicated as triggers for vulvodynia.

- Alcohol
- Apples
- Bananas
- Caffeine (coffee, tea, carbonated beverages with caffeine)
- Chemical preservatives
- Chocolate
- Citrus foods
- Dyes that contain tartrazine

- Lentils
- Lima beans
- Sharp cheeses
- Spicy food
- Sweeteners (aspartame, saccharin)
- Tobacco
- Tomatoes
- Yogurt

Preservatives in foods and even medications may present a problem if you have vulvodynia. PEG is a preservative that is put in the cream to keep it sterile. This can be used in non-compounding or even compounding pharmacies, so discuss with your physician to specify whether or not PEG is being used when the vaginal cream is being made by the compounding pharmacy.

Therapies for Vulvodynia

Conventional Therapies

Conventional therapies center around several avenues.

Lifestyle

- After intercourse apply an ice pack to the area

- Avoid activities that put pressure on the vulva like riding a horse or going bicycle riding.

- Avoid hot tubs or pools that contain chlorine

- Avoid potential irritants, such as strong soups and douches. Use mild soaps without perfume instead.

- Avoid sitting for a long time

- Avoid strong spermicides

- Do not use fabric softener

- Do not wear panty hose

- Urinate after intercourse and rinse the area with cool water

- Use only all-cotton tampons or pads

- Use only white toilet paper with no scent

- Wear loose fitting cotton underwear

Medications

- Anticonvulsants

- Estradiol cream

- Tricyclic antidepressants

- Interferon injections

- Local lidocaine cream

- Nerve blocks

- Surgery (for severe cases)

- Vestibulectomy (nerve fibers are cut)

- YAG Laser therapy

Precision Medicine Therapies

Precision Medicine therapies include ALL the conventional therapies along with a multidisciplinary approach of the following:

- Acupuncture

- Biofeedback

- Compounded estriol vaginal cream

- Compounded medications that do not include hormones

- Exercises to decrease muscle spasms

- Hormone balance. Have your doctor order a saliva test to determine levels of hormones

in the body, including sex hormones and cortisol, and treat accordingly.

- Hypnosis

- Physical therapy to strengthen pelvic tissues

WEIGHT GAIN

See Menopause; Polycystic Ovarian Syndrome (PCOS); Premenstrual Dysphoric Disorder (PMDD); Premenstrual Syndrome (PMS).

ZINC DEFICIENCY

See Osteoporosis; Premenstrual Syndrome (PMS).

CONCLUSION

Part II has been an extensive discussion of ailments and problems that I hope you have found illuminating since both conventional and Precision Medicine therapies were discussed. For treatment of these conditions, please see the reference section of this book to find a healthcare provider and/or compounding pharmacist to assist you in your care.

PART III

Hormone Replacement Therapy

INTRODUCTION

A woman's body is designed not to need hormonal therapy. If you are nutritionally sound, not stressed, you exercise, you are not overweight, and you are not toxic, your body will usually make the optimal amount of each hormone before and after menopause. However, in today's world there are very few women who fall into this category.

The good news is we now have the science to balance the hormones in your body—no matter what age you are. Whether you are suffering from PMS, PCOS, or postpartum depression, they are all hormonal imbalances. Consequently, balancing your hormones is a key component in helping you feel great. If you are infertile, optimizing and enhancing your hormonal levels may help you conceive. Additionally, if you are perimenopausal or menopausal, balancing your hormones will not only help you relieve symptoms—it will also decrease your risk of developing other diseases.

It is wonderful that you can have your hormone replacement therapy individualized and customized to meet your own personal needs. In the past, the only type of hormonal therapy available was a "one-size-fits-all" type, which meant that every woman, regardless of symptoms and severity of symptoms, received the same dosage of hormonal treatment. This is problematic, as you have discovered in this book, since two women with similar symptoms may have entirely different ailments and more than one cause of their symptoms. Now, with customizable hormonal therapy, a Precision Medicine approach, this is no longer the case. You can be prescribed medication specifically designed for your symptoms and your body.

In this part of the book, you will learn what hormone replacement therapy is. The difference between synthetic and natural hormonal replacement therapy will be explained, along with studies that show why natural HRT is the best option. Reasons you should consider HRT and information on how to get started once you have decided to do so are also provided. Different types of tests that measure hormonal levels are detailed in this part of the book as well.

Additionally, Part III will extensively discuss three major reasons why you should consider natural hormone replacement therapy, and how proper nutrition and herbal remedies can alleviate symptoms and maximize your treatment.

Welcome to the new era of medicine.

WHAT IS HRT?

Up until a few decades ago, the only hormonal therapy available in the United States and most countries was synthetic hormone replacement.

SYNTHETIC HRT

Some people may hear the word "synthetic" and think "fake," but this is not always the case. When it comes to hormone replacement, the word synthetic means "the chemical structure is not what your own body makes." Conversely, "natural," when referring to hormones, means "the exact same chemical structure that your body produces." It does not necessarily mean that the item has a plant origin, even though hormones are made from soy or yams.

If the chemical structure of the hormone matches the chemical structure of the hormone in your body, it is called "bio-identical." Therefore, even though some hormones are produced in a laboratory, they are still called natural and bio-identical if they match the chemical structure in your body. Anything else is called synthetic.

The government-sponsored Women's Health Initiative program halted its study on estrogen plus progestin (synthetic progesterone, or Prempro) on July 9, 2002. The study was conducted on 16,000 women who had not had a hysterectomy. Participants were either given Prempro or a placebo. The study was ended three years earlier than initially planned because researchers found that there was an increased risk of breast cancer in some of the women who were participating in the trial and taking the hormones. Analysis of the study also revealed that heart attack risk began increasing in the progestin (synthetic progesterone) group early in the study.

The trial revealed that the women taking Prempro, when compared to the women taking the placebo, had:

- A 22 percent increase in heart disease
- A 24 percent decrease in total fracture rate
- A 26 percent increase in breast cancer development
- A 33 percent decrease in fracture rate of the hip
- A 37 percent decrease in colorectal cancer
- A 41 percent higher risk of stroke
- Double the rate of blood clots

Additional studies, such as the "Heart and Estrogen/Progestin Replacement Study Follow-Up (HERS II)," agree with the findings of the Women's Health Initiative program. HERS II results also showed an increase in cardiovascular risk for the women taking synthetic progesterone. Likewise, several other studies have shown recently that progestins (synthetic progesterone) have an unfavorable effect on cholesterol levels and may promote cardiovascular disease.

Furthermore, a Danish medical trial has shown a link between synthetic hormone replacement and an increased risk of developing ovarian cancer. The elevated risk depends on which hormones are used, how long the person takes them, and the route of administration. In addition, as you have seen in the chapter on breast cancer, synthetic progestin increases the risk of developing breast cancer.

■ Other Possible Problems With Synthetic HRT

Synthetic HRT has also been shown to have other potential problems.

- It is estimated that one-half of women quit taking their synthetic hormone replacement therapy after one year because they are unable to tolerate the side effects.

- Synthetic hormones waste energy by giving incomplete messages to cells, which then fail to produce a balanced hormonal response.

The results of the Women's Health Initiative study brought to the forefront why synthetic hormonal therapy will become a treatment of the past. A groundbreaking article by Dr. Kent Holtorf was published in the medical journal *Postgraduate Medicine* in January 2009. Dr. Holtorf's article answered the question of whether natural hormones are safer or more efficacious than synthetic hormones. After an extensive review of medical literature, the article concluded that the "physiological data and clinical outcomes demonstrate that bioidentical hormones are associated with lower risks, including the risk of breast cancer and cardiovascular disease, and are more efficacious than their synthetic and animal-derived counterparts. Until evidence is found to the contrary, bioidentical hormones remain the preferred method of HRT."

NATURAL HRT

The results of the Women's Health Initiative study (see page 355 for more information) highlight the problems associated with "one size fits all" hormone replacement, which is when all women suffering hormonal problems—regardless of their symptoms—are instructed to take the same type and dosage of hormones. What is needed is for doctors and other healthcare providers to more carefully evaluate each woman's own unique set of environmental, genetic, and physiological risk factors to develop an HRT plan that is designed to fit her individual needs. For this, there is natural hormone replacement.

If you are taking natural hormone replacement, it means you are using hormones that are biologically identical to, or the same chemical structure as, the ones your body makes.

One size does not fit all in medicine today; it is all about a customized approach to healthcare, known as Precision Medicine. The science is here to individualize treatment for every patient. Your hormone response is as unique to you as your fingerprints are. How you respond to HRT is related to her genetic profile, stress level, health status, exposure to environmental toxins, health of her GI tract, ability of her liver to detoxify, nutritional status, and diet. Since no two women share the same lifestyle, it goes without saying that no two women should share the same HRT therapy.

Twelve Reasons You Should Consider HRT

1. Bone production (prevention of osteoporosis)

2. Growth and repair

3. Heart health

4. Improvement in sleep hygiene

5. Improvement of skin health

6. It can be tailored to your needs

7. It is a safe method of hormone replacement when prescribed in appropriate doses

8. Management of menopausal symptoms

9. Prevention of memory loss

10. Reduction of inflammation

11. Studies have shown that women who use hormone replacement live longer than those who do not.

12. Immune system support

■ Compounded Hormones

The way to ensure you receive the hormone replacement therapy you need is to use compounded hormones. With compounded hormones, your HRT therapy will be made for your own individual needs. Your hormones are mixed into different dosages, and special routes of administration are available, depending on what updated research and your personal biology have revealed. There are even different bases in which topical hormones can be placed, contingent on your own physiology. Your doctor or other healthcare provider can have a compounding pharmacist make your prescription for you and you only. Your HRT will be made from plant extractions that are an exact replica of your own hormones.

The key to effective hormone replacement therapy, in summary, is individuality. Fixed doses do not allow for customized, tailor-made treatment. Having your hormonal therapy personalized, at any age, helps you achieve and maintain the optimal hormonal symphony for your body.

CONSIDERATION

If you are considering HRT, you should thoroughly understand how your body's hormones work and interact with each other. For example, insulin resistance and hyperinsulinemia (elevated insulin levels) influence the synthesis of testosterone and the metabolism of DHEA in women. Therefore, insulin resistance is involved with increased testosterone levels and depletion of DHEA. This occurs because the increase in insulin elevates the activity of an enzyme, 17, 20-lyase, which converts DHEA to cortisol and testosterone. This encourages your body to gain weight.

To take this concept one step further, a study done at the University of Toronto revealed a 283 percent increase in the risk of breast cancer in women with elevated insulin levels. This is due to the fact that there are insulin receptors on breast cells. Cancer cells also have insulin receptors. Insulin attaches to the receptor and turns it on, which increases the growth of cancer cells. Therefore, if your blood sugar is high, you may be increasing your risk of breast and other kinds of cancer.

Estrogen and the Female Brain

Estrogen is a powerful hormone that can exert enormous influence on the female brain. Estrogen can actually alter the neurochemistry and structure of the brain in ways that improve cognition. Among other functions, estrogen:

- Coordinates the healing and regrowth of nerve cells in response to strokes and other brain damage

- Helps maintain and increase nerve connectivity and complexity in the brain

- Increases the surface area of potential "docking sites" on neurons for incoming messages

- Boosts the metabolism of the brain by promoting its uptake of glucose, its basic energy source

- Protects your nerve cells from damage by acting as an anti-inflammatory, boosting the body's natural antioxidants (which fight free radicals), and guarding against plaque deposits

- Reduces the formation of amyloid plaques, the toxic brain-destroying protein deposits implicated in Alzheimer's disease

- Stimulates the production of various neurotransmitters that are heavily involved in cognitive and memory processes, including acetylcholine, dopamine, gamma-aminobutyric acid (GABA), glutamate, noradrenaline, and serotonin

As a result, when administered as part of a hormone replacement therapy at the onset of menopause, estrogen can have the following effects:

- Acts as an upper, increasing energy and feelings of wellbeing

- Boosts metabolic activity of many areas of the brain and spinal cord within hours of administration

- Decreases distractibility

- Increases manual speed and dexterity in women

- Increases performance and speed of learning on sensory-motor tasks

- Increases sensory perception: hearing, smell, visual signal detection, and fine touch

- Increases short-term memory

- Increases verbal fluency, speech ability, articulation agility, syllable repetition, speed counting, and word reading

- Maintains central processing motor integration in tasks such as driving

THE BIG THREE REASONS TO START HRT

What does the medical literature really say about hormone replacement and cognition? What does the medical literature reveal regarding HRT and heart disease? Does hormone replacement therapy have an effect on the aging process of the skin? Let's examine each one of these individually.

■ HRT and Cognitive Function

The nineteenth century Scottish poet Alexander Smith had it right when he wrote, "A man's real possession is his memory. In nothing else is he rich, in nothing else is he poor." Your memory is you're most prized possession that God gave you. Maintaining your cognitive function is imperative. There are many things you can do to maintain rapid-fire memory as you age, and one of the main things is hormone replacement therapy.

Estrogen is one of the major hormones that help you maintain memory as you age. Many studies have suggested that estrogen has a role in many cognitive functions, including learning and memory. Estrogen not only influences memory formation and maintenance processes in some situations, but also affects the learning strategies employed to resolve a task, therefore altering what and how information is learned, not only how much is learned (for example, the strength of the memory.) Researchers in a 1996 study found a 54 percent reduction in the risk of developing Alzheimer's disease in those who had taken estrogen. These women had been tracked for up to sixteen years.

In another 1996 study, scientists found that estrogen not only reduced by 50 percent the risk of developing Alzheimer's disease but also delayed the onset of the disease, even in those at increased hereditary risk of developing Alzheimer's disease. Yet another study conducted on 1,889 older women in Utah revealed that women who had taken estrogen replacement were 40 percent less likely to develop Alzheimer's disease. Furthermore, the longer they were on hormone replacement therapy the lower was their risk. Estrogen replacement therapy has been shown to be most effective to maintain cognition if taken during the onset of menopause and the first few years afterward depending on when you lose estrogen. As you have seen in the section on estrogen (page 5), not all women lose estrogen when they stop cycling. In an animal study, eight weeks of estrogen deprivation was found to induce hippocampus-dependent memory impairment. Consequently, numerous studies have revealed that estrogen replacement therapy has been shown to help prevent memory loss.

Progesterone promotes the formation of myelin sheaths and has many positive effects on your neurons. It also helps regulate brain levels of certain neurotransmitters associated with learning and memory, including dopamine and GABA. In addition, progesterone also exerts a neuroprotective role, which can be effective to counteract the cognitive decline related to aging. Therefore, scientists are now looking at progesterone replacement to aid in the prevention of memory loss. One study found that progesterone therapy reduced the impairment in spatial, reference, and working memory in people who suffered global cerebral ischemia, a condition in which the brain does not receive enough oxygen as a result of a heart attack or stroke. In addition, progesterone was found to prevent the narrowing of the brain's memory center, the hippocampus, which is otherwise damaged by ischemia.

There is evidence that testosterone replacement can also help women's cognition. It has an enhancing effect on cognitive performance. Likewise, a small pilot study suggested that testosterone replacement might protect the memory of healthy aging women. Another study indicated that testosterone replacement improved verbal learning and memory in postmenopausal women.

Low DHEA levels are often caused by stress and the aging process and can lead to cognitive decline. In one study, researchers found that patients with Alzheimer's disease had DHEA levels that were 48 percent lower than those of their normal counterparts. A double-blind, placebo-controlled, crossover study in which DHEA was given to postmenopausal women showed that DHEA replacement therapy improved performance on a variety of visual and spatial tasks, including mental rotation, subject-ordered pointing, fragmented picture identification, perceptual identification, and same-different judgement.

When produced in normal amounts, cortisol is very useful for the maintenance of memory and brain function. In particular, cortisol helps to regulate the prefrontal cortex, the area of the brain that is responsible for working memory, personality expression, critical analysis, and decision-making. As discussed previously, stress can increase the amount of cortisol your body produces. When you are under chronic stress or long-term stress, your body churns out more and more cortisol in an ongoing attempt to manage the pressure. Cortisol levels also elevated with age. This elevation in cortisol levels creates a number of negative consequences for your memory. Studies show that excess cortisol can destroy existing nerve cells and even rewire the electrical circuits of the brain. It can also indirectly cause the destruction of brain cells by stimulating the production of free radicals.

The hippocampus, your brain's memory center, is especially vulnerable to stress; when exposed to excess levels of cortisol, cells in the hippocampus begin to die. Damage to the hippocampus as the result of stress can also lead to memory loss, as a smaller or atrophied hippocampus is often seen in individuals who suffer major depression, an independent risk factor for the onset of cognitive decline. As a result, high cortisol levels are associated with decreased cognitive function and increased risk of Alzheimer's disease and other forms of dementia and memory loss. As discussed in the section on cortisol (see page 40), there are many ways to lower cortisol levels and one of them is to replace DHEA if the level is low. When your health provider prescribes you DHEA it is important that you also take adaptogenic herbs and even calming herbs to lower cortisol. Otherwise, if you only take DHEA, the next time it is measured, your level will be lower, even though you are taking DHEA, since the body requires more than DHEA to improve cortisol levels. Stress reduction techniques are also very important.

Pregnenolone is the hormone of memory. It has many functions in the body, including promoting new nerve growth factor to help you maintain memory. Interestingly, a study revealed that pregnenolone may protect the brain from cannabis intoxication. Discuss with your healthcare provider about measuring pregnenolone levels and prescribing compounded pregnenolone if your level is low or suboptimal, provided you are a suitable candidate for hormone replacement therapy.

As you have seen, sex hormones are important in the prevention of cognitive deterioration in people going through menopause, which represents the fastest growing segment of the population in industrialized countries. Consequently, a major reason to consider HRT is to help maintain a strong memory as you age.

■ HRT and Heart Disease

Before menopause, women have a lower risk of coronary heart disease than men of the same age. After menopause, women start having an increased risk of developing heart disease. This is because estrogens produced by the body are important regulators of cardiovascular homeostasis in premenopausal women and delay the development of hypertension and coronary artery disease.

Estrogen

Epidemiologic studies have shown that estrogen replacement therapy may reduce the risk of heart disease by 50 percent in postmenopausal women. There are many mechanisms by which estrogen is heart protective.

- Menopause (natural or surgical) is commonly associated with a change in the lipid profile for the worse: elevation of LDL cholesterol, higher total cholesterol and triglyceride levels, and lower HDL, as well as the LDL/HDL ratio moving to a non-favorable ratio even if the total cholesterol level does not change. Studies have shown that estrogen replacement therapy has a beneficial effect on the lipid profile. It increases large VLDL particles and lowers remnant VLDL levels. LDL levels are also decreased due to an increase in clearance by induction of liver LDL receptors. It also raises HDL-2. A study revealed that triglycerides and blood sugar were improved in women who used transdermal estrogen versus oral estrogen. Therefore, the route of administration does matter.

- Lipoprotein (a) levels have been shown to be lowered by 15 percent with estrogen replacement therapy.

- Animal studies have demonstrated that estrogen replacement reduces the accumulation of lipids in the arterial wall even if the levels of total cholesterol and lipoproteins are not reduced.

- Studies reveal that estrogen may improve arterial function independent of lipid effects.

- Estrogen stimulates endothelial nitric-oxide synthase (eNOS) in vascular endothelial cells. This enhances endothelial dependent vasodilation mediated by nitric oxide.

- Estrogen has effects on post-transcriptional and translation modulation of proteins and enzymes positively affecting glycosylation, phosphorylation, and methylation. The post-translational actions of estrogen include the following:
  - Decreases turnover of growth factor-induced ornithine decarboxylase, which increases cell proliferation
  - Activates secretion of MMP-7, which increases paracellular permeability
  - Alters synthesis of glycosyltransferases, which increases paracellular permeability

- Increases expression of propyl hydroxylase domain 1, which decreases cellular sensitivity to hypoxia

- Increases protein binding to mRNA for AT1 receptors, which decreases expression of AT1 receptors

- Coordination of phosphorylation (the attachment of a phosphoryl group to a molecule) and sumoylation of steroid receptor coactivators, which has cell specific control of ligand-dependent nuclear transcription

- Estrogen also has actions on the mitochondria that generate most of the chemical energy needed to power your cell's biochemical reactions. Therefore, it can affect mitochondrial function in the vascular endothelium. It also has other actions on the mitochondria.

  - Increases oxidative phosphorylation while lowering reactive oxygen species (ROS) production, which decreases the rate of accumulation of mitochondrial DNA mutations over a lifetime. In other words, estrogen will protect against future mitochondrial damage but would not reverse any damage that is already present before estrogen replacement. The production of ROS by the mitochondria plays a large role in oxidative stress. Estrogen may therefore have an important impact on vascular oxidative stress. Also, when ROS production remains low, and its system is not overwhelmed, the signaling pathways may be maintained.

  - Decreases mitochondrial superoxide production

  - Decreases hydrogen peroxide production

  - Increases levels of manganese superoxide dismutase

  - The targets in the mitochondria for estrogen are unknown. Levels of nuclear respiratory factor-1, a major regulator of nuclear-encoded mitochondrial genes, increase after estrogen replacement therapy. Estrogen may also have a direct effect on the mitochondrial genome since estrogen receptors are present in the mitochondria. Several genes for mitochondrial proteins encoded by either nuclear or mitochondrial DNA are regulated by estrogen receptor alpha (ER-alpha) or estrogen receptor beta (ER-beta).

  - Estrogen also suppresses ROS through other mechanisms than the mitochondria. ERT reduces angiotensin II-induced free radical production in vascular smooth muscle cells. Estrogen decreases

NADPH-stimulated superoxide production. Estrogen also decreas strain-increased NADPH oxidase activity and intracellular gener ation of ROS. Estrogen in vascular smooth muscle cells increases protein levels of both manganese superoxide dismutase (SOD) and extracellular SOD by increasing transcription rate.

- The most prominent effects of estrogen on vascular reactivity are through its ability to influence endothelial function.

- Animal studies show that estradiol increases cardiac output by causing systemic vasodilatation. Many studies in humans have shown that estrogen promotes vasodilation through an eNOS-dependent mechanism. Estrogen stimulates increases in plasma concentrations of nitric oxide, increases in reactive hyperemia after estrogen replacement, and changes in the menstrual cycle reflective of an estrogenic effect. Several studies have shown that women using estrogen replacement therapy have more flow-mediated vasodilation if they have received estrogen in the past or all along.

- Estrogen also affects production of other endothelial factors. Estrogen replacement increases prostacyclin synthesis by elevating levels of cyclooxygenase-1 and prostacyclin synthase, which results in a shift from cyclooxygenase-dependent vasoconstriction to vasodilation after hormonally therapy.

- Estrogen increases the release of endothelium-derived relaxing factor(s) in postmenopausal woman.

- Estrogens stimulate muscarinic and B-adrenergic cardiac receptors.

- Estradiol decreases arterial impedance in the carotid and uterine arteries in postmenopausal women.

- Left ventricular systolic flow measurements are increased on hormone replacement therapy. This reflects an increase in stroke volume and preserved myocardial contractility helping to maintain optimal heart function.

- A study showed that women who used estrogen replacement in the past or present have a lower incidence of subclinical cardiac disease. Women also had reduced left ventricular mass on ECG and better E/A ratios on doppler assessment of mitral inflow, which is a measure of cardiac diastolic function on hormone replacement therapy with estrogen.

In women with coronary heart disease, estrogen receptors are absent in areas of atherosclerotic plaque. Therefore, estrogen may limit the progression of fibrofatty lesions through inhibition of proliferation of smooth muscle by receptor-mediated processes.

- Estrogen replacement therapy limits neointimal formation following arterial injury and transplant-associated acceleration of atherosclerosis in humans.

- Estrogen may also limit the progression of atherosclerotic plaque formation by cytokine-induced adhesion of leukocytes and fibroblast migration and uptake/degradation of lipids.

- Estrogen aids in the rapid repair of vascular wounds by increasing endothelial regrowth with release of endothelium-derived factors, such as nitric oxide, which inhibits smooth muscle proliferation, consequently decreasing the development of intimal hyperplasia.

- Estrogen helps with the rapid repair of vascular wounds also by modulating hematopoiesis in the bone marrow of endothelial progenitor cells.

- Estrogen aids with the rapid repair of vascular wounds also by slowing the senescence of the progenitor cells through elevated telomerase activity and increased proliferation through activation of ER alpha.

- Estriol replacement has been shown to prevent coronary hyperreactivity in vascular smooth muscle.

- Studies of carotid arteries have shown a consistent reduction in carotid intimal medial thickness in postmenopausal women using estrogen replacement compared to controls.

- Positive modulation of the quantity of arterial calcification and intimal hyperplasia show the effects of estrogen on components of the vascular wall.

- Furthermore, estrogen replacement has been shown to suppresses the stress response to both physical and emotional stresses.

- Estrogen has also been shown to lower blood pressure by several mechanisms.

  - Estrogen is a calcium channel blocker, which helps to regulate blood pressure. Estrogens affect the regulation of intracellular calcium

through hyperpolarization of the membrane of smooth muscle c
and inhibition of voltage-gated calcium channels. Estrogen ma
also regulate intracellular calcium through enhancement of calciun
efflux.

- Studies have shown that HRT decreases serum ACE activity by 20 percent.
- Estrogen down-regulates angiotensin 1 receptors.
- Estrogen also inhibits the renin-angiotensin system by reducing transcription of angiotensin-converting enzyme in endothelial cells.
- Estrogen also promotes up-regulation of endothelium-derived vasodilator factors with simultaneous down-regulation of vasoconstrictor factors like endothelin-1.

- Estrogen regulates adrenergic neurotransmission through several means. It modulates neuronal activity through binding to estrogen receptors and regulates through effects on catecholamine reuptake at the synaptic cleft, competes with norepinephrine for adrenergic binding sites, and promotes genomic regulation of alpha-adrenergic receptors.

- Women on estrogen replacement therapy had coronary calcification scores lower than women who were not on estrogen in clinical trials.

- Transdermal application of estrogen has an anti-inflammatory effect which decreases the risk of heart disease. Estrogen modulates inflammation through several mechanisms.
  - Reduces infiltration of leukocytes to arteries after endothelium denudation and cytokine-induced gene transcription in smooth muscle.
  - Lowers inflammatory proteins produced by the liver, like CRP.
  - Direct effects on the vascular wall.
  - Indirectly through the hypothalamic-pituitary-adrenal axis, including stimulating the release of corticotropin-releasing hormone, and corticosteroid hormone release.
  - Decreases IL-6, TNF-alpha, IL-1.
  - Generally, estrogen suppresses the stress response.

- Estradiol has been shown to improve insulin sensitivity in women with coronary heart disease.

Estrogen has a positive effect upon clotting as long as it is applied on the skin. Estrogen lowers fibrinogen and PAI-1. In fact, a study showed no increased risk of stroke or venous thrombosis with transdermal estrogen use. Another study also showed no risk of venous thromboembolism with transdermal estrogen. Oral estrogen, however, was associated with an increased risk. Therefore, estrogen should only be prescribed transdermally (on the skin) or vaginally as a means of hormone replacement therapy.

● The latest medical literature explores the effects of estrogen on cardiovascular function are mediated by nuclear and membrane estrogen receptors, including estrogen receptor alpha, estrogen receptor beta, and G-protein-coupled ER.

In light of the studies presented, estrogen has many beneficial effects upon the cardiovascular system. Timing of the estrogen replacement does appear to matter. The ability for estrogen to prevent or slow the progression of vascular remodeling or plaque formation may be somewhat limited if not begun at the time of menopause. The same concept holds true for the actions of estrogen on the mitochondria. This does not mean, however, that it would not be prudent to start hormone replacement therapy at the age of ninety. It would still afford the body some heart protection. In fact, one study suggests that in the future, IV estrogen may be used to treat heart attacks due to its antiarrhythmic effect protecting the body from abnormal heart rates or rhythms.

Unfortunately, many times physicians and other healthcare providers that are not trained to prescribe hormones tell patients that hormones increase the risk of heart disease. They quote the Framingham Heart Study. When you pull the actual trial there was an increase in heart disease, but it was not statistically significant. In medical terms, this means there was not an increase in heart disease. This study was published in 2000. Many studies since that time, as you have seen, shed more light on this subject and prove that estrogen replacement, if applied to the skin, decreases your risk of heart disease significantly. In fact, numerous studies have shown a 40 to 50 percent reduction in cardiovascular morbidity and mortality with hormone replacement therapy.

Progesterone

Progesterone is heart protective since it inhibits smooth muscle cell proliferation (growth). It also inhibits vascular cell adhesion molecule-1

(VCAM-1) expression in human vascular endothelial cells. In postm. pausal women, progesterone was shown to enhance the beneficial ef. that estrogen has on exercise-induced myocardial ischemia. In additic progesterone has been shown to lower blood pressure. Moreover, proges terone prevented coronary hyperreactivity in both nonatherosclerotic and in pre-atherosclerotic animals in another study. Last, the results from the PEPPI trial show that micronized (natural) progesterone yields a more favorable HDL than other progesterone medications.

Testosterone

Testosterone replacement in women that have low testosterone levels has been shown to relax coronary arteries and allow more blood to flow to the heart thus decreasing the risk of heart disease. Testosterone replacement has also been shown to decrease symptoms of angina (chest pain). In another study, testosterone replacement in postmenopausal women was found to lower lipoprotein (a) levels by up to 65 percent. Elevated lipoprotein (a) is a major risk factor for heart disease.

DHEA

DHEA replacement has been shown to have an anti-remodeling and vasorelaxant drug effect. Therefore, it has been shown to have a role in prevention of cardiovascular disease. In addition, DHEA was shown to inhibit vascular inflammation, which is a known risk factor for heart disease. A study showed that replacement of DHEA improved indices of arterial stiffness. Another trial concluded that DHEA given orally may help treat systemic vascular remodeling including restenosis. The mechanism proposed is inhibition of the Akt axis. Moreover, DHEA was shown to prevent the aggregation of platelets obtained from postmenopausal women with type II diabetes. Consequently, if DHEA levels are low, have a specialist in Precision/Anti-Aging Medicine prescribe you compounded DHEA to help prevent coronary heart disease.

Cortisol

Abnormal cortisol levels are associated with many risk factors for heart disease including:

- Dyslipidemias (high cholesterol and/or elevated triglyceride levels)
- Endothelial dysfunction

ypercoagulability: elevated fibrinogen, high von Willebrand factor, high homocysteine, elevated levels of factor XII, XI, IX, VIII, plasminogen, 2-antiplasmin, and plasminogen activating factor. (This means that you have an increased risk of having a blood clot or pulmonary embolism.)

- Hypertension

- Insulin resistance

- Obesity

- Perivascular coronary artery inflammation

Normalizing your cortisol level is a great way to decrease your risk of heart disease. We all have stress. It is about mitigating what causes us stress that reduces inflammation and lowers the risk of developing heart disease.

There is considerable evidence suggesting that hormones modulate cardiovascular physiology and function in both health and disease, and that it could potentially serve as a cardioprotective agent. In other words, the medical evidence overwhelmingly favors the use of natural hormone replacement to prevent and even treat heart disease.

■ HRT and Anti-Aging Skin Care

This section focuses on perimenopausal and menopausal women and the effects of hormones on the skin during this time in a woman's life. The skin, the largest organ of the body, is the organ in which changes associated with aging are most visible. The skin is a target organ for various hormones, and sex steroids have a profound influence on the aging process. Aging of the skin is associated with thinning skin, atrophy, dryness, wrinkling, and delayed wound healing. Many of these changes are due to hormone decline or deficiency. A decrease in sex steroids induces a reduction of those skin functions that are under hormonal control. Keratinocytes, Langerhans' cells, melanocytes, sebaceous glands, collagen content, and the synthesis of hyaluronic acid, for example, are under hormonal influence. Let's take a closer look at the intricacies of the endocrine system and its relationship to skin aging through the lens of hormones.

Estrogen and the Skin

Cutaneous aging manifests itself as a progressive reduction in function and reserve capacity of skin tissue. Collagen atrophy is a major factor in skin aging. There is a strong correlation between skin collagen and estrogen deficiency due to the menopause. Skin aging is associa with a progressive increase in extensibility and a reduction in elastici With increasing age, the skin also becomes more fragile and susceptible to trauma, leading to more lacerations and bruising. Furthermore, wound healing is impaired in older women. Estrogen deficiency following menopause results in atrophic skin changes and the acceleration of skin aging. Skin thickness is reduced by 1.13 percent and collagen content is reduced by 2 percent per postmenopausal year in menopausal women.

The effects of aging on the skin of older females correlate with the period of estrogen deficiency rather than chronological age. Another study of postmenopausal women indicated that estrogen deprivation is associated with dryness, atrophy, fine wrinkling, poor healing, and hot flashes. Epidermal thinning, declining dermal collagen content, diminished skin moisture, and decreased laxity have also been reported in postmenopausal women. The good news is that estrogen use after the menopause increases collagen content and dermal thickness and elasticity and decreases the likelihood of dry skin.

There are many skin manifestations of estrogen deficiency that occur at menopause, including:

- Decreased elastin
- Decreased skin firmness and elasticity
- Impaired wound healing
- Increased collagen
- Increased number and depth of wrinkles
- Increased oxidative stress
- Premature skin damage caused by the sun
- Skin dryness
- Thinner skin

These skin changes can be reversed by estrogen replacement, which increases keratinocyte proliferation, epidermal thickness, epidermal hydration, and skin elasticity; reduces skin wrinkles; augments the content and quality of collagen; and increases the level of vascularization. In addition, estrogen increases epidermal hydration, skin elasticity, and skin thickness. Estrogens can significantly modulate skin physiology, targeting keratinocytes, fibroblasts, melanocytes, hair follicles, and sebaceous glands, and improve angiogenesis, wound healing, and immune responses.

Therefore, estrogen has many positive effects on skin aging. In fact, e study suggested that estrogen therapy has long-term benefits on skin nd supports the use of early and continuous HRT in preventing detrimental skin changes. Let's examine further how estrogen replacement benefits each manifestation of estrogen deficiency.

Oxidative Stress. Estrogen deficiency is strongly linked to an altered oxidative state. Estrogen is a potent direct antioxidant and indirect inducer of antioxidant enzymes. Oxidative stress decreases procollagen I synthesis in human fibroblasts, while estrogen significantly increases the synthesis of procollagen I. Estrogen can increase the viability of fibroblasts and keratinocytes, which are affected by H_2O_2. Furthermore, estrogen counteracts H_2O_2-mediated lipoperoxidation and DNA oxidative damage in skin cells. The physiological concentration of estrogens also increases cell viability, which is reduced by reactive oxygen species (ROS) and protects human skin cells by decreasing oxidative damage.

Collagen. A difference in collagen subtypes has also been documented in post-menopausal women. When evaluated by immunohistochemistry, compared with premenopausal women, postmenopausal women demonstrate a decrease in collagen types I and III and a reduction in the type III/ type I ratio within the dermis. Types I and III skin collagens are thought to decrease by as much as 30 percent in the first five years after menopause. The use of topical estrogen has also been shown to increase skin collagen and has been demonstrated to promote an increase in collagen synthesis, as shown by increased type I and type III procollagen levels. Current studies have also shown that estrogen treatment prevents the loss of the collagen I peptide and increases the expression of type III collagen. Also, estrogen increased tropoelastin and fibrillin, which may be associated with an increase in elastic fibers.

Transforming growth factor β (TGF-β) is a growth factor that stimulates fibroblast proliferation and extracellular matrix (ECM) secretion, which can affect angiogenesis and epithelialization of the skin. TGF-β improves skin aging by enhancing the production of subcutaneous VEGF and thereby increasing the thickness of collagen. Estrogen can enhance the expression of TGF-β to delay skin aging through these mechanisms.

Matrix metalloproteinases (MMPs) induce skin aging by degrading (breaking down) collagen. There is increasing evidence that the expression of MMPs is controlled by tissue inhibitor of metalloproteinase (TIMP). TIMP is a tissue inhibitor that inhibits MMPs and thereby inhibits collagen degradation. In addition to its inhibitory effects on most known MMPs, the encoded TIMP proteins are capable of promoting proliferation in a variety of cell types and may also have anti-apop functions. Estrogen can upregulate the expression of TIMPs to downre ulate the expression of MMPs, which reduces the breakdown of collage to protect the skin.

Water Content. Research has shown that the positive effects of estrogens on the water content of the skin may be due to dermal and epidermal components. Estrogen maintains skin moisture by increasing acid mucopolysaccharides and hyaluronic acid in the skin and possibly maintaining stratum corneum barrier function. Dryness is also alleviated through increased water-holding capacity, increased sebum production, and improved barrier function of the skin. The increased hydration is believed to be due in part to an increase in the water-holding capacity of the stratum corneum.

Estrogen is necessary to maintain glycosaminoglycans and hyaluronic acid in the skin. Estrogen stimulation increases the levels of glycosaminoglycans and hyaluronic acid, which contribute to an increased water content in the dermis. The water content of the epidermis is related to the thickness of the epidermis and the amount of natural moisturizing factors. A study showed that estrogen induced the expression of the epidermal growth factor in keratinocytes. Moreover, the synthesis of hyaluronic acid in the dermis increased. Additionally, dermal hyaluronic acid and acid mucopolysaccharide levels were increased with estrogen replacement, which also improved hydration. In an animal study, estrogen administration increased hyaluronic acid synthesis by 70 percent in two weeks, leading to increased dermal water content.

Skin Thickness. Epidermal thinning is associated with aging, and topical estradiol has been shown to reduce epidermal thinning in aging skin and maintain skin thickness. Estrogens have moreover been shown to influence skin thickness by stimulating collagen synthesis, maturation, and turnover in animal trials.

Topical estrogens have been shown to improve skin thickness in clinical trials. Topical application is an efficient method, since estrogen easily penetrates the stratum corneum of the skin. In one study, it demonstrated an increase in keratinocyte proliferation and epidermal thickness in response to only two weeks of topical estrogen in the skin of elderly females.

Sebum. Sebum levels are higher in postmenopausal women receiving hormone replacement therapy, which helps maintain skin moisture.

Wrinkling. Skin wrinkling is synonymous with aging. It is also ...cted by environmental and hormonal factors. Wrinkling occurs due decreased skin elasticity as a result of elastic degeneration and loss of connective tissue. It has been reported that estrogen is effective in the treatment of aging skin. Improvement in skin elasticity and wrinkle depth was observed after six months of treatment in premenopausal women with skin aging symptoms in one trial. In another study of early post-menopausal women monitored for five years, skin elasticity was shown to have decreased by 1.5 percent per year, a change not seen in women on HRT. This led to the suggestion that estrogen deficiency plays a role in wrinkle formation. In a large cohort study, it was shown that wrinkling is reduced in postmenopausal women who were administered estrogen. Skin wrinkling may benefit from estrogen as a result of the effects of the hormone on the elastic fibers and collagen, and it enhances the morphology and synthesis of elastic fibers, collagen type III, and hyaluronic acid.

Photoaging. Ultraviolet (UV)-B exposure is associated with upregulation of matrix metalloproteinase (MMP) production, leading to an increase in collagen breakdown, and is also thought to decrease type I and type III collagen synthesis. Estrogen replacement therapy has been shown to offer some degree of protection against skin photoaging.

Vascularization. Estrogen has been shown to enhance the level of vascularization in the skin.

Wound Healing. Estrogen accelerates and improves cutaneous wound healing by regulating the levels of a cytokine. Furthermore, estrogen modulates local inflammation, granulation, re-epithelialization, and possibly wound contraction, which accelerate wound healing at the expense of forming lower quality scars. In wound healing models, estrogen reduces wound size and stimulates matrix deposition in both human and murine skin, highlighting the effects of estrogens on dermal fibroblasts. Likewise, physiologic studies on estrogen and wound healing suggest that hormone replacement therapy may play a beneficial role in cutaneous injury repair.

Progesterone and the Skin

Several studies have shown the anti-aging effects of progesterone that is applied to the skin or taken orally. In a double-blind study, forty perimenopausal and postmenopausal women were treated with either topically applied 2 percent progesterone cream or placebo cream every evening to the face and neck. After sixteen weeks, there was a significant increase of skin elasticity in the women treated with the topical progesterone cre[...] but not in the control group.

The positive impact of topically applied progesterone cream or[...] markers of skin aging may be due to the suppressive effect of progesterone on tissue-degrading enzymes known as matrix metalloproteinases (MMPs). For example, progesterone has been found to decrease the expression and activity of MMP-1 and MMP-9, the most important conductors of photoaging (aging of the skin due to exposure to the sun) and chronological aging, by binding to their receptors. In addition, epidermal hydration has been shown to improve with oral micronized (natural) progesterone therapy.

Testosterone and the Skin

Hormonal treatment is not usually the first option to treat female acne. However, some acne patients (30 to 80 percent) showed various degree of hyperandrogenemia (high testosterone and other androgens). Following all the suggestions in the section on PCOS to lower testosterone levels will help decrease your acne if it is related to elevated testosterone levels.

DHEA and the Skin

A placebo-controlled, randomized, prospective study was performed with seventy-five postmenopausal women between the ages of sixty and sixty-five years old. The data suggest the possibility that topical DHEA could be used as an efficient and physiological anti-aging skin agent. In another study, DHEA formulation (1 percent) or a placebo was topically applied for four months to facial and hand skin, in two groups of twenty menopausal women. DHEA treatment increased the rate of sebum, which was considered positively by the menopausal population usually affected with a declining sebum level. In addition, topical DHEA improved skin brightness, counteracting the papery appearance of skin and epidermal atrophy, a characteristic feature of hormone-related skin aging. Topical DHEA also reduced wrinkles.

Moreover, DHEA may be related to the process of skin aging through the regulation and degradation of extracellular matrix protein. A study demonstrated that DHEA can increase procollagen synthesis and inhibited collagen degradation by decreasing matrix metalloproteinases (MMP)-1 synthesis and increasing tissue inhibitor of matrix metalloprotease (TIMP-1) production in cultured dermal fibroblasts. DHEA was found to inhibit ultraviolet (UV)-induced MMP-1 production and the UV-induced ecrease of procollagen synthesis. DHEA (5 percent) also induced the expressions of transforming growth factor-beta 1 and connective tissue growth factor mRNA in cultured fibroblasts and aged skin. The authors suggested the possibility of using DHEA as an anti-skin aging agent.

Cortisol and the Skin

Long-term chronic stress can also lead to premature skin aging. The central role in cellular skin reactivity to various stressors may be attributed to dermal mast cells. Many other cells also actively take part in skin response to stress. Moreover, psychological stress has been linked to the stimulation of the autonomic nervous system, renin-angiotensin system, and hypothalamus-pituitary-adrenal system, contributing to inflammation, oxidative stress, and DNA damage, which influence all tissues, including the skin.

GETTING STARTED ON HRT

The fabulous news is that the science is here to help. You can have this individualized kind of medical care. Make sure that you see a fellowship trained specialist in Precision/Anti-Aging Medicine. These specifications guarantee your healthcare practitioner has completed an extra two to three years of training in natural hormonal therapies. For information on how to find this type of specialist, see the Resources section (page 391). Confirm that your compounding pharmacist has this specialty training as well.

HORMONAL TESTING METHODS

It is very important to have your hormone levels measured before you begin hormone replacement therapy, no matter what age you are. There are several ways to test for hormones (saliva, serum, and urine), but saliva testing is considered to be the most accurate way to assess bioavailable (the amount of hormone that is absorbed and actually reaches your bloodstream) hormone levels. Hormones are lipophilic, as they have a cholesterol backbone. Because of this, they must be bound to carrier proteins when travelling through serum, which renders them inactive. Therefore, it is paramount that the bioavailable amount of the hormone be measured and not the total hormone level.

SALIVARY TESTING

Salivary, or saliva, testing is the preferred method of hormone testing for perimenopausal women, menopausal women, and women with PMS symptoms or other hormonal imbalances. It is a non-invasive method of testing and can be done in the privacy of your own home. There are hormone receptors all over the body. For example, there are not only estrogen receptors in the breast and gonadal tissues, but also in the eyes and on your colon. In addition, saliva testing is also the optimal way to measure hormone levels because it allows for changes over an entire day or even a number of days, as opposed to a one-time blood draw that shows levels only at the time of the test.

Salivary testing is also an excellent way to evaluate infertility, since a twenty-eight-day test can be done. This test gives your doctor or other healthcare provider the ability to look at your estrogen, progesterone, and testosterone levels throughout your entire monthly cycle. Commonly stress plays a role in infertility and the twenty-eight-day saliva test also measures your cortisol and DHEA levels.

So, how does salivary testing differ from conventional serum testing? The steroid hormones in saliva are representative of the small fraction of hormones circulating in the bloodstream that are bioavailable to tissues. This bioavailable fraction represents about 1 to 3 percent of the total hormone circulating in the bloodstream that breaks away from blood binding proteins, enters tissues, binds unique receptors, and is responsible for triggering specific responses characteristic of the hormone. Blood (serum) levels measure the total level of steroid in the bloodstream, not the small fraction that is released from the steroid-binding proteins in the bloodstream into saliva and tissues, or the bioavailable fraction that is representative of the active level of hormone at the cellular level.

The actual bioavailable fraction of the steroid in serum can vary considerably depending on the level of binding proteins for a specific steroid, which may depend on the level of other hormones and the individual variability in the liver's capacity to manufacture the hormone-binding proteins. Therefore, serum is a much less accurate measurement than that of saliva when assessing functional hormone levels. Moreover, saliva testing accurately measures topically dosed hormones. The discrepancy between free and protein bound hormones becomes especially important when monitoring topical/transdermal or sublingual hormone therapy. Studies show that this method of delivery results in increased tissue hormone levels (thus measurable in saliva), but no parallel increase in serum levels. Therefore, serum testing cannot reliably be used to monitor topical hormone therapy.

BLOOD SPOT TESTING

Dried blood spot is a form of collection in which you place blood drops on a filter card after a finger prick with a lancet. Once the blood has dried, blood spot cards are extremely stable for shipment and storage. Blood spot is ideal for measuring hormones and other analytes, such as insulin, blood lipids, Vitamin D, thyroid hormones, and elements like magnesium. It offers distinct advantages over serum because it eliminates the need for a blood draw, saving you time and money. It eliminates needles, fees, and the need to see a phlebotomist. Individuals can collect their samples at home at the time that suits them. Research also shows that blood spot is more accurate than serum for measuring blood hormone levels in patients using topically applied hormones.

URINE TESTING

Urine testing also measures the downstream metabolites, or breakdown products, of the sex hormones, which include many circulating estrogens in the body, as well as other breakdown products. This is advantageous because it helps to make sure the hormones are broken down into metabolites that decrease the risk of disease and not increase the risk of other pathological processes. Hormones in the urine are reflective of the combination of both endocrine production and peripheral production of the hormones and their metabolites. In other words, urinary hormones tell your doctor the hormone levels produced by your hormonal system, and also your hormone production and conversion that occur throughout your entire body.

Therefore, urine testing reflects hormone metabolites and is the best medium for assessing the way the body is metabolizing and excreting hormones. Urinary hormones are also a good method to look at the wear and tear (catabolic) versus the rest and recovery (anabolic) balance in the body. If you are in optimal health, your anabolic state is higher than your catabolic state. A high catabolic state ages you, since your body is spending more time breaking down than building up your metabolism. Do not overhydrate if you are taking a urine hormone test because it can affect the accuracy of the testing.

BLOOD TESTING (SERUM TESTING)

Serum measures the "protein-bound," biologically inactive hormone levels in the body. In order for steroid hormones to be detected in serum, they must be bound to circulating proteins. In this bound state, they are unable to fit into receptors in the body, and therefore will not be delivered to tissues. They are considered inactive, or non-bioavailable. If you are using estrogen or testosterone, which are both applied topically, serum testing has been shown not to be accurate, since hormones that are applied transdermally (on the skin) are underestimated in the blood. Consequently, if your healthcare provider uses blood testing to measure topically applied hormones, you can be easily overdosed.

■ Blood Testing That May Be Needed

One kind of blood test that you should ask your healthcare provider to order is the SHBG test. This test measures your levels of sex hormone-binding globulin (SHBG). SHBG is a glycoprotein that binds to testosterone, dihydrotestosterone (DHT), and estradiol. (Progesterone and cortisol bind to transcortin.) Once bound to SHBG, testosterone, DHT, and estradiol circulate in the bloodstream. Only a small amount of testosterone and estradiol is left unbound or free. This unbound part is biologically active and able to enter a cell and activate its receptor. High SHBG levels decrease testosterone and estrogen's ability to do this. Therefore, the availability of your sex hormones is related to SHBG.

SHBG is produced by your liver and then released into your bloodstream. The brain, uterus, vagina, and placenta also produce SHBG. The amount of SHBG that is produced is regulated by other hormones in your body. For example, if your insulin level is too high the amount of SHBG produced is lower. In other words, if your body is producing too much insulin (as is the case with insulin resistance and type-2 diabetes) then you have more estrogen and testosterone available as free hormones for the body to use because there is less SHBG available for these hormones to bind to. Another example of the hormonal interplay that occurs with SHBG is that elevated testosterone levels decrease SHBG, and high estrogen and thyroxine (one of the thyroid hormones) levels increase SHBG levels. Recent studies have shown that an elevated level of SHBG may be associated with an increase in breast cancer risk.

■ Medical Conditions Associated With SHBG Deficiency

- Diabetes
- PCOS
- Hypothyroidism

If your level of SHBG is too low, how do you raise it? If you are overweight, losing weight is helpful. Also drinking coffee or green or black tea has been shown to raise SHBG levels.

■ Medical Conditions Associated With SHBG Excess

- Anorexia nervosa
- Hyperthyroidism
- Hepatitis
- Liver disease
- HIV
- Pregnancy

Excess SHBG is commonly linked to the body using too much estrogen, which can occur with estrogen dominance or the use of oral contraceptives or other forms of hormonally related birth control. Estrogen by mouth increases SHBG by 50 percent. Equine estrogens increase SHBG by 100 percent.

If your level of SHBG is too high, eating a high-protein diet may be helpful. Also, taking minerals such as boron, zinc, calcium, and magnesium may be beneficial. Vitamin D supplementation and taking fish oil are also recommended.

Blood testing is also used to measure thyroid hormones and insulin. A study showed that 45 percent of women on estrogen had suboptimal levels to maintain their memory and bone structure when their doctor went by symptoms only and did not measure hormone levels. This led researchers to conclude that monitoring symptoms alone was not enough. Therefore, repeated measurement of your hormone levels is needed in order for your doctor to optimize your hormone replacement therapy. Estrogen, progesterone, testosterone, cortisol, and DHEA are all hormones and should not be prescribed without measuring levels first, and then on a regular basis. (See the Resources section on page 391 for availability of testing.)

Hormones do not function by themselves. As you have been learning, they are a symphony, a web that is interrelated. Measuring the urine metabolites of your sex hormones reveals enzyme activity and facilitates a deeper level of intervention to individualize and customize your care.

■ Herbal Therapies for Hormonally Related Symptoms

Herbal supplements are wonderful to help resolve symptoms like hot flashes and night sweats. However, they may not be enough to maintain your bone structure, prevent heart disease, or help you maintain your memory. *Do not use any of the herbs in this section if you are pregnant, nursing, or if you have been diagnosed with breast cancer. In addition, all of these herbs can interfere with the efficacy of birth control pills and some HRT.*

BLACK COHOSH

Black cohosh (*Actaea racemosa*) is a flowering phytoestrogenic plant that grows in the woods of eastern North America. Black cohosh is one of the most commonly used herbs for alleviating menopause symptoms due to its effectiveness in controlling hot flashes, depression, and night sweats. Black cohosh is also called black snakeroot, bugbane, bugwort, rattleroot, rattletop, rattleweed, and macrotys.

■ Functions of Black Cohosh

- Acts as a sedative

- Acts as an anti-inflammatory

- Acts as an antispasmodic

- Has a balancing effect on estrogen (If you have too much estrogen, black cohosh lowers it, and if estrogen is too low, it enhances estrogen's effects.)

- Has antibacterial properties

- Has direct effect on the hypothalamus (brain) to decrease hot flashes

- Has antifungal properties

- Is a relaxant

- Lowers blood pressure

- Lowers LDL (bad) cholesterol

- May relieve mild depression

- Relieves muscle soreness

■ Contraindications

- Do not take black cohosh if you are taking an antidepressant or have a hormonally related cancer, such as breast, ovarian, or endometrial. Do not take if you have liver damage or drink alcohol excessively. Do not take if you are pregnant since it may stimulate uterine contractions. Use with caution if you have fibroids or endometriosis.

■ Possible Side Effects of Black Cohosh

- Abdominal pain
- Decreased heart rate
- Diarrhea
- Dizziness
- Headaches

- Impaired circulation
- Joint pain
- Nausea
- Shortness of breath

- Tremors
- Vertigo
- Vision changes
- Vomiting
- Weight gain

CHASTEBERRY

Chasteberry (*Vitex agnus-castus*) has been proven in scientific studies to help women overcome hormonal imbalance. It is used for PMS, PCOS, and menopause. In addition, it can also be of benefit to women for infertility and regulating ovulation.

■ Functions of Chasteberry

- Acts as a diuretic (reduces swelling by promoting urination)

- Decreases LH and prolactin
- Raises progesterone and facilitates progesterone function

■ Contraindications

- Do not take if you are pregnant or breast feeding
- Do not take if you have breast, uterine, or ovarian cancer
- Do not take if you have Parkinson's disease

- Do not take if you have schizophrenia
- May interfere with dopamine antagonist medications

■ Possible Side Effects of Chasteberry

- Headaches
- Itching
- Nausea

- Rash
- Stomach cramps
- Swelling

DONG QUAI

Dong quai (*Angelica archangelica*) is another herb that is commonly used to treat women's hormonally related symptoms.

■ Functions of Dong Quai

- Contains phytoestrogens

■ Contraindications

- Do not mix dong quai with some types of antibiotics, antidepressants, cancer drugs or antipsychotic medications (Check with your pharmacist or healthcare provider before taking if you are on any of these classes of drugs)

- Do not take if you have breast, uterine, or ovarian cancer

- Do not use if you have the cold or flu

- Dong quai should be avoided when taking other drugs that cause photosensitivity

- Dong quai should not be taken with herbs or supplements that may increase the risk of bleeding, including ginkgo biloba, garlic, and saw palmetto.

- Interacts with anticoagulants (blood thinners)

- It may make menstrual blood flow heavier, so do not use if your cycles are already heavy

- The use of dong quai for pregnant or nursing women is discouraged due to possible hormonal or anticoagulant properties (Dong quai may also increase the risk of miscarriage)

- This herb has a mild laxative effect and prolonged use may cause diarrhea, nausea, upset stomach, vomiting, loss of appetite, bloating, or burping

- When combined with other herbs, dong quai is known to cause headache, sedation or drowsiness, dizziness, irritability, insomnia, sweating, fever, weakness, kidney problems, or skin rash

■ Possible Side Effects of Dong Quai

- Bleeding

- Bruising

- Skin irritation

- Sun sensitivity (Therefore, stay out of the sun and protect yourself with sunscreen)

RED CLOVER

Red clover is a perennial clover plant that originates from Asia, parts of Northern Africa, and Central Europe. It has a high mineral content, containing magnesium, calcium, potassium, and chromium. Red clover is also greatly sought after in easing menopausal symptoms, such as hot flashes and night sweats. It is a clover that derives its name from its distinctive appearance.

■ Functions of Red Clover

- Contains isoflavones that raise HDL (good cholesterol)

- Contains phytoestrogens

■ Contraindications

- Do not take if you are pregnant or breast feeding

- Do not take if you have a hormonally related cancer, such as breast, ovarian, or endometrial cancer

- Red clover is a blood thinner (Do not take if you are on a medication that thins the blood.)

■ Possible Side Effects of Red Clover

Serious side effects are rare. More serious side effects may include abnormal vaginal bleeding, liver damage, and possible infertility.

SELECTIVE ESTROGEN RECEPTOR MODULATORS (SERMS)

Selective estrogen receptor modulators (SERMS) are a type of hormone replacement therapy (HRT). An estrogen receptor is a group of receptors in your body that is activated by the hormone estrogen. Estrogen effects are mediated through two different estrogen receptors called estrogen receptor-alpha and estrogen receptor-beta. Estrogen receptor-alpha increases breast cell proliferation (growth). Estrogen receptor-beta inhibits (decreases) cell growth and prevents breast cancer development.

Some estrogen receptor modulators, such as estriol (E3), are made inside your body. These are called endogenous estrogen receptor modulators. There are also exogenous estrogen receptor modulators, which are made from external sources like plants (phytoestrogens) and pharmaceutical medications like tamoxifen.

SERMs work by blocking the effects of estrogen in your breast tissue. They remain inside your estrogen receptors in your breast cells, preventing estrogen from entering and attaching to the cell. This stops the cell from receiving estrogen's signal to grow and multiply.

Of course, the cells in your body's other tissues also have estrogen receptors, which are all structured slightly differently depending on which cell they are in. Since SERMs are selective, as their name informs, they block only estrogen from one type of cell—the breast tissue cell. However, SERMs can activate estrogen's action in other cells.

■ Possible Side Effects of SERMs

- Hot flashes
- Fatigue
- Night sweats

- Mood swings
- Vaginal discharge

You should not take a SERM if you are breastfeeding, pregnant, or trying to get pregnant, or if there is any chance you could be pregnant.

BIRTH CONTROL PILLS (ORAL CONTRACEPTIVES)

What a woman should choose as a birth control method is always an interesting discussion. Nutritional depletions, like the ones discussed in this section, are one of the key issues. If you are going to take birth control pills, it is important that you supplement with a pharmaceutical-grade multivitamin to replace the nutrients that are depleted with this kind of medication.

Oral contraceptives can deplete your body of zinc and elevate copper levels in your system. This can have many side effects, including abdominal pain, anemia, diarrhea, fatigue, headaches, memory impairment, and sleep disturbances. Birth control pills contain progestin (synthetic progesterone). As you have seen in the section on progesterone (page 23), progestin use can make the symptoms of a progesterone deficiency worse. Likewise, progestins decrease the protective effects of estrogen on your heart.

Estrogen-containing birth control pills decrease vitamins B_6, B_{12}, and folate in your body. These vitamins are needed to metabolize homocysteine, an amino acid. A buildup of homocysteine in your body can predispose you to heart disease, Alzheimer's disease, breast cancer, osteoporosis, and depression. Even low-dose birth control pills contain more estrogens and progestin than the amount that is usually needed for treatment of perimenopause or menopause. Women taking birth control pills have been shown to have decreased serum testosterone and DHEA levels.

Progestins in contraceptives increase breast cell replication and growth due to the stimulation of estrogen receptors by progestins. Progestins in contraceptives have been shown in medical trials to increase the risk of developing breast cancer. For all of the previous reasons, oral contraceptives are not the optimal hormone replacement therapy for perimenopausal and menopausal women.

NUTRITION AND HRT

Proper nutrition plays an important part in maximizing your HRT, preventing disease, and general treatment of menopause.

The following nutrients and supplements can help you deal with hormonally related symptoms.

SUPPLEMENTATION TO HELP MAXIMIZE HRT		
Supplements	Dosage	Considerations
Boron	1 mg	Increases testosterone and decreases calcium loss in bones.
Fiber	30 to 50 g	Decreases your cancer risk by decreasing estrogen levels in the blood. If you are estrogen dominant this is a good thing.
Folate	800 micrograms	Repairs DNA and lowers breast cancer risk.
Vitamin A	5,000 to 8,000 IU	Helps make hormones.
Vitamin C	1,000 to 2,000 mg	Helps make hormones.
Vitamin E	400 IU, twice a day	Helps relieve hot flashes. Also protects adrenals and ovaries from free radical damage.
Zinc	25 to 50 mg	Makes your sex hormones, helps make healthy breast tissue, promotes ovarian and adrenal gland function, and maximizes estrogen receptor function.

CONCLUSION

As you have seen, in Part III of this book, there are many advantages to hormone replacement therapy. Hormone replacement therapy is a treatment that should be considered by all women who are candidates for hormone replacement. This decision should be made in conjunction with the advice of your health care provider, your pharmacist, and a specialist in Precision/Anti-Aging Medicine.

Conclusion

The science of medicine in today's world is maturing. The previous concept that one agent causes a single disease and is treated with one medication is changing. Now, medicine has progressed into a deeper understanding of the complexities of human beings—women specifically, for the purpose of this text.

I hope this book has shown you that medicine today looks at each individual molecule. It looks at cellular messengers and intercellular communication, which work to coordinate function between diversion systems. This paradigm shift in medicine is exemplified in the hormonal symphony in the body. In addition, your hormonal needs are not stagnant; they change throughout your lifetime. They are affected by age, pregnancies, medications, exercise, infections, toxins, and even your spiritual belief system. Consequently, you will need different hormones in various doses, through your life---even if you are experiencing similar symptoms to those of another woman, your needs are unique.

The Human Genome Project has helped us understand the biochemical individuality of medicine. One size does not fit all. This personalization of care is achievable through a function approach to healthcare connected to the newest and fastest growing medical subspecialty: Precision Medicine. This specialty looks at the cause of the problem instead of treating only the symptoms. With the realization in medicine that approximately 20 percent of disease is inherited while 80 percent is related to the environment in which you live, the foods you eat, and the state you put your body in, this specialty illustrates the importance of helping you, the patient, maintain a healthy terrain in your body. The goal is abatement of your symptoms, which you erroneously thought were part of your normal physiologic landscape. Furthermore, the aim of customized hormone replacement therapy is to prevent disease.

Your hormones function as a web. Ideal levels of all your hormones are required to be balanced for you to be healthy. As you have seen, hormone restoration and balance play an integral role in helping you achieve and maintain optimal health throughout your life.

Resources

In this book, I've tried to provide all the information you need to create a program that will help you achieve optimum hormone balance. Although you can put together and follow this regimen on your own, it is often helpful to work with a Precision Medicine specialist and/or compounding pharmacist who can customize your program to your special needs. This can be especially important if you are managing a health condition and are already taking various medications. As you have learned in this book, certain diagnostic tests can also be valuable in helping you be healthy and stay healthy, finding the cause of your symptoms, and aiding your healthcare professional in developing a personalized medicine approach to hormone replacement therapy. You will also benefit most if you use pharmaceutical grade supplements, which meet the highest regulatory requirements. The following lists will guide you to the resources that can help you realize your goal of achieving and maintaining optimal health through hormonal balance.

FINDING A COMPOUNDING PHARMACY

Compounding is the practice of creating personalized medications to fill the gaps left by mass-produced medicine. To meet the special needs of an individual, a compounding pharmacy can provide unique dosages, innovative delivery methods, and unusual flavorings, and can also eliminate allergens and unnecessary fillers. Professional Compounding Centers of America can help you find a PCCA Member pharmacy in your area.

Professional Compounding Centers of America
9901 South Wilcrest Drive
Houston, TX 77099

Phone: (800) 331-2498
www.pccarx.com

Alliance for Pharmacy Compounding
100 Daingerfield Rd, Ste 100
Alexandria, VA 22314

Phone: (281) 933-8400
info@a4pc.org
www.a4pc.org
www.compounding.com

FINDING A FELLOWSHIP-TRAINED ANTI-AGING SPECIALIST

American Academy of Anti-Aging Physicians
1510 West Montana Street
Chicago, IL 60614

Phone: (773) 528-4333
www.worldhealth.net

FINDING A PERSONALIZED/PRECISION MEDICINE PRACTITIONER

ForumHealth.com

DIAGNOSTIC LABORATORY CONTACT INFORMATION

Medical testing now makes it possible to measure your amino acids, fatty acids, organic acids, vitamin levels, salivary hormone levels as well as gastrointestinal function, genome, and much more. This means that your regimen can be personalized to meet your specific needs. The following laboratories can perform tests to evaluate many important aspects of your health. Before ordering any medical test, be sure to consult with your healthcare practitioner.

Access Medical Labs
5151 Corporate Way
Jupiter, FL 33458
Office: 866-720-8386 x120
Facsimile: 866-610-2902
www.accessmedlab.com

Cyrex Laboratories
2602 South 24th Street
Phoenix, AZ 85034
Phone: (877) 772–9739 (US)
(844) 216–4763 (Canada)
www.cyrexlabs.com/

Doctor's Data
3755 Illinois Avenue
St. Charles, IL 60174
Phone: (800) 323–2784
www.doctorsdata.com

Genova Diagnostics
63 Zillicoa Street
Asheville, NC 28801
Phone: (800) 522–4762
(828) 253–0621
www.gdx.net

Genomind
2200 Renaissance Blvd., Suite 100
King of Prussia, PA 19406

Great Plains Laboratory
11813 West 77th Street
Lenexa, KS 66214
Phone: (800) 288–3383
(913) 341–8949
www.greatplainslaboratory.com

Microbiome Labs Research Center
1332 Waukegan Rd.
Glenview, IL 60025
Phone: 904·940-2208
www.biomeFx.com

Rocky Mountain Analytical
105–32 Royal Vista Drive NW
Calgary, Alberta T3R 0H9
Canada
Phone: (866) 370–5227

(403) 241–4500
www.rmalab.com

SpectraCell Laboratories
10401 Town Park Drive
Houston, TX 77072
Phone: (800) 227–5227
(713) 621–3101
www.spectracell.com

Vibrant America Labs
1021 Howard Avenue
San Carlos California 94070
Phone: (866) 364-0963
Support@Vibrant-America.com

ZRT Laboratory
8605 SW Creekside Place
Beaverton, OR 97008
Phone: (866) 600–1636
(503) 466-2445
www.zrtlab.com

PHARMACEUTICAL GRADE COMPANIES

You can find many good supplement brands at health food stores. Always make sure you buy pharmaceutical grade nutrients. The following pharmaceutical grade companies offer many quality nutritional supplements. Your healthcare provider or pharmacist will help you order your nutrients from these companies.

Biotics Research Corporation
6801 Biotics Research Drive
Rosenberg, TX 77471
Phone: (800) 231–5777
(281) 344–0909
www.bioticsresearch.com

Designs for Health, Inc.
980 South Street
Suffield, CT 06078
Phone: (800) 847–8302
(860) 623–6314
www.designsforhealth.com

Douglas Laboratories
112 Technology Drive
Pittsburgh, PA 15275
Phone: (800) 245–4440
www.douglaslabs.com

Life Extension
5990 North Federal Highway
Fort Lauderdale, FL 33308
Phone: (800) 678–8989
www.lifeextension.com

Metagenics
25 Enterprise
Aliso Viejo, CA 92656
Phone: (800) 692-9400
(949) 366–0818
www.metagenics.com

Microbiome Labs
1332 Waukegan Rd.
Glenview, IL 60025
Phone: 904-940-2208
microbiomelabs.com

Ortho Molecular Products
1991 Duncan Place
Woodstock, IL 60098
Phone: (800) 332–2351
www.orthomolecularproducts.com

Vital Nutrients
45 Kenneth Dooley Drive
Middletown, CT 06457
Phone: (888) 328–9992 (toll free)
(860) 638–3675
www.vitalnutrients.net

Xymogen
6900 Kingspointe Parkway
Orlando, FL 32819
Phone: (800) 647–6100
www.xymogen.com

References

The information and recommendations presented in this book are based on over a thousand scientific studies, academic papers, and books. If the references for all these sources were printed here, they would add considerable bulk to the book and make it more expensive, as well. For this reason, the publisher and I have decided to present a complete list of references, categorized by section and topic, on the publisher's website. This format has the added advantage of enabling us to make you aware of further important studies and papers as they become available. You can find the references under the listing of my book at www.squareonepublishers.com.

About the Author

Pamela Wartian Smith, M.D., MPH, MS, spent her first twenty years of practice as an emergency room physician with the Detroit Medical Center and then spent the next twenty-eight years of her career as an Anti-Aging/Functional Medicine specialist. She is a diplomat of the board of the American Academy of Anti-Aging Physicians and an internationally known speaker and author on the subject of Anti-Aging/ Precision Medicine. She holds a master's degree in public health as well as in metabolic and nutritional medicine. Dr. Smith is currently in private practice and the senior partner for the Center for Precision Medicine, with offices in Michigan and Florida. She is also the founder of the Fellowship in Anti-Aging, Regenerative, and Functional Medicine and the past co-director of the master's program in metabolic and nutritional medicine at the Morsani College of Medicine, University of South Florida.

Dr. Smith has been a featured guest on CNN, PBS, and a number of other television networks, in addition to hosting two radio shows. She can also be seen in the PBS series *The Embrace of Aging,* the online medical series *Awakening from Alzheimer's* and *Regain Your Brain,* and the PBS/CNN special How to Maximize Your Immune System. She is the author of eleven best-selling books, including *What You Must Know About Vitamins, Minerals, Herbs, and So Much More,* and *Max Your Immunity.*

Index

Within this index, the term Precision Medicine refers to therapies that are an individualized approach for each patient; for example, compounded bio-identical hormones. Precision Medicine therapies also embrace many other treatments, such as botanical, nutritional, dietary, mind-body, and stress management. Conventional treatments include medications, laser therapy, surgery, and generalized lifestyle changes.

What You Must Know About Vitamins, Minerals, Herbs and So Much More
SECOND EDITION
Choosing the Nutrients That Are Right for You
Pamela Wartian Smith, MD, MPH

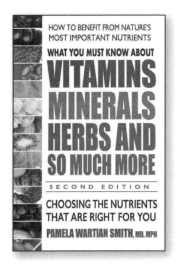

Almost 75 percent of your health and life expectancy is based on lifestyle, environment, and nutrition. Yet even if you follow a healthful diet, you are probably not getting all the nutrients you need to prevent disease. Why? There are many reasons, ranging from the mineral-depleted soils in which our foods are grown, to medications that rob the body of various vitamins and minerals. What, then, is the answer?

Now available in a fully revised edition that reflects the latest research and science-based studies, *What You Must Know About Vitamins, Minerals, Herbs and So Much More—Second Edition* explains how you can restore and maintain health through the wise use of nutrients. Part One of this easy-to-use guide presents the individual nutrients necessary for wellness. Part Two offers personalized nutritional programs for people with a wide variety of health concerns. People without prior medical problems can look to Part Three for their supplementation plans.

Whether you are trying to overcome a medical condition or you simply want to preserve good health, this new Second Edition can guide you in making the best dietary and supplement choices for you and your family.

ABOUT THE AUTHOR

Pamela Wartian Smith, MD, MPH, MS, is a diplomate of the American Academy of Anti-Aging Physicians and co-director of the Master's Program in Medical Sciences, with a concentration in Metabolic and Nutritional Medicine, at the Morsani College of Medicine, University of South Florida. An authority on the subjects of wellness and functional medicine, Dr. Smith is also the founder of the Fellowship in Anti-Aging, Regenerative, and Functional Medicine. Dr. Smith is also the best-selling author of seven books, including *What You Must Know About Women's Hormones; What You Must Know About Memory Loss;* and *What You Must Know About Allergy Relief.*

$16.95 US • 464 pages • 6 x 9-inch paperback • Health/Nutrition • ISBN 978-0-7570-0471-1

What You Must Know About Thyroid Disorders & What to Do About Them
Your Guide to Treating Autoimmune Dysfunction, Hypo- and Hyperthyroidism, Mood Swings, Cancer, Memory Loss, Weight Issues, Heart Problems & More
Pamela Wartian Smith, MD, MPH

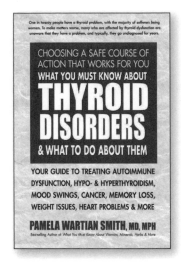

It is estimated that one in twenty people have a thyroid problem, and that most sufferers go undiagnosed for years. But it doesn't have to be that way. Written by best-selling author Dr. Pamela Wartian Smith, *What You Must Know About Thyroid Disorders & What to Do About Them* enables readers to identify common thyroid problems and seek the treatment they need. The book begins by explaining the many functions that the thyroid performs in the body. It then goes on to discuss common thyroid-related disorders and symptoms, including hypothyroidism, hyperthyroidism, excess weight gain, thyroid cancer, and more. Finally, Dr. Smith explains each disorder's cause and common symptoms, diagnostic tests, and both conventional and alternative treatment approaches.

$16.95 US • 224 pages • 6 x 9-inch paperback • ISBN 978-0-7570-0424-7

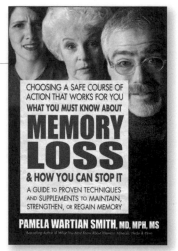

What You Must Know About Memory Loss & How You Can Stop It
A Guide to Proven Techniques and Supplements to Maintain, Strengthen, or Regain Memory
Pamela Wartian Smith, MD, MPH

Contrary to popular belief, not all memory loss is caused by the aging process. In *What You Must Know About Memory Loss & How You Can Stop It*, Dr. Pamela Wartian Smith describes what you can do to reverse the problem and enhance your mental abilities for years to come. You'll learn about the most common causes of memory loss, including nutritional deficiencies, hormonal imbalances, toxic overload, poor blood circulation, and lack of physical and mental exercise. The author explains how each cause is involved in impaired memory and supplies a list of proven remedies.

$15.95 US • 240 pages • 6 x 9-inch paperback • ISBN 978-0-7570-0386-8

Max Your Immunity

How to Maximize Your Immune System
When You Need It Most

Pamela Wartian Smith, MD

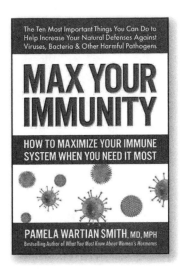

---

*"A guide, written for lay readers. . . an excellent
supplementary resource for personal health and
wellness . . . highly recommended."*

—MIDWEST BOOK REVIEW

The word immunity has unfortunately become an
all-too-common term in our vocabulary, and for
good reason. When the pandemic hit, many of the
major drug companies jumped at the opportunity
to create a vaccine that could offer us "immunity" against this specific virus.
Yet, few of us understand that almost all these vaccines work based upon their
activating our own built-in systems of defense. It is our very own immunity
to these viruses that can make the difference between illness and health. To
help clarify what each of us can do to protect ourselves and our loved one,
Pamela Wartian Smith, MD has written *Max Your Immunity*. Here is a complete
guide to understanding and maximizing your natural defenses against various
infectious diseases.

Max Your Immunity is divided into three parts. Part One explains how our innate
and adaptive immunity systems work. Our innate immunity system is based on
our built-in barriers designed to fight or separate us from infectious agents. Our
adaptive immunity, also called acquired immunity, is composed of lymphocyte
cells that are triggered when a specific pathogen enters the body. These cells
learn to identify the invading pathogens and hunt them down. In this section,
each component in both systems are clearly identified and explained. Part Two
provides ten important things that you can do to increase and strengthen all of
these components. And Part Three provides specific nutritional plans to increase
your body's immunity to help defend off the most common health disorders.

The fact is, few of us make it a point to keep our immune system in top shape.
However when our immune system is weakened, we greatly increase the odds
of our getting sick. By simply having a clear understanding of how our internal
defenses work and what we can do to increase our immunity; we can play an
important role in maintaining good health. *Max Your Immunity* can help show
you what you need to know to protect yourself and your family.

$16.95 US • 324 pages • 6 x 9-inch paperback • Health / Nutrition • ISBN 978-0-7570-0512-1

What You Must Know About Allergy Relief
How to Overcome the Allergies You Have & Find the Hidden Allergies That Make You Sick
Earl Mindell, RPh, and Pamela Wartian Smith, MD

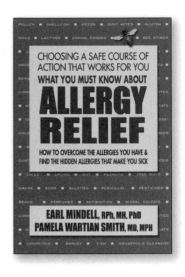

When most people have allergies, they know it. But for many others, allergies and intolerances are hidden culprits that lie at the heart of a number of health conditions. If you are an allergy sufferer or have a recurring health issue that you can't seem to resolve, this is the book for you. Written by a pharmacist and medical doctor, it provides important answers to common questions about allergies—what causes them, how they can affect you, and how you can overcome them. Up-to-date and easy to understand, *What You Must Know About Allergy Relief* offers the tools to identify hidden allergies and the means to relieve their symptoms.

$17.95 US • 288 pages • 6 x 9-inch paperback • ISBN 978-0-7570-0437-7

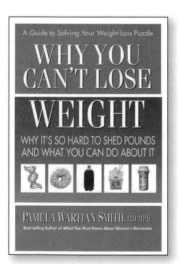

Why You Can't Lose Weight
Why It's So Hard to Shed Pounds and What You Can Do About It
Pamela Wartian Smith, MD, MPH

If you have tried to slim down without success, it may not be your fault. In this revolutionary book, Dr. Pamela Smith discusses the eighteen most common reasons why you can't lose weight, and guides you in overcoming the obstacles that stand between you and a trimmer body. It's time to learn what's really keeping you from reaching your goal. With *Why You Can't Lose Weight,* you'll discover how to shed pounds and enjoy radiant health.

$16.95 US • 256 pages • 6 x 9-inch paperback • ISBN 978-0-7570-0312-7

**For more information about our books,
visit our website at www.squareonepublishers.com**